The Coaching Process

The Coaching Process: Principles and Practice for Sport

Edited by

Neville Cross

BA (Hons) MSc (Leicester) MSc (Heriot-Watt) FISC

Lecturer in Sport and Leisure Studies, Faculty of Education, The University of Edinburgh, Edinburgh, UK

and

John Lyle

BA (Hons) MSc MEd EdD PgDipMan PgCertEd

Head of Sport Sciences Division, Faculty of Social Science, University of Northumbria at Newcastle, Newcastle upon Tyne, UK

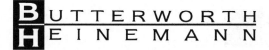

OXFORD   AUCKLAND   BOSTON   JOHANNESBURG   MELBOURNE   NEW DELHI

Butterworth-Heinemann
Linacre House, Jordan Hill, Oxford OX2 8DP
225 Wildwood Avenue, Woburn, MA 01801-2041
A division of Reed Educational and Professional Publishing Ltd

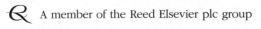 A member of the Reed Elsevier plc group

First published 1999

© Reed Educational and Professional Publishing Ltd 1999

British Library Cataloguing in Publication Data
A catalogue record for this book is available from the British Library

Library of Congress Cataloguing in Publication Data
A catalogue record for this book is available from the Library of Congress

ISBN 0 7506 4131 2

Typeset by Keyword Typesetting Services Ltd, Wallington
Printed and bound by Biddles Limited, Guildford and King's Lynn

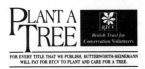

Contents

Preface

This book is about the 'coaching process'. It is a process that is multifaceted and multidisciplinary and, as such, it requires input from a variety of different areas and from a number of different specialists. These complementary contributions have to be co-ordinated by a single individual. This is the role of the coach. It is the coach who will be responsible for managing and blending the various contributions to the process into an effective strategy for improving performance. Despite their individual specialist areas of expertise and research, all of the contributors to this book acknowledge that it is the coach who will direct the process and who, in partnership with the athlete, is the key to enhanced sports performance.

Sports coaching does not exist in isolation. The social and sporting structures and the systems within which it operates will influence it to a greater or lesser extent. Although sports coaching is not yet recognized as a 'formal profession', it is an occupation with its own education and accreditation structures, membership affiliation bodies, career development and codes of conduct.

Although their experience lies in a number of different performance sports, the individual contributors to this book are united by a love of sport, a respect for coaches and athletes, and a desire to see 'coaching' given the professional recognition and status it deserves. Coaching is growing in importance as an academic discipline. Not only is coaching and coaching science being offered at undergraduate level, but there are also an expanding number of postgraduate courses in coaching studies and coaching science currently being offered at postgraduate level. However, there is no suitable textbook or 'reader' on the coaching process available at this time, and this book has been focused to address this need.

Although it is fashionable (and sometimes deserved) for the media to highlight poor coaching practice, outstanding contributions made by coaches (and there are many) often go unnoticed. All of the contributors in this book have personally coached one or more sports, some at a very high level (including the Olympics), and some for a very long time. Some have coached individual sports and others team sports. Some have most of their experience in amateur sport, others in professional sport, and some are at present involved in the current professionalization of certain sports such as rugby. Some have had most of their experience with coaching children and others with adults. All are highly respected in their particular sports and in their particular areas of expertise. Most have made significant contributions to coach education, National Governing Body development, representative coaching at national level and coaching research. All have worked or are currently working together in the same academic institution. This has allowed the group to spend many hours debating the importance and the particular significance of the various contributions for coaches, students and potential researchers.

Their contributions stress the importance of all of the areas of expertise that individually contribute to effective coaching practice, and which together constitute the essential elements of the 'coaching process'. The process is a serial combination of training and competition elements that are inter-related and interdependent, and directed towards an identified set of goals. Coaches will have to manage the process, which will include behaviours such as planning, goal-setting (often in collaboration with the athlete), leadership, communication, monitoring and feedback, and process adjustment (often referred to as 'contingency' or 'crisis' management). How these behaviours are combined will reflect the coach's experience and expertise.

Of course, the process can be implemented in a wide variety of ways. The method chosen will have to consider and reflect the context within which the coach and athlete operate. In many instances, one coach will be responsible for several athletes, sometimes in less than ideal circumstances or environments. In such cases, the context may become problematical and the delivery of certain aspects of the coaching process will be compromised.

With a group of contributors with such a diverse set of interests and expertise, one would not expect universal agreement on all aspects of coaching practice. For example, the differences encountered in coaching teams rather than individuals may cause difficulties in individualizing training, and even in the type of leadership style possible and/or recommended. These differences suggest that there may be more than one way to achieve coaching effectiveness, not only in different sports, but even in the same sport. In fact, the best method for achieving coaching effectiveness may still lie undiscovered!

As co-editors, we would like to stress the following point. Sports coaching is a normative activity. As such, it is underpinned by values, philosophies and ideologies. Consequently, it might be anticipated that we would have insisted on a 'party line' within the chapters. This is not the case. As editors, we have brought to the role two distinct approaches that are perhaps a more accurate reflection of the current state of play. For example, Neville Cross' experience is largely with the individual sport of swimming, both as a competitor and as a national coach. Over the years he has developed a strong 'humanistic' or athlete-centred orientation to his coaching and to the way he presents coach education. It is a conviction for which he strives in his coaching practice, and which permeates his writing. On the other hand, John Lyle's background is principally in team sports, first as a professional athlete and later as a national team coach. Based on these experiences, he has developed a more 'pragmatic' approach which accepts the need for more direct coach control, but within a coaching philosophy that attempts to balance concern for the individual with the practicalities of adhering to a strong achievement goal for the team. We have deliberately presented both approaches, and tried to identify advantages and disadvantages in each case.

There is a large sport-specific coaching literature. However, despite the National Coaching Foundation being a catalyst for generic coach education material, surprisingly little has been produced on performance coaching practice, or on the coaching process itself. This has been exacerbated by the general lack of attention to coaching behaviour in sports performance research. In addition, there is still no academic journal on sports coaching that deals with the 'process'. It was in this context, and in the knowledge that there was no suitable coaching text that considered coaching in a 'holistic' way, that we came to consider writing this book.

It is more than a collection of papers that are loosely related to sports coaching. As editors, we invited our colleagues to address several questions.

In what way is your specialism related to sports coaching? What impact does your specialist area have on coaching practice? Are there any particular issues to be considered in integrating your area into the coaching process? What is the balance between the knowledge and skills that you would expect the coach to have, or to develop, and the need for additional specialist expertise? Furthermore, we invited our colleagues to adopt a perspective that acknowledged sports coaching as a process and, by implication, to consider their contribution in relation to those of others.

The structure we have adopted is intended to reflect three distinctive collections of papers. In the first chapter, the emphasis is on the coaching process and is intended to crystallize the developing body of knowledge in this area. John Lyle explores the nature of the coaching process and how it might be conceptualized for better understanding and analysis. This is followed by a chapter that views coaching as an interpersonal relationship. This particular chapter focuses on the coach's philosophy and how the values encapsulated within it influence practice. In the third chapter, Neville Cross examines coaching effectiveness. He explores the various ways in which coaching effectiveness may be monitored and measured, and the implications of these for coaching practice.

In the second group of papers, four sport scientists describe how their specialisms influence the coaching process. Richard Cox uses his extensive experience as a sports psychologist working at all levels of sport to describe a number of principles that coaches should incorporate into their working practice. Andrew Maile bases his chapter on the importance of physiology in the training process. Much of his analysis is as a result of sports science support he has provided for elite sports teams. Biomechanics is a fundamental aspect of sports performance. However, it is often given less attention in sports coaching than some of the other sciences. Simon Coleman takes this opportunity to incorporate his practical coaching and research experience to describe the importance of biomechanical principles and analysis for the coach. In the final chapter in this section, Malcolm Fairweather explores how recent developments in motor skill knowledge should change traditional coaching practice; principles which he himself has incorporated into his work with elite athletes.

In the third group of papers, principles of good practice are identified in a variety of coaching contexts. In the first chapter in this section, Bob Brewer and Neville Cross combine their very extensive coaching experience with their backgrounds as educationalists to examine good practice in coaching children. This is followed by a chapter by Neville Cross which highlights the importance of individualizing the coaching process, and identifies many of the constraints which inhibit it. In the next chapter, Neville Cross and John Lyle point to the dangers of overtraining; an outcome which they attribute to lack of planning and monitoring in the coaching process. This is followed with a chapter by John Lyle, which explores how coaches make decisions, particularly in situations (such as during a match) in which the coach has little time to weigh up the options. In the final chapter, John Lyle takes an overview of the sports performance system and considers why this system should be analysed from a systems perspective.

Coming from a variety of different backgrounds, and having lived and worked in a variety of different cultures, can only have served to enhance experience and coaching knowledge. This we have tried to pass on in order to assist coaches and students of coaching to improve practice and to increase research into coaching behaviour. For some readers, we will not have given equal attention to all aspects of the coaching process. Others may perceive that we have paid insufficient attention to certain aspects. We may even be accused of a certain bias, as we are all white Anglo-Saxon males. If such bias does exist, it is not intended.

Finally, we would remind readers that this book is a contribution to a developing field of knowledge. What we have attempted to do is to bring some insight and order to this field, and to stimulate further research into coaching practice. As the chapters will have indicated, performance sports coaching is multivariable, eclectic, interpersonal and contested. Coaches are accountable for a process that is difficult to regulate, demanding in its range of contributory disciplines and subject to both internal and external monitoring procedures.

Neville Cross and John Lyle

Contributors

Neville Cross BA(Hons) MSc (Leicester) MSc (Heriot-Watt) FISC
Neville Cross is a lecturer in sport and coaching studies in the Faculty of Education at the University of Edinburgh. His former occupation as a full-time professional swimming coach included appointments at both English and British national team level. During this time, he placed swimmers on three consecutive Olympic teams. He has been involved in tutoring swimming coach education courses for many years, and is one of a select band of coaches who hold the ASA Senior Coach certificate. He continues to coach part-time at club level, and is an active researcher in the area of coaching elite athletes. He has published widely in the area of swimming coaching.

John Lyle BA(Hons) MSc MEd EdD PgDipMan PgCertEd
John Lyle is Head of Division (Sport Sciences) in the Faculty of Social Sciences at the University of Northumbria at Newcastle. He has extensive experience in sport as both a player (former professional footballer and Scottish international volleyball player) and a coach (Scotland Senior Men's International Team Coach and GB World Student Games Team Coach). He is a former Director of the NCF, and has experience of coaching consultancy with both the NCF and the Scottish Sports Council. He publishes widely in the area of sports coaching.

Bob Brewer BEdPE(Hons) MA(PE) MA(Ed)
Bob Brewer is a lecturer in Physical Education in the Faculty of Education at the University of Edinburgh. His coaching experience includes being a member of the 1988 and 1992 British Men's Olympic Basketball Coaching Staff, and being Men's Head Coach at the World Student Games in 1987, 1988 and 1991. He is the current Convener for Performance and Excellence for the Scottish Basketball Association, and is presently researching the *Sports Coaching Competencies for Teachers* initiative' (Scottish Office, 1997).

Simon Coleman BA PhD
Simon Coleman is a lecturer in Sports Biomechanics in the Faculty of Education at the University of Edinburgh. He has considerable experience of competitive sport as a player, and is also an internationally qualified volleyball coach. He was Biomechanics Chairperson of BASES (British Association of Sport and Exercise Sciences) from 1996–1998, and has published widely in the field of biomechanics.

Richard Cox PhD CPsychol AFBPsS
Richard Cox is a lecturer in psychology in the Faculty of Education at the University of Edinburgh. He is a consultant in sport psychology to the Scottish Rugby Union team, and has worked in a similar capacity with professional footballers from two Premier League clubs for more than 4 years. In addition, he has advised numerous individual elite athletes (including two world champions) from more than 10 different sports. Richard attended the

1992 Olympic Games as sport psychologist to the British Swimming Team. He has been a reviewer for the *International Journal of Sport Psychology* since 1991.

Malcolm Fairweather BA PgCertEd MSc PhD

Malcolm Fairweather is a lecturer in skill learning in the Faculty of Education at the University of Edinburgh. He has spent 7 years in the USA coaching athletics at the elite level. During this time, he guided three Olympic and World Championship gold medallists. Since returning to Scotland to take up his current position, he has become fitness and skills adviser to one of Scotland's top rugby teams and has advised several international players. He has also prepared fitness programmes for the Scottish badminton team in their preparation for the 1998 Commonwealth Games. Currently, he is a consultant to the Scottish Golf Union, where he is developing amateur international training programmes and co-ordinating research activities at the Scottish National Golf Centre. His research is recognized at international level, and he has published in the world's leading skill learning journals.

Andrew Maile BA(Hons) MA PgCertEd

Andrew Maile is a senior lecturer in Sport Science in the Faculty of Education at the University of Edinburgh. He is accredited by BASES (British Association of Sport and Exercise Science) both as a Laboratory Director and Sport and Exercise Physiologist. In addition, he is a staff tutor for the NCF (National Coaching Foundation). Andy has acted as a consultant to a number of NGBs (National Governing Bodies), with particular reference to the development of physical parameters associated with sports performance. He holds a full FA Coaching Licence and is a BASI (British Association of Ski Instructors) qualified ski instructor.

Part 1

The Concept of the Coaching Process

1

The coaching process: an overview

John Lyle

- The benefits of analysing coaching practice
- Boundaries, roles and definitions
- Assumptions about the coaching process
- The role of the coach
- The distinctions between participation and performance coaching
- Modelling the coaching process
- Analysis of coaching models from the literature
- Key principles of coaching practice

Introduction

It would be appropriate to begin this introductory chapter with a review of
the current literature on the significance of the coaching role, a summary of
the most up-to-date research on coaching practice, and an overview of the
most recent developments in the effective application of the coaching process. Unfortunately, sports coaching as a process has received far less attention than the study of the athlete's performance. In addition, it has been
treated as a non-problematical aspect of the purposeful improvement of
sports performance. However, the coach's role in the promotion of participation (rather than performance) sport is rather better appreciated.
Nevertheless it seems almost inconceivable, at a time in the UK when
coach education has been re-shaped at national level and the National
Lottery is able to support the provision of full-time performance coaching
posts, that there is such a sparse literature on coaching practice. In the United
Kingdom, the Sports Councils and the National Coaching Foundation have
promoted research on sports performance, largely within specific science
disciplines, but have failed to pay adequate attention to the coach's role in
the delivery and decision making process.

This may not be entirely surprising. The study of sports coaching as an
academic field or discipline has struggled to establish a toehold within educational institutions in the UK. Coaches themselves have often presented
coaching as an art (although they would be hard-pushed to say what they
meant by this) rather than a craft, and historically the role and status of
coaches has been diminished, often purposefully, in traditional sports such
as cricket and rugby union. The stereotypical image of the coach as under-
trained, rather authoritarian and focused on winning rather than welfare has
been promoted (perhaps with some justification) by educationalists eager to

protect the role of the school and the teacher in British sport. In addition, the different sport systems in the USA or Eastern Europe have meant that research and models of coaching practice (for example, the wealth of material on the career-orientated high-school or collegiate coach in the USA) have had limited relevance for UK coaching. One final factor has been the somewhat haphazard recruitment, training and appointment of coaches in professional sport, and the understandable reluctance of the coaches themselves to expose their situations to scrutiny.

It was partly the dearth of critical analysis on coaching that led to this book. The purpose of this introductory chapter, therefore, is to establish a starting point for understanding coaches' practice. The approach taken is two-fold: to create an integrated and cohesive description of the coaching process, and to situate this in the relevant literature. The process elements are then further illuminated in the remainder of the book, in which each chapter examines an aspect of coaching practice and how it can be enhanced. Although it is tempting to say that there is no consensus about coaching as a process, it would perhaps be more accurate to recognize that any short-comings resulting from this are caused by a failure to ask the appropriate questions. Those responsible for developments in sports performance and sports coaching have, more often than not, simply not asked themselves whether a knowledge of coaching practice, or the principles underlying it, might be beneficial for this purpose. How such knowledge might be used to improve coaching practice will be analysed in subsequent chapters. However, it would be valuable to emphasize a number of points at this stage.

First, practitioners in all occupations, particularly professions and pseudo-professions, become more expert through experience, interaction with others, and a mix of formal and informal educational and training opportunities. Without a greater knowledge of successful coaching practice, role priorities and the personal attributes necessary, those responsible for coach education, the performance development system, National Governing Body and club mentors and the coaches themselves will be less likely to be responsible for expert coaching practice. This will be more important when the coach has moved beyond the formal coaching awards system. Second, there are actually very few data to support the assumption that the coach inevitably adds value to performance development. However, the centrality of the coach's role in directing the process, and a measure of common sense and experience, reaffirms the significance of the coach's contribution. It is necessary to understand exactly what the coach's contribution to performance enhancement in a wide variety of situations might be. For example, in team sports, in sports in which the coach influences the progress of the competition (e.g. basketball, volleyball) and in managing the elite athlete's programme, there is much yet to be learned about what constitutes good practice. This will require a sophisticated insight into the coaching process and its application in a variety of contexts. Third, the coaching process clearly involves an interpersonal relationship between performer and coach, or a set of relationships. A great deal has been written about ideological or philosophical approaches to relationships in coaching, and there are some psychological and socio-psychological principles about relationships in general. However, there are few studies that have dealt with *in situ* coaching behaviour and related this to specific role interpretations and technical implementation. Once again, a more detailed knowledge of the coaching process is required. Another objective in this chapter, therefore, is to establish a vocabulary and a set of concepts about coaching and the coaching process.

These few examples serve to illustrate the point that successful performance coaching is more problematical than has been previously assumed. Its implementation implies a complicated, rather than a simple, process. Research into the enhancement of sports performance has focused almost exclusively on applied (as opposed to pure) performance research; for example, laboratory research into the efficacy of dietary supplements on performance. This has been to the disadvantage of application or implementation research, which would focus much more on the effect of such supplements as actually used by the athlete and coach. Much of the application research has been related to the work of support science personnel, but not put in the context of the coaches' role or contribution. The researcher can focus on one element of the process or of the performance, but the knowledge gained has to be integrated into the whole, or its priority balanced, by the coach, who is responsible for the entire process. It is difficult to escape the conclusion that the coach's delivery capacity, within a synoptic overview of the process, is treated as a limitation by researchers and not as the essential part of the jigsaw that it is. Research on sport performance is incomplete if implementation in a naturalistic coaching situation has not been taken into account.

Research is but one example, and there are many others. For example, coach education (this does not mean the setting of standards for coaching practice, but how to achieve these) has yet to deal adequately with the more advanced levels of coaching. Also, the recent growth in school sport development posts has again raised issues about role demarcation between teachers, coaches, sport leaders and development officers. Another example is the relationship between support personnel (such as sport psychologists or physiotherapists) and coaches, which needs to be understood as an issue of substitution (replacement) or support. Neither of these diminishes the coach's role, but the contribution of support personnel must be appreciated in the context of that role. Furthermore, the recent restructuring of the UK performance sport system to include the UK Institute of Sport, regional institutes, sport-specific centres of excellence and university elite squads has implications for the management of performance and for the coach's role as a manager of performance. It would be over-optimistic to imagine that the needs of the coaching processes of elite athletes were the basis of the network of services and structures, and not the interests of the organizations and agencies involved. The final example is the extent to which those responsible for the hiring and firing of coaches appreciate the distinctions between 'successful' and 'effective' coaches, and between effectiveness as a capacity and as a measurement of performance. These particular issues are pursued in greater depth in Chapter 3. In each of these examples, we can see the need for a clear understanding of the coaching process and what it entails.

Coaching theory

In this context, coaching theory does not imply a fully formed set of explanatory concepts and relationships. It would be strange if it did, given the dearth of research into coaching practice to which we have already alluded. The term 'coaching theory' has come to be used in two distinct ways. One is for referring to knowledge which is non-sport specific – for example, sub-discipline knowledge in sport psychology, sport biomechanics, pedagogy, sports medicine and so on has an application across all sports. Particular mention should perhaps be made of 'training theory'. Although there is a good deal of habit and fashion in the sets of principles attached to planning, periodization and training loadings, the principles themselves are based on established physiological and biological theorems, etc. Training theory is not a suitable substitute for coaching theory, and its prevalence reinforces the emphasis on performance variables. However, it is a useful reminder that the coaching process draws upon an extensive and eclectic range of disciplines and sub-disciplines.

The second use of the term 'coaching theory' is the one used in this chapter. Coaching theory refers to those generic aspects of coaching practice and behaviour that are common to all sports coaching processes. This, of course, assumes a commonality of purpose and process in sports coaching – an issue to which further attention will be given. It may be more appropriate to demonstrate the scope of coaching theory in a series of questions:

- What is the purpose of coaching? What do we mean by the use of the word?
- What is it that distinguishes coaching from other forms of sports leadership or interpersonal behaviour? When is coaching taking place, and when is it something else?
- Are there any essential elements that characterize coaching?
- What is the role of the coach? How does this role relate to those of others involved in the process?
- What is the process that takes place in coaching? How can this best be represented in order to facilitate communication and understanding?

The remainder of the chapter will be devoted to answering these questions. However, before doing so, it would be useful to summarize a number of the main themes that will emerge:

1. Sports coaching must be understood as a process. The coach, the rela-tionship between athlete and coach, coaching practice and behaviour, and the training and competition elements, are all part of the coaching process.
2. The term 'coaching process' should be the common, all-embracing term for representing and understanding coaching. The coaching process must be understood in order to appreciate the variations in scope and scale occasioned by differing circumstances.
3. There are two distinct forms of sports coaching. One is focused on initiating, improving and maintaining *participation*. This is demonstrated best in a range of roles, including those of sport animateur, teacher and sports instructor. This is normally a less intensive process than the sec-ond form, which involves specific preparation for the *performance* of sport. However, the differences may not always be as clear-cut as this implies.

4. Performance coaching is an essentially cognitive activity, with contributory elements of (skills-based) craft, which are related to interpersonal behaviour, managing the training environment, managing the competition environment, and specific sport expertise.
5. The interpersonal and technical (specific strategies for improving performance) elements of the coaching process are always present. These two elements are in a constant state of flux, and are influenced by ideology as much as by the dynamic of the process.
6. The coaching role should be interpreted as that of manager of performance. In some circumstances this role is exercised in isolation, although most often it takes the form of a partnership with the athlete(s) concerned. With the elite athlete, it may be as the hub of a network of specialists contributing to the coaching process.

Boundaries, roles and definitions

This section of the chapter deals with the 'what' rather than the 'how' of coaching. An assumption is made that the coach's role and the coaching process can be interpreted and implemented in a number of ways, reflecting style, philosophy or value framework, and influenced by a wide range of factors arising from the context in which the coaching takes place. The issue for the moment is what makes one particular social construction coaching, and another not coaching. The key assumption is that a generic process exists termed 'coaching'. The evidence for this is its widespread use in a variety of contexts. It is normal practice in music, poetry and drama to coach artistes for a particular performance. Children are often given extra coaching in preparation for examinations. In management training, the interpretation of the manager's role as a coaching role is a current fashion (Lyle, 1997). In each of these cases, there is a generic process – the improvement in performance (not basic learning) towards identifiable goals by a structured preparation or practice process, directed by a coach.

The words describing the generic process form the basis of a very simple definition of the sports coaching process. However, it would be useful to elaborate a little on the key elements within the process. The following statements could be thought of as assumptions about the coaching process. These allow the reader to question the assumptions in detail, rather than to agree or disagree with a very concisely expressed definition.

- Coaching is a form of sports leadership in which identified objectives are pursued in a purposeful manner.
- The central purpose of coaching is to improve performance in competition sport. (Other objectives, such as the athlete's personal development, may be paramount for some coaches, but must be accompanied by the central purpose.)
- Sports coaching is a process in that: (a) it is serial, (b) it has inter-related and interdependent elements and stages, (c) it has sub-processes and stages designed to contribute to an overall goal, and (d) it is incremental or accumulative in its effect.

- The coaching process is almost always framed in the context of a specific sport, and the athletes will exercise a membership/competitor role within that sport and its organizations.
- The process varies in scale and in the degree of the control exercised over the variables that influence performance. The process varies by the intensity of the involvement (duration, frequency, continuity, stability), by the coach's role in competition, by the degree of responsibility exercised by the athlete, by the contribution of other individuals to the implementation of the process, and by the requirements/constraints of the organizations within which the coach operates.
- The achievement of performance goals is constrained by the athlete's commitment and genetic disposition, the coach's expertise, the resources available, the contested and relative nature of achievement in sport, and the complexity of the variables influencing performance.
- Coaching involves one or a series of interpersonal relationships. These may vary in strength, empathy and extent. Therefore, the nature of these interactions can shape the coaching process significantly, potentially providing both positive and negative reinforcement.
- The role of the coach is to manage (including leadership and direction) the process towards improved performance, based on the athlete's aspirations and abilities. A more specific part of this role is to reduce the unpredictability of performance – that is, to help the athlete to produce an appropriate performance at the appropriate time.
- Sports coaching is an intervention programme. Neither maturation nor unstructured experience will lead to athletes reaching their full potential. A well-managed process will enhance the athletes' performances by strategic improvements in the various elements of performance crucial to the particular sport.

This catalogue of assumptions should describe the coaching process in a much more detailed fashion than any definition will do. Nevertheless, a definition will follow – if only to reinforce the terms being used. A coaching process can be defined as:

> The purposeful improvement of competition sports performance, achieved through a planned programme of preparation and competition. In normal circumstances, a coach manages this process within a time- and context-bound agreement or contract, although there will be considerable variety in the implementation of the process.

It is important to use the term 'coaching process' as the basic unit in communication about sports coaching. It is inappropriate to define what is meant by the term 'coach'; this might best be thought of as a generic role descriptor, such as social worker or architect. Although such a descriptor may provide some general expectations of the role, and some knowledge and expertise is assumed, operational definitions are useful only in the context of a specific coaching process. Another way to express this is to say that coaching practice can only really be understood from an analysis of the coaching process, and not merely from an analysis of the coach. Another point to make, and one that will be reinforced later, is that we should try to avoid using the term 'coaching' or 'to coach' to apply only to circumstances in which the coach is directing training or practice sessions.

Acceptance of the process nature of coaching has implications for the key skills of the coach. Before identifying these, however, it would be valuable to say a little more about the role of the coach. This should provide us with some insight into how a coach might interpret the key elements of the coaching process. The role can be described in a number of ways:

1. As a statement of priorities elaborating on the central purpose of coaching. An example of this would be the coach who says that 'my role is to help athletes to make decisions for themselves'. This type of statement does not suggest that the coach will fail to exercise a leadership role or carry out all of the more technical functions of the coach. However, it does reflect a value position and might be expected to influence the leadership style adopted by such a coach.
2. As a broad descriptor of the functions being undertaken by the coach. A useful categorization is to divide the coach's role into three parts: direct intervention, process management and external constraints management.
   a. Direct intervention characterizes those situations in which the coach works directly with the athlete – for example, in training sessions or at competitions.
   b. Process management relates to the management of the coaching process and how this indirectly influences the athlete. Thus, planning, organizing, counselling, selecting, monitoring and keeping records will be process management responsibilities carried out by the coach. A potentially very important function will be the management of the support science team.
   c. In external constraints management, the coach attempts to control and maximize the effect of constraints, such as finance, facilities, competition access etc., which impinge on the athlete. However, the coach is also likely to have a role in more strategic issues, such as in setting organizational goals, recruitment, performance planning, coach education, development strategies etc.

      Obviously, one would expect these three sets of functions to be interdependent. However, one might also expect the balance between the functions to differ in a number of different circumstances. Head coaches, who have a number of support personnel, may find themselves dealing with the more strategic issues to the exclusion of some of the direct intervention role. The club coach with no assistance may find that the direct intervention role precludes giving full attention to the other functions. In any performance sport context, we might express concern if the process management functions were not given sufficient attention.

3. As an issue of organizational hierarchy. This has two elements. The first refers to the coach's role in relation to the execution of the coaching process, and the second refers to the coach's relationship to support personnel.
   a. In the first, there will clearly be a number of distinctive coaching 'positions', and these will have implications for the extent to which

the coaching process can or will be implemented. The most obvious distinction is between the participation coach and the performance coach, and we will return to this shortly. However, even within performance coaching, leadership role differences will determine how the coaching process is to be implemented. The coach of national squads who meets the athletes relatively infrequently will be likely to operate only a partial coaching process. Perhaps the club coach will be the individual who will be most likely to direct a comprehensive process, given the opportunities for the greatest control over variables. There are a number of confounding factors – the player/coach, the manager/coach, professional instructors, university or collegiate coaches, and the assistant coaches, defensive co-ordinators and trainers reporting to head coaches. These positions are important because they affect education and training, accountability and expectations. It is a reasonable assumption to make that there should be a coincidence of intent between the scale of the coaching process, the athlete's aspirations, the achievements expected, the coach's accountability for this achievement, and the coach's expertise and experience.

b. The second aspect of organizational hierarchy is the relationship of the coach to non-coaching support personnel and, in particular, to sports science support teams. There is no doubt that the specialist expertise of the sport scientist can extend well beyond that of the coach in particular, discrete areas. There is a need, particularly for the elite athlete, for this expertise to be incorporated into the coaching process. The expertise of the coach is demonstrated by the metacognitive co-ordination (synergy) of each of the discrete elements of the coaching process. The most important factor is that the integration and co-ordination of the process is upset to the least extent possible. In order to appreciate the nature of the integration exercise, it is necessary to understand the role played by the support team. Is it a *supporting* role (e.g. screening, scouting, testing), in which the relevant expert provides data which is subsequently incorporated into decision making and delivery by the coach? Is it a *replacement* role (implementing training programmes, managing injury, directing tactics), in which the expert substitutes for the coach in this particular aspect of the coaching process?

It is equally important to stress that the network approach, in which the coach (or might we begin to call this person the 'performance manager'!) co-ordinates a team of specialists, is a vision of the future. The coach in this instance will require strong skills of planning, integrating and co-ordinating. However, current coaching practice is somewhat different. For the majority of coaches, networking in this way is not feasible because of having to operate in relative isolation, and with only partial support from a series of support services. It takes a strong coach to assert the primacy of integration and co-ordination (because of the multivariable and interdependent nature of performance factors) against the obviously expert, but perhaps less synoptically aware, advice of the specialist in a particular field (biomechanics, sports physiology etc.).

This analysis of the issues relating to the coach's role differentiation reinforces a point alluded to earlier. There is a key principle that is necessary for understanding and analysing the coaching practice associated with any role: it is more useful to consider the variation in the coaching process than the variation in the coach. In other words, there are coaches with differing leadership styles, value frameworks, personal characteristics and levels of knowledge and expertise. Limited insight is gained by trying to match these differences to the actual roles played by coaches, since a very wide variety of characteristics are demonstrated at all levels. It is much more valuable to analyse coaches' practice and behaviour in terms of the coaching process in which they and their athletes are engaged. An individual coach may exhibit fairly stable characteristics but play different roles – for example, club coach, teacher, representative coach and assistant to national squad coach. Understanding the particular role and coaching process enables inferences to be drawn about accountability, expectations, effectiveness and expertise. Knowledge of the coaching process – its elements, boundaries, resources, goals, scale etc. – means that the coach's performance can be evaluated (albeit with some difficulty!) within a specific role-context and with an acknowledgement that the athletes' performance outcomes are limited by the scale and scope of the process (in addition to the inherent constraints of athlete capacity, coach's expertise etc.).

Participation coaching and performance coaching

An important distinction between coaching roles must be highlighted. In order to appreciate coaches' practice and begin to identify the skills or expertise required, we must distinguish between *participation coaching* and *performance coaching*. This is fundamental to understanding the wide range of leadership roles to be found in sport. The ski instructor, the professional rugby coach, the PE teacher, the club swimming coach and the British hockey team coach may each find the term 'coach' used to describe his or her role. However, there is plainly such a significant difference between these roles that a further distinction needs to be made. *Participation* coaching best describes contexts in which the principal goal is *not* competition success. The performers are less intensively engaged in the process, and may be concerned more with improvement in order to enjoy participation and its immediate satisfactions. The emphasis is on *participation* (i.e. taking part) rather than *preparation*. The coaching process is not implemented to a systematically controlled plan, and the quality of the interpersonal relationship between athlete and coach may be emphasized beyond other goals. Not all of the performance elements will be dealt with, and the emphasis may be on learning skills.

On the other hand, performance coaching is the more appropriate term for coaching processes involving athletes who are preparing for competition and who set longer-term goals. Their involvement is almost entirely characterized by detailed planning and monitoring of progress, and their commitment, in terms of time, effort and emotion, is significant. The coaching process is understandably more extensive, and there is an attempt to control the variables that influence performance improvement. In performance coaching, the athlete is likely to come into contact with a number of individuals (assistant coaches, managers, sponsors, physiotherapists, etc.) because of the scale of the coaching process. Once again, it is worth emphasizing the point that participation and performance coaching are two very distinctive roles, and not two stages on a continuum. The roles differ in terms of purpose, goals, occupational circumstances, athlete aspirations, expertise and relationship to competition sport structures. The beginner performance coach is not a participation coach. The experienced participation coach is not a performance coach. This is an area of research that has been largely neglected. We need to understand better how coaches are recruited into performance coaching. It seems likely that they will move, in a number of ways, from competition sport into assisting roles, and thence into positions of greater coaching responsibility (Lyle *et al.*, 1997).

We have already noted that the expertise demanded of the participation coach and performance coach may differ in emphasis. The participation coach concentrates more on single episodes or sessions, whereas the performance coach may need to engage to a greater extent in planning, monitoring and managing. These skills are necessary because of the process element. The attempt to control the factors influencing the improvement and exhibition of sports performance is so complex, and the process so extensive, that the coach's capacities in planning, regulating, integrating, co-ordinating, managing, leading and problem solving will be crucial. These skills will be in addition to the delivery skills required for direct intervention (i.e. directing training sessions). All coaches will have developed, to some extent, the skills of communicating, teaching and organizing, which are complemented by a capacity for interpersonal social skills. When sports-specific knowledge, sub-discipline knowledge (sports psychology, physiology etc.), previous performer experience and desirable personal qualities are added to the list, the result is a formidable range of expertise. Of course, all coaches will not necessarily consistently exhibit all of these qualities, and questions can be raised about the quality of the coach education intended to develop such capacities. For the moment, the message is that coaching expertise ought to be developed in relation to the particular process in which the coach is engaged or wishes to be engaged. There may be a danger that, in concentrating on the immediacy of practice, process skills are neglected in favour of technical knowledge and delivery skills.

Failing to understand the difference of emphasis between essentially problem solving and decision making skills on the one hand, and the craft-based delivery skills on the other, has resulted in unnecessary debate about the 'art' and 'science' of coaching (Woodman, 1993). Coaching may not always be applied in a systematic fashion (Lyle, 1992), and some sports (particularly interactive team sports) are so multivariable that the complexity may overwhelm the coaches' capacity to plan adequately for and control the variables. It is also true to say that the enhancement of athlete performance has a strong research-based science discipline basis, whereas the coaching process as a whole, despite many statements of principle, has been investigated much less rigorously. Coaches sometimes operate on an apparently intuitive application of their experiential knowledge. Their procedural knowledge (how to) is not always easily verbalized, although it may be quite sophisticated. The result of this dilemma is a recourse to art form as an explanation for what is really the under-investigated practice of coaches. Any process that involves human beings, is very complex, contested and essentially cognitive, and involves a high degree of integration and co-ordination, will appear unique and idiosyncratic. Coaching practice may not be as systematic as it could be, but this is no excuse for substituting the inexplicable for the unexplained.

Summary

This section has attempted a concise and cohesive explanation of the coaching process. The result is a set of constructs about coaching, which are open to challenge. This is the intention – to generate debate about the coaching process, and to stimulate research into coaching practice. The following section is in two parts. In the first, there is a review of some of the coaching process literature. The second part examines previous attempts to model the process.

Describing and modelling the process

There has been relatively little literature that has explored the conceptual development of the coaching process and treated the coaching process as a problematic aspect of the research. Researchers have preferred to focus on observable behaviour and on the direct intervention aspect of the coach's role (for example, Solomon *et al.*, 1996). In addition, studies that have tried to go beyond observation have used very limited interpretations of coaching tasks (Jones *et al.*, 1997). The outcome is that there is a great deal of literature on matters such as leadership, feedback and coaching style, etc., but these have largely been restricted to descriptive studies or have used measures of athlete satisfaction as criteria of appropriate outcomes. The reduction in the scale and complexity of the coaching process, and the failure to situate the coaching boundary variables, have reduced the value of such studies. These direct intervention studies, and the concomitant emphasis on coaching episodes, have served to marginalize the coach's planning, monitoring, decision making, contingency, integration and managing skills, at the expense of instructional, pedagogical and motivational skills. The result is that coaching behaviour is emphasized, but coaching practice is sadly under-researched.

The coaching process has been recognized as such for more than a decade (Lyle, 1984). This early work pointed to the distinction between extended professional practice and coaching behaviour involving athletes directly. This was followed in 1986 with a paradigm paper for the VIII Commonwealth Conference (Lyle, 1986) in which it was suggested that coaching theory 'lacked an underpinning conceptual base'. The intention had been to stimulate debate and invite contributions from around the world, some of which would focus on developing that theory. Disappointingly, writers are still able to say, more than 10 years later, that progress has been slow. For example, Sherman *et al.* (1997), who adopted a rather narrow interpretation of coaching in their instructional model and used a very limited article (Fairs, 1987) to exemplify what they said was the coaching process, nevertheless claimed that coaching was under-conceptualized.

Lyle (1996) attempted to address the conceptualization of the coaching process. This paper was the precursor of much of the thinking behind the earlier parts of this chapter. One of its principal suggestions was that research papers should make clear their assumptions about the coaching process(es) under scrutiny. The boundaries of the coaching process should always be identified. This would help the reader to distinguish between episodic teaching variables and the more complex performance coaching *process*. The paper also explored in some detail the extent to which coaching practice could be said to be systematic. Drawing on earlier research (Lyle, 1992), it was suggested that coaches have a systematic planning 'shell', but that their implementation and regulation of the process relies on a series of trigger or threshold mechanisms. Planning, which is at the heart of coaching practice, differs between the seasonal target sports (e.g. athletics) and those sports (such as league sports) with an emphasis on weekly performances. Contingency planning is much more prevalent in the latter instance.

A clear message that has begun to emerge in the literature is the acknowledgement that coaching is a cognitive enterprise, although it also relies on practical implementation skills. Abraham and Collins (1998) provide a very timely critique of behavioural assessment research and current coach education provision. They support the contention that coaches' expertise is about making 'correct decisions' and is a 'cognitive skill'. Disappointingly, the paper does not add to this analysis of the process, and lapses into the teaching paradigm interpretation of the coaching process. Nevertheless, their exhortation to produce research that is more usable and applicable is valuable.

A recent approach to coaching research has been to acknowledge that the knowledge and practice of expert coaches needs to be investigated by qualitative approaches that ask the coaches for their personal insights (Bloom *et al.*, 1997). Several useful contributions have been made in this way, but these have tended to be in isolation. Given the conceptual framework described in the earlier part of this chapter, and the difficulty of educating coaches' decision making, it is not surprising that Gould *et al.* (1990) found that coaches' knowledge developed through situated learning from other coaches and that it was difficult to identify general principles for practice. Similarly, Salmela's (1995) interviews with expert coaches revealed that they were expert teachers. However, the most important finding was that the coaches integration skills (a reflection of the coaching process) were paramount – 'a metacognitive form of knowledge which experts possess and are able to verbalize. Academics cannot compete with these integrated concepts'. Cote *et al.* (1995) attempted to take these concepts further into a conceptual model, and this will be evaluated in the second part of the section.

This has been a very selective review of a small selection of the literature, and these and other articles are discussed further in Chapter 3. The overall conclusion is that, despite the research into observable coaching behaviour, little of it has tried to embrace the entirety of the coaching process. From the researchers' point of view this is understandable, since the experimental design parameters are more controllable. What is more disappointing is that there are few attempts to offer a conceptual appreciation of the coaching process with which to provide a framework for analysis and understanding. One way of doing this is to model the coaching process. The next section examines some examples.

Models are a means of representing the structure and function of, in this case, a process. They identify the dimensions of the process and how these interact in practice. A good model will describe the phenomenon appropriately, have explanatory power when applied to specific cases, allow inferences to be drawn about its application and have some predictive power when particular values or weightings are inputted. There are two different types of models – a model *of* something, and a model *for* something. Any model *of* coaching practice should be based on empirical research into expert or successful coaching practice from which a common process is deduced. This has the value of being based on (expert) practice, but is clearly limited by the capacity of researchers to embrace the process in all its variety and context. In addition, it may perpetuate traditional practice if used in coach education. Models *for* coaching are more idealistic representations of the process. They are devised by identifying a set of assumptions about the process and creating a structure and function based on rational, logical application of these assumptions, or on sets of existing principles (e.g. pedagogical, sports training theory, problem solving, etc.). Such models are useful for coach education and training and for analysis, but may not necessarily represent existing good practice. Difficulties may occur if a model *for* is introduced into practice, since its assumptions may not be matched by the existing parameters.

Models are normally presented in two dimensions, and this restricts the capacity of the modeller to fully represent a process. There is also a tendency to emphasize structure rather than function. This is a problem in modelling a continuous and interactive process such as that which exists in coaching. A number of issues specific to processes have to be addressed:

1. Although it is possible to identify the variables that apply to coaching, these interact and co-act in a dynamic fashion.
2. The process is based on bringing about change in individuals, and is driven by individuals. There is, therefore, a high degree of dependence on human factors – emotion, cognition and motivation. In practice, this leads to an untidy and unique process.
3. There is a difficult decision to be made between representing the generic core of the process, which may be neither useful nor sufficiently descriptive of practice, or elaborating to include significant variation (degrees of freedom). The coaching process is very context specific, and we have already noted the strong element of 'how' the process is implemented.
4. Representations of processes have particular requirements. What is the central purpose of the process, and how is it operationalized? How is the process regulated (i.e. monitored and measured)? How does the process deal with change, both intentional and unintentional?

Obviously, there is a demanding set of problems for the model builder. What follows is a brief review of a number of individuals who have attempted to address these problems.

Fairs' (1987) model is referred to here because it is cited in many reviews (for example, Woodman, 1993). Fairs' model is a five-step 'objectives' model, which is intended to represent a process. It is a model *for* coaching and employs 'orderly, inter-related steps' – data collection, diagnosis, planning, execution, and evaluation. The model is continuous in the sense that evaluation leads to reassessment and revision. The assumptions on which the model rests emphasize a teaching, episodic approach, which may result in a lack of attention to long-term planning. There is no recognition of the complexity of performance, or of the interpersonal nature of the coaching relationship. However, it is important not to criticize the model for what it did not attempt to be. Although it is a very simplistic objectives model, which could be applied to any process, it does illustrate a number of useful stages. However, the model is not sufficiently descriptive of the coaching process in practice, and the absence of context, complexity and regulation limits its explanatory and predictive capacity.

The model by Franks *et al.* (1996) is also quoted extensively (for example, Woodman, 1993; Sherman *et al.*, 1997; Abraham and Collins, 1998). Their model of the coaching process has to be inferred from a paper that deals with coaching effectiveness. The most important assumption identified is that, once again, coaching is conceptualized as episodic skill learning–in other words, an instructional model. The model is an objectives model, but there is a suggestion that quantification should be introduced to measure progress. Analysis of competition performance is recognized as one of these measures, and there is an emphasis on key performance factors. The ideas encapsulated in this model have been used to devise a computer-based system for analysing coaching behaviours (Johnson and Franks, 1991; More *et al.*, 1994), although with limited success. The model might better be termed an instructional delivery model, and this is reflected in its behavioural emphasis. However, the attempt to use quantifiable performance measures as progression and regulation mechanisms is useful. It is a model *for* coaching, in which the cyclical use of key performance factors may usefully be employed to describe team sport coaching practice. Once again, there is a limited interpretation of the coaching process *per se*, but it is a potentially valuable analytical tool.

There are few models *of* coaching practice. However, Cote and colleagues (1995) have devised a model from interviews with 17 expert gymnastics coaches. Their model is useful for recognizing the difference between contributory contextual factors and what they term the 'core process'. The core process is facilitated by a 'mental model' developed by the coach. The model has also acknowledged the complexity of the process and the need for 'constant monitoring and adjustment'. Although the authors acknowledge that the representation in their paper does not fully convey all the detail elicited from the coaches in their interviews, a complete understanding of how the process operates is not clear, and this limits the model's descriptive powers. In addition, the nature of the relationships between the constructs identified is not described, and this limits its predictive capacity. Although the paper addresses many of the difficult issues raised in this chapter, the final outcome is perhaps illustrative of the problems involved in aggregating and synthesizing coaches' practice, and in representing such a complex process.

Before moving on to one final model, passing reference should also be made to examples of models which, although tangential to the coaching process itself, do provide some useful analytical tools. For example, MacLean and Chelladurai (1995) devised a 'dimensions of coaching performance' model. This was an occupational and organizational model that included an unproblematic set of assumptions about the coaching process. Nevertheless, it contains some useful constructs describing direct and indirect coaching behaviours. In addition, in acknowledging the occupational context of coaching, it highlights the relevance for a developing profession in the United Kingdom. Another example is that of Sherman and colleagues (1997), who acknowledge the difficulty of conceptualizing and modelling the coaching process, but whose re-conceptualization into a sports instruction model is too limiting. This model fails to distinguish between participation and performance coaching, adopts the episodic teaching approach and largely ignores the interpersonal relationships developed. As such, it is a useful illustration of the dangers of partial answers (however valuable) failing to provide an holistic analysis of the coaching context, which is claimed but not delivered in this particular case.

Before moving on to the final example, a future model is predicted in which the coaching process is treated as a complex, dynamical, self-regulating system (Barton, 1994). In complex, adaptive systems, the system learns to adapt; in this case, coaching behaviour emerges that will bring the greatest reward for the most appropriate amount and type of work. Perhaps the most important contribution will be the identification of the most important attractors (key elements) around which the system functions (for example, competition performance, the mental attitude of the performer, coach's mental model, etc.). The coach will focus on these and seek to provide the context within which incremental progress occurs. However, the interplay between the vast array of variables involved in the coaching process will be treated as a self-regulating system. The coach will focus on a small number of key attractors that exert the most influence on progress, and use trigger or threshold mechanisms to contingency manage any others that are disturbing the system.

As a final example, I have invoked an author's privilege to describe my own attempts to model the coaching process. The ideas have developed over an extended period of time, and are intended to address a number of the limitations evidenced in other models. These ideas were brought together in a paper and more recently in a coach education workbook (Lyle, 1996; Lyle, 1998). Although there is a diagram to illustrate the relationship between the elements of the process (Figure 1.1), the model consists of three further stages: prior assumptions about the coaching process, identification of the building blocks on which the process is constructed, and a conceptualization of how the process operates. Despite it being a model *for* sports coaching, its roots lie in an extensive experience as a coach, and it has been modified during research on coaches' behaviour (Lyle, 1992). Its constituent parts have begun to be researched (for example, the basis for Chapter 11 in this book).

The assumptions on which the model is based were outlined earlier in the chapter; the significant words used are process, instrumental pursuit of performance goals, interpersonal relationship, competition sport (or an explicit reference to developmental/participatory goals), control of variables, purposeful intervention, and control of outcome related to scale and scope of process. In their elaborated form, these assumptions provide the principles within which the model should be understood. Criticisms of models or conceptual analyses should first address these assumptions, prior to concentrating on the detail of the process and sub-processes. Failure to provide the

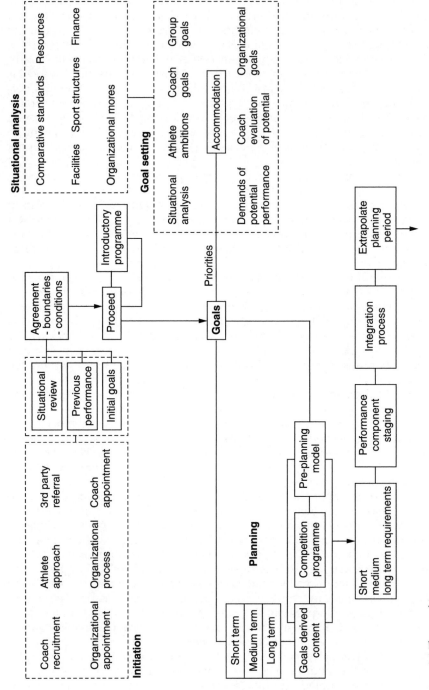

Figure 1.1 The coaching process

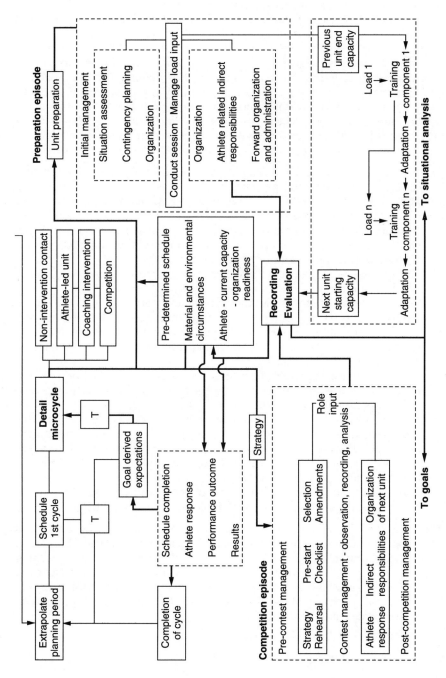

Figure 1.1 (*Continued*) The coaching process

assumptions on which the analysis is based is a major criticism of a great deal of research into coaching practice and behaviour.

The building blocks, or starter concepts, for the model were identified in each of the sources cited above (Lyle, 1996; Lyle, 1998). These are: an information base, knowledge and skills of the coach, athletes' capabilities, performance analysis, regulatory mechanisms, systematic progression, operationalization (programme management, practice management, competition management), goals setting, planning, a preparation programme, a competition programme and individualization. These building blocks are then interwoven into the process, which is represented in Figure 1.1. What is more important is how the process actually operates. A number of principles will assist the reader to conceptualize how the model will operate in practice:

1. The process is cyclical and operates around a set of goals, which exert a continuous influence on progress.
2. The process is serial, and consists of an aggregation of performer and coach behaviours. The performer's practice is varied – training sessions, more informal preparation (e.g. mental rehearsal at home), competitions etc. The coach's practice embraces direct intervention, indirect responsibilities and management of the process.
3. The process operates within a specific set of external constraints, some of which are more controllable than others.
4. The specificity of the goals, the expectations generated within these, improvements (or decrements) in performance, and the time-bound nature of competition seasons, resource allocation and athlete maturity, create a process dynamic, which should lead to regulatory (monitoring and planning) mechanisms.
5. A number of the relatively discrete elements in the process (preparation episodes, competition episodes, goal setting, planning) have sub-processes operating within them.
6. The process is a continuous series of interpersonal interactions. This dependence on individuals enables the process to be interpreted, managed and delivered in a wide variety of ways. Therefore, the overall process is subject to personal philosophies, styles, leadership orientations, characteristics, and motivations etc.
7. There is a cultural dimension to the process, and this brings with it a series of ethical, moral, and legal implications and responsibilities.

This is a model *for* coaching, and is therefore subject to the limitations (described earlier) that apply to such models. Its potential usefulness is in its attempt to embrace a much more holistic interpretation of the coaching process, and to redress a little the attention paid in other models to the instructional role of the coach. It is intended to be a catalyst for research. There are still questions about how coaches' practice relates to the model, and this is dealt with in the final section.

Coaching practice

There is no doubt that an ideally implemented coaching process would be extremely demanding indeed. Completely systematic practice implies a constant process of data gathering, compiling player profiles, monitoring progress in all performance components, analysing all competition performance data, planning and re-planning, individualizing all programmes, managing player lifestyles, recording all observations during interpersonal interaction, and ensuring a relationship between training cycles. These recording and regulating functions are in addition to the delivery functions in training and competition, and other organizational and administrative tasks. This has to be set against a number of factors:

- The difficulty of making accurate measurements of (some) workloads and characteristics, and the expectation of natural fluctuations in performance.
- The changing nature of the environment (facilities, weather, availability, injury, illness).
- An absence of evidence (from naturalistic research) on the effect of subtle changes in workloads on eventual performance.
- The psychological benefit to performers of a stable work pattern.

Given the sheer volume of data management implied by systematic practice, the coach has to weigh up the cost–benefit of very detailed regulation of the process against time spent on other direct intervention strategies. There is a need to find a balance between appropriate monitoring and regulation and workable practices for the athlete and coach. This will be exacerbated or alleviated by the presence of a support team, and the extent to which the coach is full or part-time. It may also be influenced by the coaching style adopted.

Coaches often operate within a pattern of professional short cuts. When taken to extremes (no recording, no written planning, short-term contingency and crisis management, use of traditional programmes), coaching practice can appear to be unregulated, by the 'seat of the pants', and completely intuitive. On the other hand, the analysis of the coaching process presented throughout this chapter can be aggregated to provide a set of propositions about coaching practice. Although there is tremendous variety in coaching practice, and this is compounded by the uniqueness and complexity of each coaching process, performance coaches:

1. Operate, more or less systematically, within a fairly detailed planning umbrella.
2. Implement more detailed exercise loadings within target sports (such as athletics), and less detailed or exact workloads in more cyclical sports (team sports in leagues).
3. Play a central role in direct intervention, particularly in interactive-skill based sports with high levels of coach-led drills. They constantly balance priorities between performance components and relatively imprecise workload management.
4. Make extensive use of mental models of day-to-day expectations about athletes' performance in both competition and training.
5. Develop sports-specific, personal cognitive matrices, which are derived from experience and facilitate decision making.
6. Exercise what is apparently intuitive decision making, but is simply an efficient mechanism for reducing decision making options.

7. Supplement subjective data gathering by objective testing and monitoring at selected times in the programme.
8. Use contingency planning as a normal and expected part of coaching practice. There is constant fine-tuning of schedules, and major adjustments are made to accommodate injury, illness and recruitment changes.
9. Operate a system of crisis thresholds (i.e. recognize and deal with problems only when they reach a threshold of under-achievement). This takes into account fluctuations in performance.
10. Solve short- and long-term problems ranging from competition management (strategy, selection) to resource management and personnel integration. Coaches have a bank of coping strategies to deal with common problems. (This has implications for coach education.)
11. Make use of support staff, as available, to provide component specific (biomechanical analysis) or function specific (pre-competition psychological preparation) assistance. This assistance is either integrated into the coach's decision making, or is an integral part of the process.

It becomes clear that coaches' practice is a largely cognitive enterprise, from the immediate decision making of the training session and the competition, to communication with performers and more long-term planning and programme building. This has obvious implications for coach education; in particular, for the way in which knowledge and experience are translated into practice routines. Little is known about the stages through which novice performance coaches pass on the way to expert status. Much more research is needed on coaches' use of mental models, scripts and schemata, and their impact on decision making. This is explored at some length in Chapter 11. It will also have become obvious that this description of coaching practice has focused on performance coaching rather than participation coaching which, it was stressed earlier, is a related but different process.

Summary

The purpose of this introductory chapter is to provide a conceptual framework for the coaching process. In doing so, it might not only contribute to what is currently an under-developed field, but also become a template to which subsequent chapters can be related. Nevertheless, this is only one chapter, and it cannot be expected to embrace all that there is to say about the coaching process. The emphasis here has been on delimiting the process itself and examining attempts to model it. The intention was to furnish the reader with analytical insights, which might prove useful for future research. It is important to note that subsequent chapters will address other aspects of the process. If this chapter described the 'what' of coaching, other chapters will describe the 'how'. In particular, the next chapter will deal with coaching philosophies.

There is no doubt that there has been insufficient research, or at best inappropriately directed research, on the coaching process. There are at present no detailed models of the process (bearing in mind that the search is for generic models of the coaching process that apply, at least in principle, to all sports). This has so far proved too difficult to achieve when a realistic interpretation of the expert performance coaching role is the objective. The model offered in this chapter is intended to be comprehensive and process-related, and is a contribution to delimiting the research field. Very little has been learned from the teaching/instructional paradigm when applied to performance coaching. As with many developing fields, there is a catch-22 situation. There is a need for research into coaching practice. However, analytical tools have not been developed to assist this endeavour, largely because there has been so little investigation into coaching practice! As this review of the coaching process suggests, coaching is a cognitive activity, interspersed with practical delivery skills, and the cognitive activity involved in implementing the coaching process is not well researched.

In some ways, it is surprising that a leadership role such as coaching, which has such a potentially significant and all-embracing impact on performers, is so under-developed in conceptual terms. However, the process element has now been acknowledged, and this is the precursor to appropriate coach education. Thus far, we have undervalued the coach's skills by not being able adequately to describe them. In addition, not having conceptualized the cognitive and integrative elements of the performance coach's role, we have been too quick to pass them off as intuitive and therefore not subjected them to systematic analysis. In bypassing these fundamental skills of the performance coach, the secondary skills of delivery and teaching have been over-emphasized. Even in trying to understand the recruitment of, and motives for, coaching, information on performance coaching has been masked by data gathered on participation coaches.

The coaching process is at the heart of the phenomenon called coaching. In practice, this is found in its applied and widely varying forms. Personal philosophies, organizational and occupational contexts, resources, specific sports, performer aspirations and many other environmental features individualize the process. This whole set of factors contributes to the uniqueness and complexity of the coaching process, which makes research such a challenge. Nevertheless, improvements to coach education and to coaching practice depend on a sound understanding of the coaching process. This chapter and those that follow are a contribution to this quest.

References

Abraham, A. and Collins, D. (1998). Examining and extending research in coach development. *Quest*, **50**, 55–79.

Barton, S. (1994). Chaos, self-organization and psychology. *Am. Psychol.*, **49**, 5–14.

Bloom, G. A., Durand-Bush, N. and Salmela, J. H. (1997). Pre- and post-competition routines of expert coaches of team sports. *Sport Psychol.*, **11**, 127–41.

Cote, J., Salmela, J., Trudel, P. *et al.* (1995). The coaching model: a grounded assessment of expert gymnastic coaches' knowledge. *J. Sport Exer. Psychol.*, **17(1)**, 1–17.

Fairs, J. (1987). The coaching process: the essence of coaching. *Sports Coach.*, **11(1)**, 17–19.

Franks, I. M., Sinclair, G. D., Thomson, W. and Goodman, D. (1986). Analysis of the coaching process. *Sci. Period. Res. Technol. Sport* (January).

Gould, D., Giannini, J., Kane, V. and Hodge, K. (1990). Educational needs of elite US National Team, Pan-American and Olympic coaches. *J. Teach. Physical Ed.*, **9(4)**, 332–44.

Johnson, R. B. and Franks, I. M. (1991). Measuring the reliability of a computer-aided systematic observation instrument. *Can. J. Sport Sci.*, **16**, 45–57.

Jones, D. F., Housner, L. D. and Kornspan, A. S. (1997). Interactive decision making and behaviour of experienced and inexperienced basketball coaches during practice. *J. Teach. Physical Ed.*, **16**, 454–68.

Lyle, J. (1984). Towards a concept of coaching. *Scot. J. Physical Ed.*, **12(1)**, 27–31.

Lyle, J. (1986). Coach education: preparation for a profession. In *Coach Education: Preparation for a Profession*. VIII Commonwealth and International Conference on Sport, PE, Dance, Recreation and Health. Glasgow, pp. 1–25. EFN Spon.

Lyle, J. (1992). Systematic coaching behaviour: an investigation into the coaching process and the implications of the findings for coach education. In *Sport and Physical Activity: Moving towards Excellence* (T. Williams, L. Almond and A. Sparkes, eds), pp. 463–9. EFN Spon.

Lyle, J. (1996). A conceptual appreciation of the sports coaching process. *Scot. Cent. Res. Papers Sport, Leisure Soc.*, **1(1)**, 15–37.

Lyle, J. (1997). Management training and the sports coaching analogy: a content analysis of six management training products. In *Conference Proceedings: Fifth Congress of the European Association for Sport Management, Glasgow, Scotland* (I. Davies and E. Wolstencroft, eds), pp. 211–21. EASM.

Lyle, J., Allison, M. and Taylor, J. (1997). *Factors Influencing the Motivations of Sports Coaches: Research Report No. 49*. Scottish Sports Council.

Lyle, J. (1998). *The Coaching Process* (NCFB2001). National Coaching Foundation.

MacLean, J. C. and Chelladurai, P. (1995). Dimensions of coaching performance: development of a scale. *J. Sport Man.*, **9**, 194–207.

More, K. G., McGarry, T., Partridge, D. and Franks, I. M. (1994). A computer-assisted analysis of verbal coaching in soccer. *J. Sport Behav.*, **19**, 319–37.

Salmela, J. H. (1995). Learning from the development of expert coaches. *Coach. Sports Sci. J.*, **2(2)**, 3–13.

Sherman, C., Crassini, B., Maschette, W. and Sands, R. (1997). Instructional sports psychology: a reconceptualization of sports coaching as sports instruction. *Int. J. Sport Psychol.*, **28(2)**, 103–25.

Soloman, G. B., Striegel, D. A., Eliot, J. F. *et al.* (1996). The self-fulfilling prophecy in college basketball: implications for effective coaching. *J. Appl. Sport Psychol.*, **8**, 44–59.

Woodman, L. (1993). Coaching: a science, an art, an emerging profession. *Sports Coach*, **2(2)**, 1–13.

2

Coaching philosophy and coaching behaviour

John Lyle

- Differences in coaches' practice
- Factors influencing coaching styles
- Characteristics of a coaching philosophy
- An example of a coaching philosophy
- A content analysis of a sample of coaching philosophies
- A humanistic approach to coaching
- Characteristics of humanistic coaching practice
- Coaching philosophy and sporting context
- Coaching and ethics

Introduction

None of us expresses surprise at the range of styles adopted by managers in dealing with their employees or the variety in bedside manner demonstrated by doctors. It is unlikely that the competence of either professional would be called into account on this basis alone, although it would be acknowledged that some approaches were more appropriate in certain situations than in others. This chapter deals with a similar variation in coaching behaviour. It is immediately obvious that not all coaches operate in the same fashion, have the same beliefs about coaching or treat their athletes in the same way. This might be interpreted as differing in the 'how' of coaching, rather than the 'what' of coaching.

It should be established at the outset that the purpose of the chapter is not to suggest that all coaches should operate in the same way. The differences that are present in coaching practice allow for the individuality of the coach, the preferences of performers and the demands of different organizational settings. On the other hand, the coach's behaviour will often reflect more deep-seated values, and these will be subject to societal scrutiny. Where there is a mismatch between behaviour and context, or where societal expectations are not met, the coach's behaviour may be considered problematical. On a more positive note, the education and training of coaches, along with recruitment and selection, will want to take behaviour patterns into account. As part of their training, coaches should become aware of their beliefs about coaching and, in particular, how this influences their practice. Of course, this is a process that should continue throughout a coaching career. Although beliefs and values are fairly stable, there will be some changes over time.

When invited to, coaches are able to express their thoughts about coaching practice in a set of inter-related statements. The drawing together of these value statements about how they practise coaching is what we term 'coaching philosophies'. These value frameworks indicate to the reader what the coach believes is important in coaching, and are a guide to the coach's behaviour. It should be obvious that differences between what coaches report as their beliefs and how they actually behave in practice is a very fertile area for research. When there is a consensus in values (and in patterns of behaviour) between significant numbers of coaches, and particularly when it is promulgated within the literature of professional bodies, we might call this an ideology of coaching practice. This can be exemplified in what is generally referred to as 'a humanistic approach to coaching' (illustrated in some detail later in the chapter). However, it is important to note that terms that are synonymous, such as coaching philosophy, coaching ethos, coaching approach or coaching style, are not just general descriptors of beliefs and values. The 'how' of coaching is not an optional extra. All coaching practice involves an interpretation or application of the coaching process (whether participation or performance), and it should be possible to delve into this practice to find the beliefs and values that drive it. In other words, the core philosophy may not always be manifest or verbalized, but its effects are ever present. For example, communication styles, decision making, feedback, goal setting, counselling, disciplinary behaviour and management will all individually and collectively reflect the coach's belief system. In the context of this book, which seeks to understand the principles underpinning the coaching process and how these affect practice, it is essential to provide a framework within which the application and delivery of the coaching process can be understood.

Coaches' practice can be expected to vary on the following bases:

1. Coaching involves an interpersonal relationship, and the vagaries of human behaviour in terms of commitment, motivation and effort lead us to expect a range of approaches. This will apply to both coach and athlete. The coaching role goes beyond that of technical expert. The improvement in competition performance, which is at the heart of performance coaching, can be thought of as a change in behaviour. When this happens over an extended period of time in an individual human being, with all the physical, psychological and emotional responses to training and competition, and is complicated by issues of power, self-image, and personality, it is hardly surprising that different approaches are adopted to achieve the end purpose. Again, this range of potential responses applies to both coach and athlete.

2. Coaching practice cannot be value-free; values will always be represented in coaches' behaviour. This is partly because we are dealing with people, and partly because the purpose of coaching involves constructs about which society has views (or a range of views). For example, the importance placed on winning, levels of commitment to sport, individuality, abuse, cheating, harassment, discrimination, violence and over-pressurizing young people are all issues that will provoke a societal

response (if considered excessive, inappropriate, or against the prevailing ideology!). Each coach will have developed a personal set of views on coaching, sport, and interpersonal relationships, which will have evolved over time, and will be derived from experience and other kinds of education.

3. The purposes of coaching cannot be assumed to be one-dimensional. Individual athlete aspirations range from the recreational to the Olympic, and the coach will be subject to the same range of objectives. A common, although rather simplistic, exemplification of this range is the emphasis often put on the athlete's personal development or on competition success. Adopting any one of this range of purposes for coaching brings with it a further set of expectations about how its goals can best be achieved, and what this will mean for the coach's behaviour.

The principal objective of the chapter is to examine in some depth what is meant by a philosophy of coaching. Some common features in coaching philosophies are identified by evaluating the results of a content analysis of a sample of coaches' value statements. This will be preceded by a more general account of coaching styles, and followed by a discussion of the potential difficulties faced when attempting to implement one particular approach known as a humanistic approach to coaching. It is inevitable when describing 'what is' in coaching that we invoke consideration of 'what ought to be'. One example of an ideology which has a pre-eminent place in the coach education literature, and against which values are often compared, is the set of constructs which, when taken together, is termed a humanistic approach. The values inherent in this approach have a self-evident appropriateness, and no other set of constructs (other than 'pragmatism') has been packaged and promoted so coherently. Nevertheless, a view is presented here which suggests that the reality of implementing this approach is more difficult than it seems, and may lead to a rather superficial adoption of its important values.

Coaching style

Coaching style can be defined as a descriptive categorization of the individual's aggregated coaching behaviours. There will be patterns in the coach's behaviour that can be differentiated and represented in a typology. The most obvious of these differentiates between autocratic and democratic coaching styles. The reason for beginning with coaching styles is that it is a common term throughout the literature, and there is an assumption that it reflects the coach's philosophy or values. There is a need to examine critically this assumption.

It would be valuable to begin with some general points:

● Once again, it is necessary to distinguish between participation and performance coaching. In the first chapter, an argument was developed which pointed out that these were two quite distinctive processes. It is extremely important, therefore, that any research carried out into coaching styles should establish the precise nature of the sample being used. It is even more important that comparisons are not made between research findings across this divide – unless, of course, this is an explicit objective. There is a danger that behaviour characteristic of more episodic participation coaching is compared only to the direct intervention behaviour of the performance coach. For the performance coach, of course, this represents only a small part of the overall process.

- There are a great many factors that influence behaviour. Abraham and Collins (1998) provide a review of the literature which identifies, amongst others, gender, team/individual, age, type of sport and athlete aspirations as factors. Research into leadership styles (often used as a synonym for coaching styles) has identified many contributing variables. Kuklinski (1990) summarizes these under player, situational and coach variables, citing examples such as gender, level of experience and environmental demands. However, there is little or no evidence with which to evaluate the contribution of the coach's value system against these other environmental factors. In other words, the coach's values may be important in shaping behaviour – indeed this is a very reasonable assumption – but how important? This is exacerbated by the dearth of effectiveness research, which does not merely use performer satisfaction as the measure of effectiveness. (Moving beyond athlete satisfaction to the efficacy of various styles and other factors on the coaching process as a whole is discussed in Chapter 3.)

- Most of the discussion on this topic will assume that the coach is free to allow a value framework to influence coaching behaviour. This may not be the case, particularly when the coach is working within a formal organization with its own ethos, rules etc. The influence of the organization may be very obvious, and part of a formal or informal policy. An example of this might be a non-elitist selection policy in a youth sport club, or a code of discipline in a professional sport club. In each case the attendant behaviour will be dictated by the organization's values. The coach may accede willingly or unwillingly. It is also possible that the coach will come to adopt the organizational values and their attendant behaviour through a process of occupational socialization. Research is required on the extent to which coaches may only appear to accept organizational values but may subvert these in practice. A more general point is that the identification of factors such as coaching role, belief system, personal characteristics and contextual variables has been less valuable than establishing their relative precedence in specific cases.

Coaching 'style' is the terminology that has been used to categorize the coach's behaviours. How this style has been established, and any difficulties in assuming the validity of research using such measures, will have implications for our discussion of coaching philosophies. Not only do we make the assumption that the philosophy is observable in behaviour, but we will stress that statements of values by coaches *should* be translated into implications for coaching practice. It is important, therefore, that any limitations in our current understanding of coaching behaviours should be recognized.

A particular limitation is the emphasis within the literature on research using behavioural observation instruments. Abraham and Collins (1998) offer a useful critique of this approach, although they acknowledge that such research has identified a number of the factors that influence behaviour.

Despite this, the emphasis has been, of necessity in such research, on the direct intervention aspect of the coach's role. This has underplayed the planning, regulatory and management aspects of the coach's role. Perhaps more importantly, it has failed to deal adequately with the subtlety and scope of the athlete–coach interpersonal relationship. A further limitation is the tendency in the literature to focus on samples of coaches (particularly in the US literature) who operate within either youth sport or educational settings, rather than performance coaches of elite athletes. Although there are significant difficulties of access, the scale and intensity of the coaching processes in elite athlete coaching circumstances might be thought to provide a more fertile ground for highlighting the potentially problematic relationship between values and social context. This is not to deny that the excesses of youth sport coaching behaviours have provided many examples of inappropriate behaviour.

It is also difficult to disentangle the 'model for' writing of coach education materials (for example, Crisfield *et al.*, 1996; Martens, 1997) from the reality of coaching practice. There is no doubt that there are coaching behaviours, commonplace in much of sport, that might be considered to be contrary to the prevailing sporting ideology, or to popular perceptions of ethical standards (e.g. partiality in selection policy, intimidation of opponents, psychological harassment or pressurizing injured players). This may put pressure on coaches to espouse rather more politically correct statements of values than might actually be observed in their practice. Respondents giving answers that they think the researchers want to hear, or those that they think will portray them in a better light, must be guarded against in all research.

Perhaps the most well used constructs in linking values and coaching practice are those associated with the autocratic–democratic distinction. It is reasonable to question whether, as normally portrayed, these are two extreme ends of a continuum of behaviours, or whether they are based on such different assumptions that it is not appropriate to compare them. Thus, the terms 'more or less democratic', and 'more or less autocratic' may be more apt. The real issue is that the individual constructs used to aggregate behaviours into a category (e.g. democratic) do themselves embrace a range of behaviours. It is therefore perfectly possible to be more democratic in communication style, but more authoritarian in decision making. What seems clear is that a full appreciation of style categories is not made any easier by researchers simplifying this complexity for the sake of efficient research design. Aggregation into styles may mask important variations across constructs such as role orientation, decision making, competition role and instructional behaviour.

Several additional points must be made before moving on to deal with coaching philosophies themselves. These points relate to the link between values and behaviour, but suggest that there are some unresolved issues:

- Kuklinski (1990) and Douge and Hastie (1993) have alluded to the limited relevance of leadership research for understanding coaching behaviour. Coach-related factors are one set of variables in determining leadership style, and there is a need to specify more clearly the nature of the coach–athlete relationship. An example of this is the power relationship conferred on the athlete/coach by the context in which they operate (age, status, selection, rewards, contract). This needs to be investigated as an environmental feature rather than as a consequence of a leadership style. This does not negate the value of leadership research, but attests to its limitations as an all-embracing explanation.

- There is a general acceptance in much of the literature and coach education material that the coach's behaviour is changeable. While this may be the case over an extended time period, it is much less obvious that the coach can alter style at will. There is little evidence that a range of behaviours is congruent with a set of values about coaching. This suggests that coaches may self-select situations in which they will be more comfortable, or perhaps make only superficial changes in behaviour.

- The emphasis on preferred behaviour and performer satisfaction (for example, Dwyer and Fisher, 1990) in leadership and effectiveness research has failed to address more realistic and difficult issues. Let us assume that athletes cannot always have exactly the coaching behaviours they prefer. How do they deal with this? What degree of choice is available to athletes, and which factors influence them most? Is it possible that some coaches use such situations to perpetrate their preferred style? Coach education and training obviously intends to provide the coach with a range of possible behaviours, and to raise awareness of values, but is there any evidence that coaches are screened on the basis of their value frameworks? Should there be?

- What seems clear is that too many studies have adopted a quantitative survey approach (for example, Lacy and Martin, 1994; Salminen and Liukkonen, 1996). In addition, the need for control of variables and reliable operationalization of constructs has militated against a more insightful and interpretive investigation of values, behaviours and context. There is a need for more naturalistic studies (for example, of conflict resolution during competition), more qualitative studies (Salmela, 1995; Bloom *et al.*, 1997) and more autobiographical or case study approaches (Hemery, 1986).

This may appear to have been a rather negative approach to the study of coaches' behaviour. However, it was important to demonstrate that the coach's value orientations are only one influence on coaching behaviour, and that the link between a coaching philosophy and observed coaching behaviour may not be a simple one.

Coaching philosophies

A coaching philosophy is a comprehensive statement about the beliefs and behaviours that will characterize the coach's practice. These beliefs and behaviours will either reflect a deeper set of values held by the coach, or will be the recognition of a set of externally imposed expectations to which the coach feels the need to adhere. It is normally assumed that individuals identify beliefs that are a true reflection of what they feel, but this need not always be the case. Of course, this then raises the issue of a potential conflict between stated beliefs, actual practice and personal values. There is a temptation to characterize the philosophy as 'this is what I think coaching should be like', but this is not appropriate. Such a statement would be a statement of aspiration, and would say nothing about the reality of the coach's practice. Therefore, it would be more appropriate to think of the philosophy as 'these principles guide my coaching practice'. This raises an interesting speculation: is it possible to have a philosophy about coaching if you are not a practising coach (or does it lose value by being merely uncontextualized aspiration)?

The essence of this book is the multifarious sets of principles that underpin coaching practice. With knowledge and awareness of these, we are in a much better position to understand coaching practice, both individually and collectively. This is particularly the case if there are some common patterns to beliefs about coaching. There is a view that insufficient attention in coaching research has been paid to coaches' thoughts and feelings (Bloom *et al.*, 1997). It might also be said that coach education has focused on practical skills and knowledge, and that the development of a coherent set of beliefs about coaching and (as the section on coaching styles has demonstrated) how to operationalize these should be an essential aspect of the coach's maturity.

Coaching philosophies are, quite rightly, susceptible to critical evaluation by employers, athletes and other coaches. However, far more knowledge is needed about how much notice is taken of the coaches' value statements. We have already queried the range of choices available to athletes who feel uncomfortable with the values and behaviours of those coaches who may be the gatekeepers to advancement in their sport. Those responsible for appointing coaches may feel that statements within coaching philosophies are easy to make but harder to keep, and focus, therefore, on behaviour itself. The danger is that the focus may move onto the success of the athletes' performances, and that the coach's practice will be masked by rhetoric and competition results. Another danger is that coaches may be evaluated by their technical model for the sport (how the game should be played), and this be mistaken for their philosophy and principles about the coaching process. It does seem likely that there will be a fairly strong correlation between the nature of the post or position held by coaches and the values expected of them. The achievement, intense commitment and 'ends justify the means' of professional sport would not be appropriate for young age-groups in amateur sport or community recreation. However, voluntary coaches, often operating in isolation, are rarely accountable to anyone for their behaviour.

Before moving on to an example of a coaching philosophy, two questions should be addressed. First, what should we expect to find in a statement of beliefs such as this, and second, how should philosophies be evaluated? At its most basic level, a coach's philosophy is likely to consist of a list of statements about various aspects of the coach's practice, presumably those that are the most relevant and pertinent to the coach at the time. Although the philosophy may be a coherent set of statements and may be strongly defended by the coach, it will, in many cases, change over a period of time. Each statement will contain a declaration of belief about an aspect of the individual's practice, and an indication of the practical manifestation of this belief. (My considerable experience in coach education suggests that the latter is not always present, but it is to be encouraged.) For example, a coach may say 'I will be open and honest with my athletes'. The values are clear, but the circumstances in which they will be evident are not specified. Will the coach always be open and honest about selection matters, opinions on performance and organizational objectives, or are there some circumstances in which the coach will be less honest 'for the greater good'? The underlying value itself is not always identified in statements of intent (more of this later in the chapter). It would be difficult to give an exhaustive list of all of the aspects of coaching practice likely to be identified by coaches. Undoubtedly some will be derived from interpersonal behaviour (degree of athlete autonomy, collaboration), direct intervention (communication, decision making, selection), the social context (competition ethics, professional standards) and the nature of the coaching role (lifestyle control, objectives).

When evaluating a philosophy statement, a number of questions should be considered. The relationship between rhetoric and practice has already been mentioned. The philosophy should reflect practice, and it may be advisable to have corroborating evidence (if you are an employer) or the assistance of another coach to critique your practice (if you want to understand your practice better). One useful mechanism is to catalogue a series of critical incidents and reflect on how these were handled. Another approach is for the coach to express an opinion on the most significant aspects of coaching practice (for example, for the performance coach it might be decision making, lifestyle control and goal setting). Have these been accorded due prominence in the coach's statement of beliefs? The values evident in any philosophy can be evaluated from a number of perspectives. Imagine that a coach has made a statement about coaching practice that implies either *control* or *empowerment*. How does one decide whether either, or neither, is appropriate? Judgement can be made on the basis of the following:

• Reflection of the expressed beliefs and behaviour of other high status coaches
• Consonance with the wishes of the athletes
• Accord with prevailing practice in that social and sporting context
• Potential efficacy in achieving the goals of the coaching process
• Comparison with socially accepted moral principles.

It is obvious that these categories are not mutually exclusive and that there is sufficient scope for any particular value to be accepted or rejected, and for different beliefs to be defended for different reasons. Many of these criteria will be used to justify in the prevailing ideologies (such as a humanistic approach to coaching), and a more general evaluation, therefore, will be whether or not the coach's philosophy and practice is congruent with such an ideology.

An example of a coaching philosophy would be appropriate at this point. I have resisted the temptation to attempt to distil many different examples into one generic standard, as this would be to fall into the trap of creating a wish list or a model for coaching practice. The example that follows was not written specifically for this chapter; it is my own coaching philosophy, and was used for coach education purposes. You may wish to critique it using the suggestions in the paragraphs above. This is a performance coach operating in a team sport, and with national and international level players.

Coaching philosophy

1. The most important team goal is competitive success.
2. Individual player goals are secondary to this.
3. Players will not be asked to behave in ways that are known to be harmful in the longer term.
4. Players will be given different amounts of attention. This will be commensurate with short- and long-term goals.
5. All players will be advised on matters relating to their participation in the team.
6. All players will be offered the opportunity for advice on matters not directly influencing participation.
7. Players will be treated as if they are self-directed. Peer-group encouragement will be used for immediate task motivation.
8. Players will be encouraged to be aware of a wider responsibility as representatives of a team, nation, their sport, and me.
9. All possible legal advantage will be sought to win important matches. Players will rarely, if ever, be expected to cheat.
10. Non-violent intimidation will occasionally be employed.
11. I will be totally loyal to the team and the players. I will not put any personal ambition before that of the team.
12. My sport philosophy will encourage players to strive to be satisfied with their own levels of performance rather than measure this against other players. Players will be encouraged not to humiliate defeated opponents and to appear gracious in defeat.
13. Players have the right to be consulted on all matters relating to team development.
14. Final decisions and the absolute right to make on-the-spot decisions must be my prerogative. These decisions can be challenged later.
15. Disciplinary matters will, if possible, be left to peer-group pressure.

You may, having reviewed this example, feel that the beliefs are clearly expressed but the behaviours and contexts are less well articulated. Do you feel that this coach is trying to mitigate the desire for control with a measure of player involvement? Is the philosophy sufficiently all-embracing to give you a good picture of this coach's practice? Against which of the categories identified earlier do you feel that the coach would attempt to defend his beliefs?

A content analysis of a selection of coaching philosophies

There is a very limited literature that has taken an analytical perspective on actual coaching philosophies, although reading autobiographies of coaches provides a valuable source of examples. What follows, therefore, is an attempt to illustrate the beliefs and values of a range of coaches by carrying out a content analysis of a set of 43 coaching philosophies. This is intended to give a very practical flavour to the discussion thus far. Each of the coaches involved was taking part in the NCF Diploma in Sports Coaching course. This is a generic coach education course for which there is a selection process, and the stated minimum level of qualification is a senior coach or comparable experience (acknowledging the variety of award nomenclatures and individual sport award systems). Few of the coaches involved were top level performance coaches. They were involved with the full range of athlete groups. This was an opportunity sample, in which six (14%) of the coaches were female, reflecting the general lack of highly qualified women coaches (White *et al.*, 1989; West and Brackenridge, 1990).

Three forms of analysis were carried out:

1. Allocation of Meaning Units (distinct statements, identified from the coaches' presentations of statement, and coherence of subject matter) to aspects of coaching practice
2. Content analysis of key words used in the coaches' statements
3. Identification of values inherent in each Meaning Unit.

It will be clear that there is a significant degree of interpretation on my part in analysing the coaches' statements. In each case, the raw data have been aggregated and sorted in order to bring some analytical clarity to the findings. The data are presented for illustrative purposes only.

The value in Tables 2.1 and 2.2 and Figure 2.2, used to illustrate the data, is simply to raise awareness of the content of the coaches' statements. However, some analysis is appropriate. Perhaps not surprisingly, the coaches paid considerable attention to why they were engaged in coaching and 'what it was about' (Table 2.1). This was complemented by attention to perceptions of their role. A good deal of emphasis was also placed on the coach–athlete relationship and on the way that the individual athletes should be/are treated. The focus is on meaning and purpose, with attention to personal characteristics and appropriate standards (or perhaps better interpreted as principles). For this reason, there is less content dealing with the operational practice of the coaches. This aspect of the philosophies is dominated by a very clear position on not cheating and working within the rules. (Although

Table 2.1: Meaning Units by aspect of coaching practice (n = 306)

Aims, goals, purposes	43			
	+	Athletes' personal development	17	
		Safety and wellbeing	11	= 71
Coach–athlete relationship	34			
	+	Athlete behaviour, expectations	14	
		Equality, individuality, respect	16	= 64
Coaches' characteristics	26			
	+	Self-improvement	19	
		Professional conduct	15	= 60
Role of the coach	41			
	+	Nature of coaching	15	= 56
Operations				
		Cheating, rules, ethics	22	
		Intervention, style	11	
		Ethos, spirit	10	
		Discipline, standards	7	
		Planning, evaluation	5	= 55
		Total		306

not obvious to the reader, and I must ask you to accept my interpretation on this, one of the main criticisms of the value statements in their coach education context was that many of the coaches wrote their statements in an aspirational style. Despite their many years of experience, a sense of 'a coach should' pervaded the statements).

Figure 2.1 attempts to bring some order to an analysis of the keywords used by the coaches. The words themselves are dependent on the vocabulary of the coaches, but reflect the more commonly used terminology in this area. Having grouped the keywords by their common association, they were aggregated into very similar categories to those evident in Table 2.1. What immediately becomes clear is that the overall impression is of a person-centred approach in which the personal development of the athlete is paramount. It is also clear that the coaching process is intended to be a partnership with the athletes. Although a place for winning is recognized, there is a more balanced approach to achievement. A leadership role is acknowledged, but a wide range of behaviours accompanies this. The individual keywords receiving most mention were enjoyment, professional, fair play, winning, wellbeing, respect, individuality, honesty, loyalty and personal improvement. If the contents of this Table were used to draw a picture of coaches in general, they would be characterized as hard working, well-organized and caring individuals, with a keen sense of purpose and a very obvious sense of appropriate standards and goals. They are clearly in the 'people business'.

This is confirmed in Table 2.2, in which there has been an attempt to identify the values underpinning the coaches' statements. The table speaks for itself, and reinforces the message from Table 2.1 and Figure 2.1. The interpersonal and developmental aspects of coaching are emphasized. This reflects a concern for the rights of the individual and the types of behaviour

Table 2.2: Identification of values by Meaning Unit

Personal growth
  Concern for wellbeing,
  Education
	30	Instrumentality
		  Goal direction, planning,
		  efficiency, quality
			9

Respect for others
  Consistency, loyalty,
  trust, honesty, integrity
	20	Independence	6

		Equality of treatment	6
		Adaptability	5

Partnership
  Co-operation, agreement,
  democracy, consultation
	19	Team work	5

		Application Commitment, discipline	5
Self-improvement (coach)	17	Non-extreme behaviour	4

Self-determination (athlete)
  Autonomy, understanding,
  empowerment, ownership
	17	Reward for effort	3

		Accountability	2
		Responsibility	1
Fairness	16	Conformity	1
Professionalism	14	Control	1
Enjoyment	13		
Individuality	11		
Openness	10		
Leadership Role model	10		

Supportiveness
  Empathy, accessibility,
  facilitation, help, giving
	10		

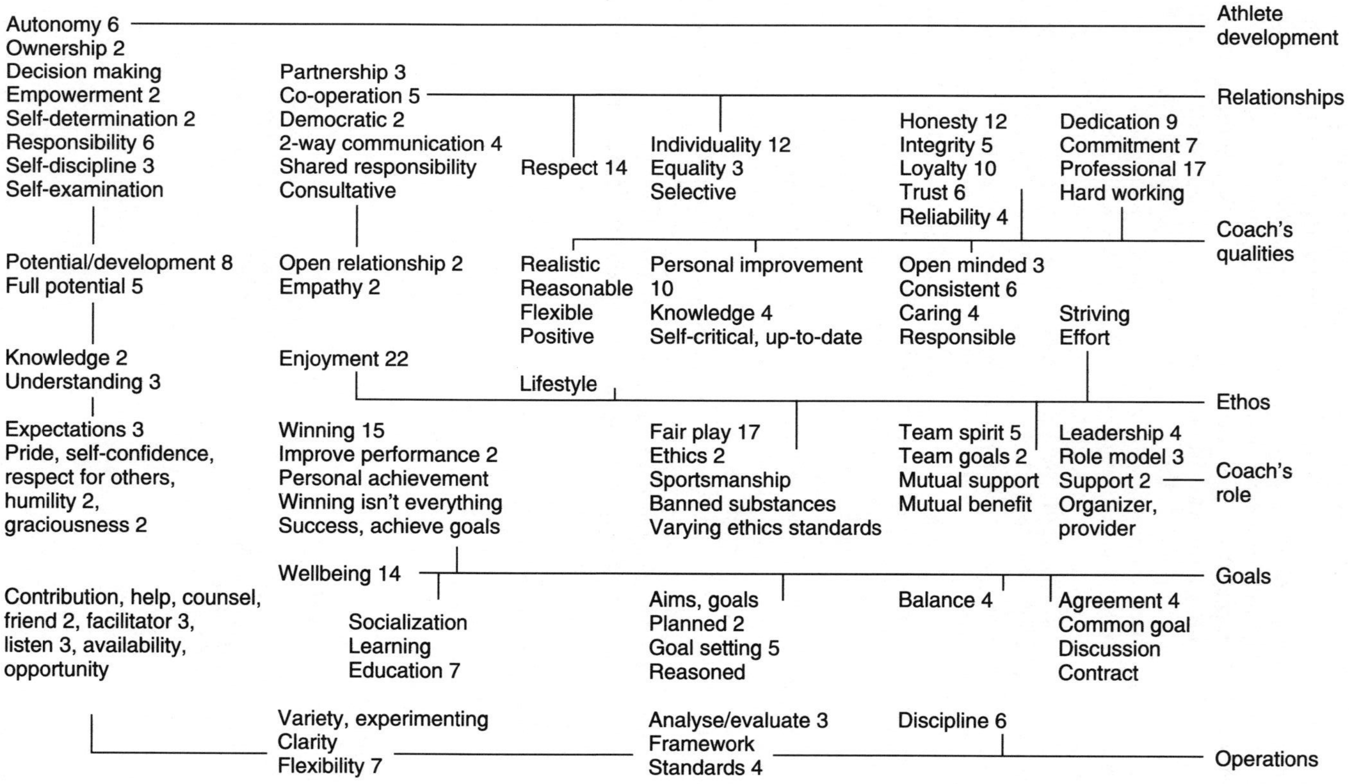

Athlete development
- Autonomy 6
- Ownership 2
- Decision making
- Empowerment 2
- Self-determination 2
- Responsibility 6
- Self-discipline 3
- Self-examination

- Potential/development 8
- Full potential 5

- Knowledge 2
- Understanding 3

- Expectations 3
- Pride, self-confidence, respect for others, humility 2, graciousness 2

- Contribution, help, counsel, friend 2, facilitator 3, listen 3, availability, opportunity

- Variety, experimenting
- Clarity
- Flexibility 7

Relationships
- Partnership 3
- Co-operation 5
- Democratic 2
- 2-way communication 4
- Shared responsibility
- Consultative
- Respect 14
- Individuality 12
- Equality 3
- Selective

- Open relationship 2
- Empathy 2
- Realistic
- Reasonable
- Flexible
- Positive

Coach's qualities
- Honesty 12
- Integrity 5
- Loyalty 10
- Trust 6
- Reliability 4
- Dedication 9
- Commitment 7
- Professional 17
- Hard working

- Personal improvement 10
- Knowledge 4
- Self-critical, up-to-date
- Open minded 3
- Consistent 6
- Caring 4
- Responsible

Ethos
- Enjoyment 22
- Lifestyle
- Striving
- Effort

- Winning 15
- Improve performance 2
- Personal achievement
- Winning isn't everything
- Success, achieve goals
- Fair play 17
- Ethics 2
- Sportsmanship
- Banned substances
- Varying ethics standards
- Team spirit 5
- Team goals 2
- Mutual support
- Mutual benefit

Coach's role
- Wellbeing 14
- Socialization
- Learning
- Education 7
- Leadership 4
- Role model 3
- Support 2
- Organizer, provider

Goals
- Aims, goals
- Planned 2
- Goal setting 5
- Reasoned
- Balance 4
- Agreement 4
- Common goal
- Discussion
- Contract

Operations
- Discipline 6
- Analyse/evaluate 3
- Framework
- Standards 4

Figure 2.1 Analysis of key words (n = 395)

required to adhere to the most common values. In the context of this book, the list of most common values reads like a set of coaching principles. Having been derived from practising coaches, they might be said to be a model of coaching values.

As with any empirical work, it is necessary to acknowledge the limitations in the data collection and its analysis, and we must therefore exercise a note of caution in placing too much reliance on these figures. This itself is a useful exercise, since it will draw attention to a number of the points made earlier in the chapter. The philosophies were compiled as an exercise on a coach education course, and we should perhaps anticipate that they would have an element of 'what others want to hear' or 'how I want to present myself'. As already noted, many of the statements were what these coaches aspired to, or written as if to apply to coaches in general. More importantly, perhaps, very few of the coaches operated exclusively with top level athletes, or in professional sport. The stereotypical perception that coaches working with elite level athletes (particularly in team sports) are less person-centred, rather more authoritarian and more concerned with an instrumental approach to competition success could not be tested. In any case, Salmela's (1995) data tends to suggest that this is a much over-simplified view.

Another weakness in all coaching philosophies is that they are self-reported indicators of behaviour. The focus is largely on interpersonal aspects of the coaching role and many of these (e.g. developmental goals, personal growth and independence) may take a long time to achieve, and via a very diverse range of behaviours. This highlights the potential lack of consonance between the coach's statements and the coach's behaviour at any particular time. Although there are significant limitations in trying to understand, for example, the subtlety of interpersonal and non-direct intervention behaviour in systematic behavioural observation studies, it would be valuable in future studies to situate them in the context of the coaches' declared philosophies.

Nevertheless, the message from the coaching philosophies was clear. A person-centred, developmental approach was commonplace. The chapter now goes on to examine this approach in a little more detail, and to consider the issue of how easy or difficult it is to implement such a philosophy.

A humanistic approach to coaching

This is a particular set of beliefs and values that stresses the centrality of the individual athlete's personal growth and development through an active engagement in the coaching experience. Even if this approach is not commonplace at all levels in sport (Coakley, 1993), its significance is that it tends to be used as a marker for the evaluation of coaching behaviours. For example, it is the basis of codes of ethics and codes of conduct and policy from official agencies (see NCF, 1996; NCF/NSPCC, 1998). It is clear from the survey of coaching philosophies described earlier that its principles underpin the coaches' perceptions of the nature and purpose of sports coaching. It has the potential, therefore, to provide a set of principles to guide coaching practice.

The humanistic approach to coaching views the sporting context and the athlete's training and performance as a vehicle through which the athlete can be influenced to develop and grow. The technical aspect of improving performance and taking part in competition is perceived to be just one aspect of a process involving interpersonal relationships, social meaning, relationships to other parts of the athlete's life and an emotional and psychological engagement in and commitment to the process. The whole process has the potential to enable the individual to grow and develop in ways that are considered to be positive. For example, if the individual (young or old) becomes more independent and self-directed, more mature, adaptable, able to deal with difficulties, self-disciplined, aware of and concerned for others, and has an increased sense of self-worth and individuality, these qualities would be regarded by almost everyone as beneficial developments. It is assumed that individuals have the capacity to 'grow' if their involvement is appropriate (for example, active, inner-directed, challenging). The coach's role is to ensure that the coaching process and all that it entails facilitates rather than prevents this happening. For these reasons, the coach's emphasis is much more on the process of coaching than on the products of coaching. This raises a number of interesting issues about how the performance of a professed humanistic coach might be evaluated. For which aspects of the process and the product do they feel themselves to be accountable? For a development of these ideas and their basic principles, see Sage (1978), Whitson (1980), Danziger (1982), Lombardo (1987), Orlick (1990) and Hogg (1995).

It is difficult to argue with the moral rectitude of these ideas, but the implication from the exhortations to humanistic practice is that it is either difficult to achieve or that there are other ideological/social pressures, or both. There are certainly elements of the sporting environment that constrain such practice. There is a good deal of top level sport, particularly professional but not exclusively, in which television-led commercialism and the high status afforded to the outcomes have produced a reward environment that emphasizes competition results. This has brought with it a singular focus on the production of improved performance through selective recruitment, extensive commitment and scientific application. It has also resulted in a values culture which stresses an 'end justifies the means' approach, and an overwhelming emphasis on product rather than process. The outcome for the individual athlete is an externally evaluated achievement ethos in which an extensive commitment is expected, success is measured (but also limited) by competition with others and where personal choice is restricted. The production process and winning are the principal and only focus.

The case has been deliberately overstated. Nevertheless, there are two further ramifications. Young people's role models are often drawn from this sporting environment. Athlete behaviour is imitated and spread throughout other levels in sport. There will also be a significant proportion of talented young performers (often termed developing athletes) who are on the fast track to top level sport. They may be subject to the same values culture (early selection, early specialization, emphasizing results) with perhaps a more damaging effect, given their lack of maturity. The implication here is that it is difficult for coaches in such a situation to implement a coaching process orientated to humanistic principles, particularly if the coaches are themselves subject to the same pressures. Coaching practice that is more directive in leadership style may even stifle the development of the athlete and militate against independence. There is a danger that focusing only on performance may undervalue the interpersonal relationship and its contribution to individual growth. Perhaps the more worrying aspect of a means/ends results orientation is that a sense of fairness and respect for others can be lost.

The basis of the humanistic psychology that informs this approach to coaching is that human beings have the capacity to learn from their experiences, if they have been actively involved in determining and evaluating these experiences. It is also important that individuals feel that they have support for making this investment in their development, and that it is valued. Individuals can develop in many situations, but sport has the potential to invoke many of the qualities required for this – self-discipline, co-operation, challenge, emotional highs and lows, success and failure, independent action, adherence to goals, etc. Many of the keywords identified in Figure 2.1 illustrate the coaching practice that would be appropriate to facilitate an athlete's development. Hogg (1995) provides a very detailed and practical application of humanistic principles to coaching practice. He stresses the variation in empowerment practices required to support athletes as they move from adolescence into maturity. A degree of control is exercised in the early years, but this is replaced gradually by a shared responsibility as the coach exploits opportunities for self-determination by the athlete. Greater and greater responsibility is taken by the athletes as their role in the coaching process increases. This would be evident in goal setting, planning, and competition strategy. Perhaps the most important aspect of empowerment (and in many ways the most difficult for the coach) is the responsibility for ultimate control of the process. The coach's role in controlling the athletes' lifestyle management, adherence to schedules and goal setting diminishes as the athlete assumes greater control. This transfer of power should be a planned process. Another interpretation of the growth in the athletes' independence is that they develop a capacity to confront the decisions of the coach, without necessarily challenging the coach's ultimate authority (see Cross, 1991).

We must acknowledge that there can be arguments put forward by coaches to mitigate their lack of attention to humanistic principles. Some of these refer to the difficulty of implementation, and others to the efficacy of such practices in the context in which they operate. We will return to these arguments shortly. First, we have to acknowledge that a truly humanistic approach may make considerable demands on interpersonal relationships. The following list is derived from the literature already cited and from Rogers' (1961) seminal work. Truly humanistic coaching practice would be based on the following principles:

1. Allow the athlete to exercise self-discipline in matters relating to application, adherence, behaviour and quality of effort. Do not use the threat of disapproval or punishment to coerce athletes to behave in a way that the coach perceives to be appropriate.
2. Value each individual's contribution equally (this does not mean that they each make the same contribution to performance, just that the coach values each of them as representative of what any individual athlete can offer).

3. Set goals with the athlete regularly, and use only these goals to evaluate progress.
4. Adopt an approach to preparation and competition that is based consistently on fairness and respect for opponents. This implies actively discouraging all forms of cheating or seeking an advantage that was not intended by the rules or spirit of the sport.
5. Allow the athletes to express their evaluation of preparation, performance and progress. Coaches should base their evaluations on those of the athletes.
6. Do not allow the athlete to become too dependent on the coach. Athletes must be allowed to resolve problems by themselves at times, even if this results in a reduced performance level in the shorter term.
7. Adopt a facilitating, reinforcing role rather than a directing one. This implies questioning and listening, rather than the assumption of a coach-directed decision making approach. Coaches use their greater knowledge and experience as a resource. This is offered to, rather than imposed on, the athlete.
8. Performance is always understood as an emotional and psychological experience as much as a physical and technical one. All monitoring and assessment and the evaluations which follow take into account the full range of outputs.
9. Allow the athlete to develop an identity that is not dependent on the coach. Allow a degree of distance or separateness, which encourages independence. Encourage the athlete to seek assistance from a range of facilitators.
10. Never fail to exercise a caring, athlete-welfare centred approach to practice. Assume that an educating role is always being exercised.
11. Agree standards of behaviour, and use these to express approval or otherwise for athlete behaviour. Express feelings of satisfaction, disapproval, frustration, etc., but always specify the cause of the emotion.
12. Maintain an open approach to information, feelings and standards. These need to be consistently applied and evident to all athletes.

This is a demanding set of requirements and, as we have noted previously, many of them are related to the ways in which coaches interact with athletes. Much of this interpersonal behaviour is not obvious to third parties, and the 'how' of a coach's practice is not always scrutinized for this reason. Perceptive readers will also have noted that it is easier to proscribe inappropriate activity than it is to specify appropriate behaviour, and this too makes coach education and training more problematic.

We must also recognize that some coaches often adopt a less humanistically orientated approach. The experience of many individual athletes will be of a much more directive style, which emphasizes performance outcomes and is less concerned with developmental, person-centred goals for the athlete. Coaches whose practice is characterized by a more authoritarian, performance orientation, may argue that:

1. The sporting context in which they operate has a different set of expectations and assumptions. Performance outcomes are valued very highly (although perhaps never explicitly at the expense of personal welfare), and this determines priorities in practice.

2. They are evaluated by shorter-term performance goals and, in the context of changing personnel, they have less incentive to attend to personal development, which is a longer-term and more incremental process. This encourages an instrumental approach that evaluates humanistic principles for their direct effect on immediate performance variables.

3. Coaching team sports requires a form of collective activity in which it is difficult (perhaps even counter-productive) to allow athletes to be completely independent and to share decision making. Chelladurai and Arnott (1985) and Chelladurai *et al.* (1989) show that team sport performers prefer a more autocratic approach in their coaches' leadership.

4. The requirements of a humanistic approach make demands on interpersonal skills for which they are not equipped. It also assumes a degree of humility and security in order to exercise leadership through co-operation, and to be open with feelings and emotions.

5. The athletes are more comfortable with a directive style.

6. They have a different philosophy about coaching.

The purpose of this chapter is not to champion any particular approach to coaching or its attendant philosophies. We have already noted that individual philosophies can be defended or justified from a number of perspectives. If a coach says 'I am driven by pragmatism and not by humanism in order to accommodate my personal beliefs or preferences, and in order to cope with my perceptions of the external environment', we may not all agree that it is necessary, acceptable or appropriate. However, the coach's recourse to arguments such as those above helps to explain how these beliefs have come about. Once again, more research is required to investigate the source and development of performance coaches' belief systems. However, another approach is to argue that there are considerable benefits not only to the athlete but also to the coach and the performance itself. It could be argued that the coach's role is made more effective by not being solely responsible for direction, motivation and knowledge. In addition, a much more comfortable atmosphere is generated when the coach eschews a blame culture. There can be little doubt that athletes, particularly elite athletes, who are self-directed, cope better with perceived pressure, and having self-confidence will be likely to perform better in competition.

The humanistic approach to coaching requires a transfer of priorities from performance to the person, and implies a leadership style based on co-operation and athlete autonomy. Developmental and educational processes are paramount. It is clear that this is not an easy task, and the intrinsic priorities are not those encouraged by much of modern sport, in which comparative success is valued very highly. It can also be interpreted as 'hard to do'. Coaches may perceive the interpersonal principles to be very demanding, and additional to the technical aspects of training and competition. Many of the goals of humanistic coaching may not come to fruition for many years, and are easier to ignore or give low priority. Some coaches may simply take the view that they are motivated by competitive success and have much less interest in the personal qualities and longer-term development of the performers (although we must not interpret this as necessarily implying a negative or impersonal approach).

One scenario that we must consider is that coaches use the rhetoric of humanism (this was apparently the case in the analysis carried out for this chapter), but that this is either not applied in practice or only applied to the 'easier' parts of the coaching process. This requires further research. Certainly Hemery (1986) notes the potential for coaches to exercise a directive style during direct intervention (i.e. training and competition), and for that to be accepted by athletes because of the coach's empathetic, supportive, person-centred approach in their indirect intervention. Cross' (1995) research with elite swimmers also confirmed that some elite athletes want the coach to make all of the important decisions because they have come to trust the coach. This principle of consensual authority has much to commend it, since it may allow the benefits (effectiveness, efficiency) of technical leadership to be exercised in concert with a more developmental approach overall. Thus a coach's practice may not adhere to the full range of humanistic coaching principles all of the time, but the developmental intentions go beyond the superficial, and personal development may still be a priority.

A distinction should be drawn between the more directive style in coaching practice in two different sets of circumstances. In the first, the coach in elite or high level sport may be directive in technical terms and give a high priority to performance outcomes, but the athlete has sufficient maturity to accept or reject this approach and to maintain an overall control of aspirations and progress towards them. In these circumstances, coach and athletes may be able to find an accommodation between the demands of external pressures and actual coaching practice that is mutually acceptable. In the second, coaching in participation sport, particularly with young people, which is directive in style with no athlete autonomy or involvement, has much less to commend it. An autocratic style exhibited in some young people's sport which is more extensive in scale and intensive in character (e.g. swimming, athletics, gymnastics) is potentially more limiting in development terms than in more intermittent, recreative contexts. In all cases we must be careful of attributing acceptance of authority to performers who have no experience of the alternative. However, this raises an interesting point. Coaches who have experienced an authoritarian regime as performers, and who have witnessed other coaches with similar approaches, need to have the expectation that coach education, both formal and informal, will help them to adjust to a different style. Indeed, part of coach education as a whole may be the responsibility to promulgate humanistic (or other agreed alternative) principles.

This brief analysis of humanistic coaching practice has identified a number of principles against which coaching practice can be compared. A humanistic approach to coaching was highlighted because it exemplified a particular, and frequently advocated, coaching ideology. The individual coach formulates a set of beliefs and preferred behaviours which reflect more or less strongly this (or, of course, another) set of values. We go on now to examine briefly a specific set of codified values for appropriate behaviour in coaching.

Coaching and ethics

Expectations of coaching behaviour can be fashioned into a particular set of value statements and associated practices which is intended to provide a coherent framework of 'rules' for coach behaviour in a professional context (see NCF, 1996). This framework needs to be acknowledged in this chapter because it is designed to influence the 'how' of coaching, and some elements in a code of ethics are closely linked to coaching philosophies.

A code of ethics deals with those aspects of coaching practice that can be agreed to have a sense of right or wrong about them – a sense of moral or social acceptability. Therefore, they deal with issues of 'ought to' and 'ought not to'. A code of ethics identifies, contextualizes and describes the values involved. These are normally expressed as a set of 'should do's or 'should not do's. An example might be that the coach should not cheat or encourage athletes to cheat; more specifically, that proscribed performance enhancing substances should not be administered to or used by athletes. Codes of ethics are supplemented by codes of conduct, which elaborate on practice that is considered to be acceptable. Other examples might be an injunction against sexual harassment or discrimination on the basis of gender or race. These two examples illustrate the distinction between those aspects of the code of ethics that are rooted in the law and those more general aspects of human behaviour about which there would be little dissent. These latter standards, for example about the exercise of leadership, or personal characteristics (trust, honesty etc.) are similar to the values expressed in many coaching philosophies. Whilst many behavioural standards are best understood as right or wrong and present or absent (for example, with racial discrimination), this is not the case with issues relating to leadership style, openness in relationships, sportsmanship or the welfare of the individual. These may require further interpretation, and might be better thought of as matters of degree. This suggests that monitoring and evaluating such standards in behaviour will be problematical.

Many of the specific coaching practices relate to an underlying value, which is that those in positions of power should not abuse that power. This is a general point that applies to the codes of ethics of doctors, dentists, lawyers, etc. We have to recognize that sport is a context in which dilemmas about appropriate conduct are likely to occur. Coaching involves an interpersonal relationship, and this brings with it the potential for an absence of empathy with or care and concern for the wellbeing of the other person. In addition, sport, by definition, is bounded by rules, and the rules of the specific sports are supplemented by more general rules about conduct, eligibility, doping limitations and finance. There is also potential for the sport performance itself to be the focus of attention and for the athletes to become secondary. This is exacerbated by the use of science to assist performance. Sport is a contested arena, and the purpose of the contests is generally to achieve a victory over opponents. Once again, this provides opportunities for excesses of behaviour in relation to victory and defeat. Finally, coaching is a form of leadership, and the sporting context creates situations in which the coach is able to exercise power in the relationship. This may be based on greater knowledge and experience, on age or gender, or on control of resources and access to opportunities for advancement. In these circumstances, abuse of that power may occur, ranging from physical, mental and psychological abuse and harassment through to absence of concern for the performer's welfare and a dictatorial dominance of the coaching process. In such a potentially problematic arena, the code of ethics says 'you may have a

different perspective on what coaching is about, but here are some behaviours that are not considered acceptable'.

Nevertheless, we have to acknowledge that codes of ethics and practice
are socially determined and will reflect a particular ideology, in addition to
legal concerns and matters of human and civil rights. The section on a
humanistic approach to coaching outlined an ideology which is standard
in codes of ethics and conduct (see the National Association of Sports
Coaches guidelines, NCF (1996) and any of the sport-specific examples). It
is obvious, however, that not all of these standards are applied in actual
sports practice (McNamee, 1998). This is a fruitful area for further study,
for it would appear that at least two distinctive codes are in operation.
There is a party line, which most coaches are concerned to see applied to
youth sport and coaching behaviour in general, and a second ethical code
which, because it is more achievement orientated, has a means/ends value
system that is much less person-centred. In this second code, the legal
requirements may be acknowledged, but there would appear also to be an
esoteric behavioural code fully understood only by those within that particular sub-culture (usually professional sport). This is a speculation on my
part. However, it does raise the spectre of coaches employing the wrong
code in inappropriate situations.

This is an issue that has implications for the development of the coaching
profession. Professions are self-regulating bodies in which membership con-
fers a set of benefits, but with it, accountability and expectations of appropriate behaviour. In developed professions, the professional body monitors
and regulates membership and can dismiss members for serious breaches of
ethical codes. Coaching is not yet a formal profession; access/gateway
requirements, a professional body with specific requirements for membership, self-regulation, the need for a licence to operate, and career structures
and training are not yet in place. There are codes of ethics and conduct but,
in the absence of a professional body, these are not implemented in any
universal or systematic fashion. Nevertheless, this is a part of coaching practice that cannot be ignored. The 'how' of coaching involves coaches' behaviour that reflects a philosophical position on what coaching is, and how it
should be implemented. How it is implemented can also be evaluated as
morally and ethically acceptable.

Summary

It has been established that coaching practice cannot be understood without
first identifying the particular interpretation the individual coach places on
the role and patterns of coaching behaviour that are found in any particular
coaching context. It has also become clear that, when it comes to the 'how' of
coaching, it is much more difficult to establish principles than to reflect them
in actual practice. Nevertheless, the coach's behaviour is susceptible to social
interpretation, monitoring and appraisal. This leads to acceptance of a coaching ideology reflective of acceptable coaching practice and, in turn, this
influences coach education and official literature. This was illustrated in
this chapter by the humanistic approach to coaching. In addition, we have
to acknowledge that there are sub-cultures in sport (many of which are

powerful in their diffusion) which have an often unwritten ideology that is less wholesome than that of the humanistic approach. The principles in such a set of values are determined by the social (and often commercial) value placed on achievement. The personal reward system that follows from this has implications for a very focused and sometimes impersonal coaching process.

It has been demonstrated that coaches can articulate a set of beliefs and values. There is a danger that these manifest value frameworks may represent aspirations and public statements of intent rather than being reflections of actual coaching practice and behaviours. A number of issues have been raised about which there has been insufficient research; the relationship between coaching style or philosophy and effectiveness, the relationship of philosophies to motivations for coaching, and whether or not coaches can easily adapt their coaching behaviour in varying circumstances. The subtlety of interpersonal behaviour, on which a good deal of interpretation rests, is not dealt with in the systematic observation procedures which characterize much of research on coaching behaviours. Indeed, there are few studies in which the coaches' value frameworks have even been identified.

In the analysis carried out for the chapter, there was a useful identification of the keywords used by a range of coaches. These coaches were certainly in the 'people business', and their terminology resonated with the language of the humanistic values and principles identified later in the chapter. On the other hand, it became clear that a truly humanistic approach to coaching practice was often difficult to implement. The demand on personal skills, the extent of the 'sharing' approach and the reliance on self-generated goals and appraisal suggested that a more superficial implementation was a potential outcome. In performance coaching, it is more than likely that an accommodation is negotiated between athletes and coaches (which we called a consensual authority). This is a rich mixture of coach-led direct intervention and planning, a person-centred developmental concern for the athlete, and a compromise between an achievement-led sub-cultural ethic and the demands of public accountability. Proving or disproving this speculation requires much increased attention to research into the subtlety of coaching values and practice.

References

Abraham, A. and Collins, D. (1998). Examining and extending research in coach development. *Quest*, **50**, 59–79.

Bloom, G. A., Durand-Bush, N. and Salmela, J. H. (1997). Pre- and post-competition routines of expert coaches of team sports. *Sport Psychol.*, **11**, 127–41.

Chelladurai, P. and Arnott, M. (1985). Decision styles in coaching: preferences of basketball players. *Res. Q. Exer. Sport*, **56**, 15–24.

Chelladurai, P., Haggerty, T. R. and Baxter, P. R. (1989). Decision style choices of university basketball coaches and players. *J. Sport Exer. Psychol.*, **11**, 201–15.

Coakley, J. (1993). Social dimensions of intensive training and participation in youth sports. In *Intensive Participation in Children's Sports* (B. R. Cahill and A. J. Pearl, eds), pp. 77–94. Human Kinetics.

Crisfield, P., Cabral, P. and Carpenter, F. (1996). *The Successful Coach: Guidelines for Coaching Practice*. National Coaching Foundation.

Cross, N. (1991). Arguments in favour of a humanistic coaching process. *Swimming Times*, **LXXII(11)**, 17–18.

Cross, N. (1995). Coaching effectiveness and the coaching process. *Swimming Times*, **LXXII(2)**, 23–5.

Danziger, R. C. (1982). Coaching humanistically: an alternative approach. *Physical Ed.*, **39(1)**, 121–5.

Douge, B. and Hastie, P. (1993). Coach effectiveness. *Sports Sci. Rev.*, **2(2)**, 62–74.

Dwyer, J. and Fisher D. (1990). Wrestlers' perceptions of coaches' leadership as predictors of satisfaction with leadership. *J. Percept. Motor Skills*, **71**, 511–17.

Hemery, D. (1986). *The Pursuit of Sporting Excellence*. Willow Books.

Hogg, J. M. (1995). *Mental Skills for Swim Coaches*. Sport Excel Pub. Inc.

Kuklinski, B. (1990). Sports leadership – an overview. *NZ J. Health Physical Ed. Rec.*, **23(3)**, 15–18.

Lacy, A. C. and Martin, D. L. (1994). Analysis of starter/non-started motor skill engagement and coaching behaviours in collegiate women's volleyball. *J. Teach. Physical Ed.*, **13**, 95–107.

Lombardo, B. J. (1987). *The Humanistic Coach: From Theory to Practice*. Charles C. Thomas.

McNamee, M. (1998). Celebrating trust: virtues and rules in the ethical conduct of sports coaches. In *Ethics and Sport* (M. J. McNamee and S. J. Parry, eds), pp. 148–68. EFN Spon.

Martens, R. (1997). *Successful Coaching* (2nd edn). Leisure Press.

NCF (1996). *Code of Ethics and Conduct for Sports Coaches*. National Coaching Foundation.

NCF/NSPCC (1998). *Protecting Children: A Guide for Sportspersons* (2nd edn). National Coaching Foundation.

Orlick, T. (1990). *In Pursuit of Excellence* (2nd edn). Leisure Press.

Rogers, C. (1961). *On Becoming a Person*. Houghton Mifflin.

Sage, G. H. (1978). Humanistic psychology and coaching. In *Sport Psychology: An Analysis of Athlete Behaviour* (W. F. Straub, ed.), pp. 148–61. Movement Publications.

Salmela, J. H. (1995). Learning from the development of expert coaches. *Coach. Sport Sci. J.*, **2(2)**, 3–13.

Salminen, S. and Liukkonen, J. (1996). Coach–athlete relationship and coaching behaviour in training sessions. *Int. J. Sport Psychol.*, **27**, 59–67.

West, A. and Brackenridge, C. (1990). *A Report on the Issues Relating to Women's Lives as Sports Coaches in the UK*. PAVIC Pub.

Whitson, D. (1980). Coaching as a human relationship. *Momentum*, **5(2)**, 36–43.

White, A., Mayglothling, R. and Carr, C. (1989). *The Dedicated Few: The Social World of Women Coaches in Britain in the 1980s*. West Sussex Institute of Higher Education, Centre for the Study and Promotion of Sport and Recreation for Women and Girls.

3

Coaching effectiveness

Neville Cross

- Introduction to the concept of 'coaching effectiveness' and the coaching process
- Problems encountered in describing and defining coaching effectiveness
- The importance of 'value added' in determining the degree of effectiveness
- What are the components of effective coaching?
- Principles of effective coaching
- Coaching philosophies and effective coaching behaviours
- Leadership styles relevant to effective coaching
- Effective according to whom? Different stakeholders and their points of view
- What does the research show us?

Introduction

More than 30 years ago, Batty (1965), describing coaching in football, stated that 'A coach must be God'. A decade or so later, Weir (1977: 99), in discussing the coaching of field hockey, suggested that a coach 'must be infallible, indispensable, independent, intelligent, influential and invigorating'. She went on to describe a coach as 'a leader whose role is to create a suitable framework in which a player and a squad can develop the potential that is inherent'. Does a combination of these statements accurately reflect the characteristics of effective coaching and therefore constitute a suitable definition of coaching effectiveness? Will the qualities Weir identifies ensure effectiveness? Is a prescribed type of coaching behaviour effective in all situations? This chapter will address these and other coaching effectiveness-related questions using a combination of research findings and conceptual analysis. Whilst some clarity emerges, no single objective measure of coaching effectiveness can be identified which is appropriate in all coaching situations. Although it might be argued that the 'principles of coaching remain the same' (Howe, 1990), different contexts such as participation sport and competitive sport, or age-group coaching (novice/intermediate) and national team coaching (elite), require somewhat different approaches in order to be effective. Note that Howe's article, despite referring to 'principles', in fact identifies only one principle; that which he calls the 'primary principle' of the coaching process. This principle suggests that the coach should be a facilitator rather than a director. Having identified this principle, Howe then goes on to discuss purposes and behaviours which are pertinent to effective coaching, rather than principles *per se*. Several coaching principles have also been identified by Rushall (1985a, 1985b), and these are discussed later in the section on components of effective coaching. In addition, Sherman and Sands (1996) have suggested that coaches should also consider what they call the 'principle of consequence' as a central component of the process of coaching. This principle demands that coaches plan for and consider the possible outcomes of (at both physiological and psychological levels) any intended training stimuli.

Are coaches even aware that there are defined concepts and principles for them to use? For example, Gould *et al.* (1990), although not identifying the principles concerned, were disconcerted to find that only 46 per cent of the 130 American National, Pan-American and Olympic team coaches they investigated believed that a well-defined set of concepts and principles for coaches existed. In addition, a majority of their respondents reported that the two most important knowledge sources contributing to their coaching styles and the practices they engaged in were experience and other successful coaches, rather than any established principles. Information is available to describe both the concepts of the coaching process and the principles that govern it. For example, Lyle (1996) has described the key concepts or elements as: an information base; the knowledge and skills of the coach; the performer's capabilities, performance analysis, mechanisms for regulating the process; systematic progression; operationalization; goal-setting; planning; the preparation programme; the competition programme; and individualization. Principles of coaching are also available, with seven identified by Rushall (1985a, 1985b), and a further seven principles of training identified by Bompa (1994). In this context, a question that needs to be addressed is whether our coach education programmes are failing to provide the information (despite it being available) that coaches need in order to enhance their effectiveness in a practical way.

Although there is an 'increasing academic respectability afforded to the examination of effective coaching' (Howe, 1990), and the academic coaching literature is increasingly identifying the need for coaching to be treated as a systematic, multifaceted process (see, for example, Fairs, 1987; Lyle, 1996), many coach certification courses and sport education programmes continue to concentrate much more on the episodic nature of coaching behaviour (e.g. communication, teaching, etc.) and/or the identification of individual areas for treatment (skills, tactics, physiological requirements etc.). Such an approach is not unexpected. After all, as Abraham and Collins (1998: 59) noted, there are many similarities between teaching and coaching. For example, they have noted that a teacher is someone who 'orchestrates learning activities and mediates social climate while diagnosing and remediating student performance – all actions that mirror the role of the coach'. In addition, a great number of sports coaches work with participation standard or improver level athletes, where instruction is often the most appropriate descriptor. The number of coaches actually working with elite athletes is understandably small. Thus, the effectiveness of many coaches at the participation level may be judged solely on their ability to teach a particular aspect of the coaching process, and not on their ability to attend to and manage the coaching process in its entirety.

Many sports not only appear to ignore the process aspect of coaching but also fail to define effective coaching. For example, Cross and Ellice (1997) noted that not only is coaching often treated in an episodic way in the sports literature, but that effective coaching *per se* does not attract much attention either. Certainly this was true of the field hockey literature, and it may very well be true for most sports. Cross and Ellice found that, while no definition or description of coaching effectiveness in field hockey is offered in the coach education literature, there is continual reference to 'good coaching and leadership' in all of the SVQ (Scottish Vocational Qualifications) hockey manuals (see Scottish Hockey Union, 1994). Good coaching may not always be the same as effective coaching, and the omission of effective coaching in the coaching education literature may indicate a lack of appreciation of the effectiveness concept and a lack of understanding of the coaching process mechanisms. While not denying the importance of individual aspects of the coaching process, Cross and Ellice (1997) noted that to concentrate on the episodic nature of coaching practice, rather than considering the need for a more holistic approach, may inadvertently result in less than optimal coaching effectiveness. (Note that 'leadership' will be discussed further on in this chapter.)

This type of criticism can be aimed at most, if not all, sports. However, it is team sports that most encourage coaches to take a more episodic approach. One of the reasons for this is that the individualization of training that might reasonably be considered a prerequisite for optimal coaching effectiveness is often easier to carry out in individual sports (such as swimming, tennis and athletics etc.) than in team sports (such as rugby, football and field hockey etc.), where the individual's needs may sometimes be subsumed by the team's needs. Whitaker (1992: 24) attested to this difficulty when he noted that 'One of the greatest challenges to a team coach is that of promoting both individual performance and teamwork to the highest level'. Indeed, even spending quality time on team dynamics in certain sports can sometimes prove almost impossible. In amateur team sports, in particular, it is often difficult to get all of the players together with sufficient regularity in order to practise team strategies, formations and tactics. Reasons for this vary, but many amateurs have to earn a living outside sport, and this can interfere with their ability to train as much as the demands of their sport and their goals dictate. Certainly this proved to be the case with the Scottish women's field hockey team when research was carried out with them in 1995 (Cross, 1995a). In fact, the inability of the whole team to get together for training sessions was identified as extremely frustrating for some players and a major constraint to effectiveness by the players interviewed. In addition, the coaches interviewed in the same study identified the players' social circumstances (study, work, family commitments) as a major constraint to their coaching effectiveness. Constraints such as these can, and often do, encourage a more episodic and fragmented approach. In the case of coaches working with representative teams, difficulties are often exacerbated by problems of regular access and availability.

Problems of description and definition

How is coaching effectiveness therefore to be defined? If coaches are to be accountable to employers (the professionalization of coaching is fairly well advanced in some sports) and appointed to national teams because of their proven expertise and effectiveness, and if coach education programmes (designed to produce effective coaches) are to be evaluated and approved, a definition needs to be agreed that provides a yardstick for meaningful evaluation. For example, with many of the governing bodies of sport currently embracing the vocational qualifications-based (NVQ, SVQ etc.) coach education route, coaches are increasingly being qualified to various levels of competence. Lyle (1998a) reminds us that 'competent' may not mean 'effective' at all, and may be better described as an appropriate term for 'not ineffective'. Competence in such a context may actually refer to a minimum level of acceptable capacity, rather than to the product orientation that is implied by the term 'effective'. 'Effective' therefore relates more to how the process is integrated and managed. Effectiveness displayed over a prolonged period of time will be a mark of the coach's applied expertise, and may result in the coach being labelled an expert (Salmela, 1995).

Thus a superficial or simplistic description or definition of coaching effectiveness that merely identifies it as contributing to enhanced performance (Cross, 1995b) or the competitive performance (Franks *et al.*, 1986; Mathers, 1997) of the athlete or team, or being synonymous with success (however that is measured!) in one form or another, does not, in fact, do the concept justice. For example, merely describing coaching effectiveness in these terms may not take into account the dynamic nature of the coaching process. In a dynamic coaching process, coaching effectiveness is not only contingent on the different pressures and/or constraints acting on the process, but these also occur over time. Thus, it may be possible to be effective in some parts of the process and ineffective in others, and it will be necessary to ensure that any improvement in performance that takes place does so in the context in which it is actually intended. An additional consideration is whether the improvement in performance was optimal. Could it have been better than that achieved? Can the improvement be attributed to the coach and the process that he or she directs? For example, an improvement in a personal best time (PB) in swimming may not be the result of effective coaching behaviour at all, but because of swimmer maturation, intrinsic motivation, an ideal physical environment or indeed any one of a number of other reasons. Some of these reasons may, or should, be embraced in a good coaching process. However, despite some good aspects of the process being in place in some cases, coaches of younger athletes in particular may wrongly attribute success or effectiveness to their own coaching style or practice when the real reasons for improvement may lie elsewhere in the process.

Even the use of the word 'success' in the context of coaching effectiveness is problematical. Lyle (1998b) has suggested that successful coaches are most often considered successful by association with successful performers, which does not necessarily equate with them being personally effective. In fact, 'successful' here may only be a measure of a single criterion such as output, whereas coaching effectiveness should relate to how the process is managed and whether this leads to the realization of potential performance in the particular circumstances and with the particular constraints and/or enablers. In addition, and perhaps because coaching effectiveness is so difficult to measure and agree upon, coaches are often appointed to positions of responsibility (such as to national teams) on the basis of association with already successful performers. This is certainly true of swimming, with at least some of the British Olympic team coaches being selected on the basis of how many athletes they have on the team. The question here is not whether this is right or wrong (most swimming coaches would agree that those with the most swimmers on the team should be part of it), but whether these coaches are, at the time, in actual fact any more effective than many of their contemporaries.

It is almost certain that there is no one 'best' method of coaching (despite the continued success of some of our top coaches and role models), but that different coaches, all striving to be effective, will employ different methods, practices and behaviour that are appropriate at different times and in different circumstances. For example, different sports, sports in different cultures, different kinds of athletes (such as men/women, boys/girls, amateurs/professionals, athletes at the top of their form and those recovering from injury) and even the same athletes at different phases of their careers may elicit a different coaching response. However, the overriding intention may, in each case, still have been 'coaching effectiveness'. Such a view is supported by Mathers (1997: 24), who concluded that 'definitions [interpretations] of coaching effectiveness, ... remain specific to individual sport situations'. Not only are they specific to the individual sport situation, but they are also specific to the evaluation context. For example, employers, parents, athletes and coaches themselves may all gauge and/or rate effectiveness differently. This is an area that will be pursued later in this chapter.

Lyle (1998b: 172), in an attempt to consider all of the important factors, has suggested the following definition:

> Effective coaching performance is a measure of output over input and can only be understood in relation to 'external factors' – material context, goals and performer capabilities. Like successful coaching performance, it is bounded by time and circumstances. The effective coach is one whose capacity for effective coaching performance has been demonstrated over time and circumstances.

Value added

Although it is difficult to construct an all-embracing definition of coaching effectiveness, it is possible to identify crucial factors. One of the principal factors is the 'value added' (referred to as output over input in Lyle's definition) by the effective intervention of the coach (i.e. the positive effect of the coach's contribution to the coaching process). This is central to the success of the coaching process, and is therefore crucial to an understanding of the effectiveness equation. Adding value suggests that the decisions made and the direct intervention strategies adopted by the coach will affect output and, hence, coaching effectiveness. However, it should be stressed that effectiveness cannot really be measured merely in terms of outputs, or indeed inputs, but should be measured in terms of the relationships between them. These, as already noted, may vary over time, place and circumstance, and good decision making or intervention by the coach that result in enhanced athlete/team performance or even customer satisfaction (i.e. value added) may only indicate coaching effectiveness at that particular time and in those particular circumstances. Thus it is not only difficult to describe coaching effectiveness meaningfully for all occasions, but even more so to measure and evaluate it, particularly when it is considered in terms of the contextual constraints within which it is operationalized (Lyle, 1998b). For example, a small improvement in the competitive performance of an individual or team operating in a less than adequate training environment (poor facilities, inadequate time for training etc.) may suggest more coaching effectiveness on the part of the coach than a larger improvement in an ideal environment. Or does it? Should coaches' effectiveness be, in part, a measure of the environment they provide for the athlete(s)? Many practising coaches would be happy to be evaluated in this way provided that it was in their power to change the environment to one of their choosing. However, with the exception of national or regional institutes of sport, it is unlikely that the majority of coaches are ever going to be working in an ideal environment. Even when they are, managing the environment itself may detract from the amount of time necessary to ensure optimum effectiveness in other areas of the coaching process. Certainly managing the external circumstances of the coaching process with a relatively large number of athletes (as is common in most swimming clubs, for example) may, by limiting the amount of individualization possible, actually constrain effectiveness. In some sports (such as golf) coaches seldom, if ever, have to contend with more than one athlete at a time, and can easily operate on a much more individualized basis. The concept of individualization is the subject of Chapter 9, and will be discussed more fully at that point.

Components of effective coaching

A number of characteristics have emerged from various observation systems to identify effective coaches (Douge and Hastie, 1993). These include:

1. Frequent provision of feedback and incorporation of numerous prompts and hustles
2. Provision of high levels of correction and re-instruction
3. Use of high levels of questioning and clarifying
4. Predominantly being engaged in instruction
5. Management of the training environment to achieve considerable order.

Douge and Hastie (1993) have suggested that this list is, in fact, not exhaustive, and that it should be acknowledged that observable coaching behaviours are not the only components of effective coaching. They suggested that recent developments pointed to effective coaching being not just a product of an established set of coaching behaviours, but also needing to include a coach's ability to observe, analyse, synthesize and modify his or her coaching 'to fit the situation and the needs of those involved'. At a sport-specific level, Cross' (1995a, 1995b) research indicated that elite athletes also sought coaching behaviours such as 'protecting the athlete', 'the coach having confidence in his/her own ability' and the coach 'being honest and realistic'.

In an early paper critical of coaches emphasizing and concentrating on only a few features of the coaching process, Rushall (1980) suggested that there is a need for coaches to assess their 'performance in terms of the macro concepts associated with effective coaching'. In order to assist coaches to do this, he provided a list of the 10 characteristics of effective coaching that, in his opinion, are together essential to maintain coaching quality. These he labelled as:

1. The provision of a totally planned system
2. The maximization of productivity
3. The maximization of direction
4. The maximization of intrinsic motivation
5. The maximization of the instructional process
6. The maximization of positive experiences
7. The maximization of social experiences
8. The maximization of progress information
9. The transfer of control to the group/self
10. The maximization of content variety.

All of these, it could be argued, are desirable elements of an effective coaching process, and several are supported by the sports coaching literature (see, for example, Douge, 1987; Bompa, 1994; Lyle, 1996).

Douge (1987: 31) has summarized the views of prominent coaches from Australia, Europe and America, and compiled a long list of the qualities of successful coaches and the characteristics necessary for and contributing to their coaching effectiveness. He stressed the importance of coaches realizing 'that competent coaching is a learned trade, requiring hours of experience and gathering of knowledge'. Many of the characteristics he identified support those of Rushall listed above.

The identification of principles for (or of) coaching centres on two distinct areas of the coaching process. First are the principles of training to which coaches should adhere, such as the 'principle of progressive overload' and the 'principle of modelling training' etc. (for example, Bompa (1994: 29–48) identifies seven of these principles). Second are those principles more akin to a philosophy of coaching, and hence the coaching behaviours that coaches should adopt in order to be effective. For example, Hogg (1995: 12.3) has described a coaching philosophy as having guiding principles such as 'honesty, integrity, fairness, dignity and excellence', which together enable the coach 'to behave with consistency and credibility in any coaching setting'. The opportunity also exists for principles based on a combination of the two areas, and Rushall (1985a, 1985b) has suggested seven principles for modern coaching along these lines. These he labels as follows:

1. The principle of specificity (the more a task is practised, the better the performance)
2. The principle of individuality (coaching should be individualized for each athlete)

3. The principle of self-control (the athlete should perceive himself/herself to be in control, which leads to higher motivation)
4. The principle of involvement (the higher the goals, the greater the volume of training needed)
5. The principle of program [*sic*] consolidation (coaching should be based on sound scientifically justified criteria with monitoring and feedback)
6. The principle of self-involvement (coaches should constantly seek to update their knowledge, learn from others and be professional)
7. The principle of balanced preparation (all of the training and preparation factors should be attended to).

Some of these principles are obviously based on, and developed from, his earlier characteristics of effective coaching (Rushall, 1980). Finally, Sands and Alexander (1987) have identified coaching principles on the socio-psychological dimension, such as knowledge, supportive environment, diagnosis, self-improvement, individual needs and self-determination. That adhering to principles such as these is beneficial is undeniable. However, whether such practice will guarantee coaching effectiveness for all concerned is another matter. With many athletes interpreting coaching effectiveness in terms of their personal success (often based on winning) rather than considering the coach's attention to the coaching process as a whole, it is inevitable that misunderstandings will occur.

Principles and coaching behaviours such as these suggest that an appropriate coaching philosophy is an important stage in the coaching effectiveness process, and that modern effective coaching may require athletes to be involved to the extent that they are partners in the process and not merely customers. Thus action will have to be taken by the coach that will have knock-on implications for leadership style, and that will almost certainly advocate and support a more humanistic coaching style (Lombardo, 1987; Cross, 1991) in which the athlete is either an active collaborator or makes a conscious decision not to contribute to the process decisions. Howe (1990) has discussed the need for a philosophy of coaching which has the following 'purposes':

1. To assist the athletes in reaching their optimum performance level
2. To enable the athletes to gain control of and take personal responsibility for their performances
3. To become the best coach possible which, in Howe's view, 'implies a continuous commitment to studying the process'.

The second of these has obvious parallels with a humanistic approach that, in seeking the maximization of potential and working towards peak performance, will encourage the athlete to be independent. The coach will adopt a much more facilitative rather than a directional role. Although the humanistic approach to coaching might be considered subversive inasmuch as it encourages autonomy and self-reliance (Cross, 1991) rather than the athlete always relying on the coach for direction, it is not intended to undermine the coach's authority but rather to encourage athletes to think for themselves and assume a measure of responsibility for their own performance. Howe's third purpose is an extremely important one for coach education and the way in which it is presented. With coach education often taking place without any input from the most effective coaches (perhaps because they are too busy!), it may suggest the need for some kind of mentoring scheme in order to learn from the best role models we have. Certainly the best way to learn about a coaching philosophy is to witness it in action. However, Salmela (1995: 12) has demonstrated that, although expert coaches consider mentoring to be highly beneficial, 'mentoring isn't happening because people are too busy'.

Does coaching effectiveness depend to any extent on the coach's leadership qualities? For example, earlier in the chapter we identified that the field hockey coach education literature referred to 'good coaching and leadership' as one of its aims, and later it was suggested that a successful humanistic coaching style is dependent on a particular type of leadership which encourages collaboration and autonomy. The adoption of a collaborative coaching leadership style such as this is advocated by both Lombardo (1987) and Cross (1991), and has been recognized as an important principle of effective coaching (Mathers, 1997). Mudra (1980) suggested that the kind of approach that encourages collaboration and autonomy can give athletes the confidence to achieve their goals. In addition, Hogg (1995: 12.6), who has also advocated a humanistic approach (particularly with mature athletes), stated that 'when they [athletes] are treated responsibly they will be happier and more productive'. Certainly, coaching behaviours are often referred to as leadership styles (Terry and Howe, 1984), and Cox (1994) has suggested that good leadership is one of the most important, yet complex, characteristics that a coach must possess. Although leadership has been defined in a variety of ways, most of the definitions refer to the leader influencing one or more group members towards their goals. For example, leadership was described by Hemphill and Coons (1957) in terms of 'the behavior [*sic*] of an individual when he/she is directing the activities of a group towards a shared goal', and by Roach and Behling (1984) as 'the process of influencing the activities of an organized group toward goal achievement'. Obviously, either of these descriptions would be suitable for describing leadership in the coaching context. Chelladurai (1978) has taken the concept of coaching leadership a step further with his Multidimensional Model of Leadership (cited in Kuklinski, 1990), where leadership is directed at the two main aims of athlete satisfaction and effective athlete performance (see also Chelladurai, 1993). Adopting leadership styles from organizational management and using organization theory to explain leadership behaviour may have very positive benefits for coaching analysis (the work of Chelladurai is an obvious example). For example, Fiedler's (1967) contingency leadership model, which is concerned with best fit between task-orientated concerns and relationship-orientated concerns (i.e. best fit between task and people), has obvious lessons for coaching leadership. So too does Adair's (1990) strategic leadership model, which identifies the core requirements of strategic leadership as direction (a visionary dimension), team-building capability and creativity (including innovation and delegation). With the coaching process requiring attention in several different areas, management skills such as these have much to offer the aspiring coach.

It is important to note that the humanistic approach or style of leadership is neither universally applied nor exclusively equated with successful or effective coaching. For example, an alternative leadership style adopted by some apparently successful coaches is the autocratic approach, sometimes incorrectly described in the same terms as the behaviourist approach (Lombardo, 1987). In fact, Mathers (1997) has reminded us that it is also possible to provide and adopt a collaborative and caring coaching stance (although not necessarily associated with coaching effectiveness!) through psychological approaches other than the humanistic approach (where collaboration is a fundamental requirement). For example, coaches employing intervention strategies which are based on different psychological approaches (such as behaviourist, cognitive and psychobiological), may all also encourage a collaborative strategy. In the case of coaching practice adopting a behaviourist perspective, a coach and an athlete might agree, after consultation, on a particular course of action in order to bring about desired changes in behaviour. This change in behaviour would be achieved by changing the contingencies of reinforcement operating on that athlete at that moment in time (Cox, 1991). In the cognitive approach, the coach and the athlete would agree and hence collaborate on activities to improve information-processing abilities (in which athletes are encouraged to solve problems for themselves). For example, the practice environment might be structured to promote understanding of both extrinsic (weather, competitors, etc.) and intrinsic (proprioception, auditory, visual, etc.) information. The overriding strategy in such cases would be to promote independence in the athlete as a result of acquiring more advanced and flexible information processing skills. Similarly, a coach using the psychobiological approach might discuss a range of alternatives with an athlete and then agree upon an intervention that should change both the physiological state and subsequent behaviour of the athlete (Collins, 1995). Examples include encouraging pre-performance routines conducive to certain rhythms of movement, and the use of imagery cues. Using these techniques, the coach encourages the athlete to generate brainwave activity (e.g. slow wave alpha) associated with good performance.

Each of the psychological approaches described above will have more or less of an impact on different aspects of the coaching process. For example, one might expect the benefits of humanistic coaching practice to be more evident in interpersonal relationships and motivation, whereas psychobiological practices might be more appropriate in pre-competition routines. Good coaches seeking to be more effective might well benefit from incorporating a variety of approaches. Indeed, it is inconceivable that this will not be common practice for many experienced and expert coaches.

In the autocratic or authoritarian leadership approach, the coach often seeks a greater degree of control in an 'I know best' manner (Cross, 1991). This approach has been described as limiting choices and opportunities for self-determination (Hogg, 1995). In addition, Lombardo (1987: 42) has noted that 'Research has shown again and again that the goals of the athletic leader too often conflict with those of the athletes', and that this is most often associated with non-humanistic coaching behaviour. Despite the obvious drawback for personal autonomy there is little, if any, coaching research which actually compares coaching style (e.g. humanist v. autocratic) with coaching effectiveness. In addition, an autocratic approach is sometimes easier to implement than a more democratic and collaborative style. Anshel (1978) noted that, with the autocratic type of approach, the coach could work with 'tangible objectives and observable behaviours' and thus be more objective.

On the other hand, relating to and building a rapport with the unique and often variable moods and characteristics of athletes might take much more time. Taking a long time to make decisions might complicate the process to the extent that effective decisions become compromised. Consequently, one would expect to see coaches operating in the autocratic, rather than humanistic, mode fairly often. However, while the autocratic approach might well be effective in the short term, it is unlikely to be so in the longer term. As athletes become more mature, they are unlikely to continue to tolerate an approach which denies them any degree of personal control.

It should be clear that the adopted leadership style of the coach depends on the particular coaching context. Therefore, coaches will need to be flexible, and Cross (1991) has suggested that a more humanistic style might be more applicable when coaching older athletes than when coaching younger ones. Hogg (1995) suggested that it might be beneficial to move along a 'leadership style continuum' (see also Kuklinski, 1990) as athletes develop. The coaching style adopted would move from more autocratic with younger and more inexperienced athletes to fully democratic and collaborative with mature elite athletes. In terms of improving coach effectiveness, different approaches will be effective for different performers. For example, Anshel (1978) suggested that it is possible for both autocratic and democratic styles to be combined effectively within the same situation, and this was confirmed by Cross (1995b) in his research with elite swimmers. He found that some mature elite athletes actually wanted the coach to make the majority of the important decisions, thus allowing them to concentrate on the physical and technical aspects of training. Not only is it possible for elite athletes to differ in their preferred approach, but it should also be noted here that there may be differences in the way participation athletes and elite athletes view coaching leadership styles. For example, Terry (1984) found that the skill level of the athlete is an important variable in preferred leadership behaviour. In his study, elite athletes preferred more democratic behaviour and social support than did club athletes. On the other hand, club athletes preferred more rewarding/reinforcement behaviour than the elite athletes. However, Terry concluded that both groups, club and elite, favoured coaching behaviour which included occasional democratic and social support, regular rewards and very little autocratic behaviour. In addition to the above, Chelladurai *et al.* (1987) have reported cross-cultural differences in perceived leadership athlete preference. It would appear, therefore, that further research needs to be carried out with different sports and in different cultures before firm conclusions can be drawn as to which, if any, leadership approach is the most effective. In fact, it may be that preferred coach leadership styles (judged by client satisfaction) only contribute to effectiveness inasmuch as they lead to a match between coach behaviour and athlete expectation. If coaching effectiveness is measured in terms of winning or improved competitive performance, preferred coaching leadership style may not be a major factor.

Effective according to whom?

Effective coaching means different things to different people (Cross, 1995b). Effectiveness may not only be monitored by the coach, but also by the athlete and the coach's employers, whether they be parents, the governing body, a club or any other organization. Determining whether the coach is effective will depend upon the criteria against which effective coaching is measured, and the goals and aspirations of 'significant others' in the process. All three of the individuals/groups identified above may have different ideas of what the best measure might be. In addition, Douge and Hastie (1993) recognized that the modifications that coaches adopt to satisfy the needs of their athletes may, in some cases, also be affected by the need to consider the expectations of their employers. These expectations may or may not always be the same as, or in the best interests of, any or all of the athletes concerned. Examples in swimming include the need for coaches to cater for a larger number of athletes than they would wish, occasions when swimmers have to swim in relay teams against their best individual interests, and those instances of financial or budgetary constraint that result in the provision of less than optimum facilities, etc. Obvious examples in professional football include playing a not fully fit or injured player (sometimes with no more than strapping applied to the injury or the application of a pain-killing spray), or where players are made to play too many matches in too short a period.

Athletes too will evaluate the coach's effectiveness in different ways. To some extent, the way that this takes place will be goal-orientated. For example, athletes with coach approved process goals such as working on improvements in technique, training more frequently or for longer periods of time or applying themselves more assiduously etc. (all aimed at improving PBs) will be assessing effectiveness in areas which are not completely outside their own control. Athletes assessing effectiveness based only on outcome goals (such as winning) may in fact be evaluating the coach unfairly inasmuch as the performance of competitors is, almost certainly, outside the athlete's or coach's control. Hence the athlete may in fact perform well but still get beaten, and consequently interpret the coach's performance as ineffective. In team sports, owners and directors often tend to operate in this fashion. Coaching effectiveness is inevitably measured in terms of how many times the team wins. Thus the coach is deemed effective if the team is successful, despite the fact that sometimes a poor performance will result in a win and other times a good performance will result in a loss.

Examples of employers who may be guilty of assessing the coach's effectiveness based solely on winning (unfairly in many people's view) are governing bodies, clubs and institutions which operate using a managerial-type structure where the product is valued more than the process. Danziger (1982: 123) stated that, in this type of scenario, 'athletes are viewed as necessary cogs in the chain of production that must be properly efficient in order to produce the needed success'. Pressure is put upon the coach to produce winning athletes whatever the circumstances, and without recognition of all of the difficulties within which the coach and athletes have to work. In reality, many coaches in a variety of sports are only as successful as their coaching circumstances allow. Far from giving enough consideration to the circumstances in which the coach has to work, some employers, blinded by the need to be seen to be winning, interpret the constraints incorrectly, and consequently label the coach ineffective. This is particularly true of many professional team sports, with football a typical example in the United

Kingdom. However, even supposedly amateur sports (such as field hockey) are increasingly guilty of assessing coaching performance in this way.

Even coaches evaluate their own effectiveness in different ways. For example, it is possible for some coaches to measure the degree of their effectiveness against the number of their athletes who improve in performance and others by the amount of success or improvement made by a particular individual or individuals. Still others evaluate their own effectiveness by the rewards available for consistent successful or effective coaching, and these might include selection to the national team coaching staff, promotion or financial reward, etc.

In seeking to be effective, coaches may therefore be influenced and pressured from three different directions (athletes, employers and personal desires), and will have to adopt an approach that will change as the different agents (significant others) apply pressure with varying significance and power. Not all of these pressures are obvious or always recognized. One such pressure is that which can be put on coaches by athletes who are themselves influential in some way. This may be due to personal success in the sport, experience and/or skill gained over a number of years, latent or potential ability as perceived by the coach (sometimes described by coaches as 'talent') or indeed by any other means. For example, Sinclair and Vealey (1989), in an investigation of hockey coaches and athletes over a season, discovered that the coaches gave more specific and evaluative feedback to athletes they considered to have more ability and whom they rated as 'high-expectancy' athletes. Whether these athletes were in turn also more demanding is not clear, but some athletes, just as in any other walk of life, are extremely demanding and coaches do not always, as a result, spend enough time with those who are not. In such cases it is unlikely that those athletes receiving too little of the coach's time and effort are likely to consider him effective. The fact that some coaches devote more time and energy to high-expectancy athletes raises the issue of recruitment as an effectiveness measure. With winning or individual athlete's success often used as an effectiveness measure, coaches who are able to recruit talented athletes to their programmes would appear to have some considerable advantage. On the other hand, if 'value added' is the measure of effectiveness to be used (as has been suggested in this chapter), recruiting already very successful athletes may even be a disadvantage. With such athletes, the improvements possible are often very small and time-consuming, and are often difficult to attribute to the coach.

Some additional research findings of interest

Gould *et al.* (1990), in a study of 130 elite coaches from more than 30 different sports, found that many of the strategies coaches adopted that were aimed at coaching effectiveness were common to all the sports in their research sample. Some differences were found between strategies for team and individual sport approaches, but this is not really surprising, as this chapter has already highlighted many of the differences that exist between coaching team and individual sports. For example, the difficulty of attending to the individualization of training in team sport situations was recognized as a major problem. The need for team coaches to be heavily involved with team strategies, tactics, team building, etc., was identified as a constraint to personalized individualization practices. This is not something that is often experienced in individual sports. Thus, if adequate and appropriate attention to individualization strategies is a necessary part of any coaching process aimed at 'value added' (coaching effectiveness), team coaches will often be at a disadvantage because of other competing responsibilities.

Cross' (1995a, 1995b, 1995c) research into what constituted coaching effectiveness for elite field hockey players and coaches and elite swimmers and coaches identified some important differences. For example, the research highlighted the apparent significant importance of hockey coaches having good crisis management skills, not something that was considered necessary for effective swimming coaching. Good crisis management skills were described in terms of 'making successful intuitive decisions at the time they were needed'. Intuition in this context was based on the knowledge accrued from previous experience, and having been in the same sort of position before. As Cross and Ellice (1997) have reminded us, field hockey is a game based on problems, strategies, chance factors and tactical play. During the play, coaches can substitute players at will (rolling subs) in order to change their strategies or to combat opponents' strategies. The time taken to decide what to do and when to do it is at a premium. This has resulted in the coach's role on the bench being dramatically increased in importance. Effective intuitive decision making in such a context can often make the difference between success and failure. Whether this type of action is best described as crisis management (Cross, 1995a) or contingency management (Lyle, 1991) is not the issue; *any* unconventional strategy (Schon, 1983) is important in the quest for coaching effectiveness in this type of scenario. Schon has labelled the intuitive form of action that experienced professionals engage in as 'reflection-in-action'. Decision making is discussed at greater length in Chapter 11.

Salmela (1995), in analysing interviews with expert coaches from four different team sports, concluded that expert coaches were able to combine a number of complex coaching issues into a 'metacognitive form of knowledge', which could then be verbalized. Using this expert knowledge, various facilitative strategies based on prior experience were brought into play, which allowed 'their decision making and operational styles to be precisely formulated into effective ways of coaching' (Salmela, 1995: 13). Although Salmela did not identify this ability as intuition, what he described is very similar to the intuitive form of crisis management that Cross' (1995a) analysis of Scottish expert field hockey coaches identified.

In fact, the use of a dual or complementary coaching strategy based on scientific training theory principles and sports science back-up on the one hand and an intuitive process based on experience, knowledge and practice from dealing with a former multitude of unique situations on the other has resulted in some descriptions of 'the art of coaching' (Whitaker, 1986) and coaching as an 'artful science' (Dick, 1977). Scientific training principles, in addition to those suggested by Bompa (1994), might include those from biomechanics (Norman, 1975), physiology (Wilmore and Costill, 1994) and psychology (Rushall, 1985a, 1985b). In order to pay adequate attention to these sports science principles, coaches may need to seek help from a variety of different specialists, and not only from these particular fields. Other areas for consultation might include nutrition, medical and remedial matters, physiotherapy, massage, acupuncture, etc. Thus, while coaching practice should be built upon a solid foundation of the coaching process and its associated principles, elements and features, it may require an 'artist' with creative flair to implement it effectively, especially in team sport situations. The swimming coaches in Cross' research (1995b, 1995c) were much more 'scientific principle' orientated, both in terms of planning training and in feedback, than were the field hockey coaches. With the obvious need for individualized training programmes in swimming (in order to encourage value added, and hence coaching effectiveness), one would expect a more scientific approach. In addition, swimming in Britain has traditionally always embraced a comprehensive coach education programme (which highlights the importance of sports science), whereas field hockey has only recently adopted a similar system. Finally, many swimming coaches in Britain are full-time professionals (all of the coaches in Cross' study were), while most of the field hockey coaches also have to earn a living and may therefore be unable to devote as much time to the planning and scientific preparation of their programmes as they might wish.

Summary

It has been identified in this chapter that the current coaching literature is increasingly treating coaching as a process. In addition, a number of sources have been identified in which principles of coaching are suggested that can be used to analyse and evaluate coaching processes and inform coaching practice. Despite these steps forward in the development of coaching theory, defining and interpreting coaching effectiveness remains problematical. It is extremely difficult to construct an all-embracing definition of coaching effectiveness (and its attendant performance criteria) that satisfies all coaching situations. As Lyle (1998b) has noted, effective coaching performance is not merely a measure of output over input, but has to be understood within its own particular context and timeframe. Thus facilities, performer capabilities, goals (including those of athletes, parents, employers and other stakeholders such as sponsors), competition environment, etc., will all have an impact on how coaching effectiveness is judged. Having reviewed a number of alternatives, 'value added', or the positive effect of the coach's contribution to athlete performance (or perhaps more accurately to the coaching process as a whole), was identified as a crucial factor in determining whether coaching effectiveness has actually been demonstrated.

Various coaching behaviours have been identified which may contribute to a more effective process. Some of these have focused more on the coach's communication and interpersonal skills than on process-related skills such as planning, monitoring, etc. For example, it has been suggested that good leadership skills and a humanistically orientated coaching philosophy may have positive benefits for improving coaching practice and enhancing athletic performance and, as a consequence, increasing coaching effectiveness. Despite these assumptions, it has been acknowledged that there is little evidence as yet to show that is the only way, or even the best way, to ensure optimal coaching effectiveness. There is some evidence that this style of coaching may result in more satisfied and contented athletes. However, this could be due to the research using athlete satisfaction rather than improved performance as an output measure of coaching effectiveness (increasingly common in coaching research). Nevertheless, recommendations have been made in the chapter that coaching strategies and behaviours which are collaborative, facilitative, delegate authority and are athlete centred are significantly preferable to more autocratic types of approach. This is especially true in the case of mature elite athletes. This type of philosophy does not, of course, exclude those circumstances when a more directive style may be recognized by all of the participants as more appropriate. This is a common occurrence in many team sports.

Finally, it has been recognized that coaching effectiveness, both at participation and elite competition levels, means different things to different people. It also appears that even the same individual's interpretation of its assessment may change according to factors such as the stage in the athlete's career, current success or lack of it, perceived potential, environmental constraints, and influence and pressure brought to bear by significant others (such as coaches, parents, selectors, employers, national governing bodies of sport, etc.). Thus, issues of selection, grading, appraisal, etc. will all influence its interpretation. Not only will it be interpreted differently, but also the terms used to describe it by the different agencies (such as competent, successful and expert) often confuse rather than clarify the situation. It is clear, however, that 'effectiveness' implies value added to the process which is the contract between the athlete and the coach. When the goals set at the start of the contract, the personal and material constraints acting on the process and the period of time over which the process is demonstrated have all been taken into account, the extent of the value added is the only really meaningful measure of whether or not coaching is effective. Unfortunately, this does not reduce the difficulty of implementing measures to guarantee coaching effectiveness in a practical way. Having identified the principles concerned, the challenge is to identify meaningful criteria with which to monitor the coach's contribution and to calculate any resulting value added.

References

Abraham, A. and Collins, D. (1998). Examining and extending research in coach development. *Quest*, **50(1),** 59–79.

Adair, J. (1990). *Great Leaders*. Talbot Adair Press.

Anshel, M. H. (1978). Behaviourism versus humanism: An approach to effective team leadership in sport. *Motor Skills: Theory Pract.*, **2(2),** 83–91.

Batty, E. (1965). *Soccer Coaching the Modern Way*. Faber.

Bompa, T. O. (1994). *Theory and Methodology of Training* (3rd edn). Kendall Hunt.

Chelladurai, P. (1978). A contingency model of leadership in athletics. Unpublished doctoral dissertation. University of Waterloo, Ontario.

Chelladurai, P. (1993). Leadership. In *Handbook of Research on Sport Psychology* (R. N. Singer, M. Murphey and L. K. Tennant, eds), pp. 647–71. Macmillan.

Chelladurai, P., Malloy, D., Imamura, H. and Yamaguchi, Y. (1987). A cross-cultural study of preferred leadership behavior and satisfaction of athletes in various sports. *J. Sport Psychol*, **6,** 27–41.

Collins, D. (1995). Psychophysiology and sports performance. In *European Perspectives on Exercise and Sport Physiology* (S. J. Biddle, ed.), pp. 154–69. Human Kinetics.

Cox, R. H. (1994). *Sport Psychology, Concepts and Applications* (3rd edn). Wm. C. Brown Communications Inc.

Cox, R. (1991). Motivation. In *Sport Psychology: A Self-Help Guide* (S. J. Bull, ed.), pp. 6–30. Cromwell Pubs.

Cross, N. (1991). Arguments in favour of a humanistic coaching process. *Swimming Times*, **LXVIII(11)**, 17–18.

Cross, N. (1995a). Coaching effectiveness in hockey: A Scottish perspective. *Scot. J. Physical Ed.*, **23(1)**, 27–39.

Cross, N. (1995b). Coaching effectiveness and the coaching process (Part 1) *Swimming Times*, **LXXII(2)**, 23–5.

Cross, N. (1995c). Coaching effectiveness and the coaching process (Part 2) *Swimming Times*, **LXXII(3)**, 23–4.

Cross, N. and Ellice, C. (1997). Coaching effectiveness and the coaching process: Field hockey revisited. *Scot. J. Physical Ed.*, **25(3)**, 19–33.

Danziger, R. C. (1982). Coaching humanistically: An alternative approach. *Physical Educator*, **39**, 121–5.

Dick, F. (1977). Coaching – an artful science! *Momentum*, **2(3)**, 1–3.

Douge, B. (1987). Coaching qualities of successful coaches. *Sports Coach*, **10(4)**, 31–5.

Douge, B. and Hastie, P. (1993). Coaching effectiveness. *Sport Sci. Rev.*, **2(2)**, 14–29.

Fairs, J. (1987). The coaching process: The essence of coaching. *Sports Coach*, **11(1)**, 17–19.

Fiedler, F. E. (1967). *A Theory of Leadership Effectiveness*. McGraw-Hill.

Franks, I., Sinclair, G. D., Thomson, W. and Goodman, D. (1986). Analysis of the coaching process. *Science Periodical on Research and Technology of Sport*. Paper A, The Coaching Association of Canada, Ottawa.

Gould, D., Giannini, J., Krane, V. and Hodge, K. (1990). Educational needs of elite US National team, Pan-American and Olympic coaches. *J. Teach. Physical Ed.*, **9(4)**, 332–44.

Hemphill, J. K. and Coons, A. E. (1957). Development of the leader behaviour description questionnaire. In *Leader Behaviour: Its Description and Measurement* (R. M. Stogdill and A. E. Coons, eds), pp. 6–38. Ohio State University Press.

Hogg, J. M. (1995). *Mental Skills for Swim Coaches*. Sport Excel Publishing.

Howe, B. (1990). Coaching effectiveness. *NZ J. Health Physical Ed. Rec.*, **23(3)**, 4–7.

Kuklinski, B. (1990). Sport leadership: An overview. *NZ J. Health Physical Ed. Rec.*, **23(3)**, 15–18.

Lombardo, B. J. (1987). *The Humanistic Coach: From Theory to Practice*. Charles C. Thomas Pubs.

Lyle, J. (1992). Systematic coaching behaviour: An investigation into the coaching process and the implications of the findings for coach education. In *Sport and Physical Activity* (T. Williams, L. Almond and A. Sparkes, eds), pp. 463–9. EFN Spon.

Lyle, J. (1996). A conceptual appreciation of the sports coaching process. *Scot. Cent. Res. Papers Sport Leisure Soc.*, **1**, 15–37.

Lyle, J. (1998a). Coaching effectiveness and the teaching paradigm. In *Active Living Through Quality Physical Education* (R. Fisher, C. Laws and J. Moses, eds), pp. 40–45. 8th European Congress, ICHPER.S.D. P.E.A.UK.

Lyle, J. (1998b). Coaching effectiveness. In *The Coaching Process* (Workbook NCFB2001), pp. 157–174. National Coaching Foundation.

Mathers, J. F. (1997). Professional coaching in golf: Is there an appreciation of the coaching process? *Scot. J. Physical Ed.*, **25(1)**, 23–35.

Mudra, D. (1980). A humanist looks at coaching. *J. Physical Ed. Rec.*, **51(8)**, 22–5.

Norman, R. W. (1975). Biomechanics and the community coach. *J. Physical Ed. Rec.*, **46(3)**, 49–52.

Roach, C. F. and Behling, O. (1984). Functionalism: Basis for an alternative approach to the study of leadership. In *Leaders and Managers: International Perspectives on Managerial Behavior and Leadership* (J. G. Hunt, D. M. Hosking, C. A. Schriesheim and R. Stewart, eds), pp. 51–61. Pergamon Press.

Rushall, B. S. (1980). Characteristics of effective coaching. *Sports Coach*, **4(2),** 3–5.

Rushall, B. (1985a). Several principles of modern coaching. *Sports Coach*, **8(3),** 40–4.

Rushall, B. (1985b). Seven principles for modern coaching: Part II. *Sports Coach*, **8(4),** 21–3.

Salmela, J. H. (1995). Learning from the development of expert coaches. *Coaching Sport Sci. J.*, **2(2),** 3–13.

Sands, R. and Alexander, K. (1987). *Sports Science, Theory into Practice and Coaching: A Practical Coaching Model*. Paper presented at the Sports Management Conference, Melbourne.

Schon, D. A. (1983). *The Reflective Practitioner: How Professionals Think in Action*. Temple Smith.

Scottish Hockey Union (1994). *Scottish Vocational Qualification Coaching Award Manuals 1–3*. Scottish Hockey Union,.

Sherman, C. and Sands, R. (1996). Thinking ahead – a new perspective. *Sports Coach*, **19(1),** 31–4.

Sinclair, D. A. and Vealey, R. S. (1989). Effects of coaches' expectations and feedback on the self-perceptions of athletes. *J. Sport Behaviour*, **12(2),** 77–91.

Terry, P. C. (1984). The coaching preferences of elite athletes competing at Universiade '83. *Can. J. Appl. Sport Sci.*, **9,** 183–93.

Terry, P. C. and Howe, B. L. (1984). Coaching preferences of athletes. *Can. J. Appl. Sport Sci.*, **2(4),** 188–93.

Weir, M. (1977). *Hockey Coaching – A Psychological Approach to the Women's Game*, p. 99. Kaye and Ward.

Whitaker, D. (1986). *Coaching Hockey*. The Crowood Press.

Whitaker, D. (1992). *The Hockey Workshop – A Complete Game Guide*, p. 24. Crowood Press.

Wilmore, J. H. and Costill, D. L. (1994). *Physiology of Sport and Exercise*. Human Kinetics.

Part 2

The Application of Sports Science in Coaching

4

Psychological considerations of effective coaching

Richard Cox

- The relationship between winning and success
- Changing behaviour for success
- Ten characteristics of excellent coaching sessions
- The importance of detailed planning and communication
- Simulating the demands of competition in training and practice sessions
- Considerations of the nature and delivery of feedback
- Detecting athletes' problems early

Introduction

This chapter concerns how psychology can help coaches to succeed in their work. It is written from a mix of pertinent research findings on the one hand, and my firsthand experiences on the other. As such, it is almost exclusively concerned with coaching elite athletes, most of whom are now either full-time or professional (or both), and much the same can be said of their coaches. Thus, conceptual discussions about what is a coach and what it is to coach effectively are not entered into here. This is not to say that such discussions are unimportant. On the contrary, they are inevitable at some stage in the developing career of all coaches, regardless of their sport. Rather, it is to say that full-time professional coaches of elite athletes know that their effectiveness will be judged on results over a stipulated period of time, for this is precisely the main criterion their employer(s) will write into their contract.

This said, it has to be acknowledged that some aspects of the professional coach's role are problematic. Some coaches in professional sport have experienced a less formal education than others – they may have been appointed 'coach' due to an exceptional competitive career from which they have now retired. This has to be taken into consideration in relation to their use of other experts to implement part of the coaching process. Coaches whose effectiveness is judged by association with successful per-formers will have to take a particular perspective on the coaching process, and their priorities will be different to those of others. Short-term psychological issues allied to recruitment and selection will be more important than the longer-term, developmental aspects of the coaching process.

At the time of writing, the final stages of the 1998 Football World Cup ended in France just 3 weeks ago and the 16th Commonwealth Games will be held in Kuala Lumpur in 6 weeks' time. Together these two major sporting events offer an opportunity to assess the progress a country such as Scotland has made in its standards of sporting excellence over a 4-year period. The results of France '98 are now known, and Scotland's team was eliminated for the seventh time in seven qualifications at the end of the first round. Whatever the thoughts and feelings are about this result, it inevitably raised debate about the standard of football in Scotland and the quality of its coaches. Significantly, the two biggest clubs in Scotland, Glasgow Rangers and Celtic, each now have a coach in charge who is neither Scottish nor British, though it must be added that no change has been made to the personnel in charge of the Scottish National team. (However, it is worth noting that at least five national coaches were sacked during the France '98 tournament.) Similar debates will take place with considerable passion about the results of the 16th Commonwealth Games. Inevitably, they will be accusatory if Scotland's athletes win fewer medals than the 20 they won at the 1994 Games in Victoria, Canada, and complimentary if they win more (if they double that total the response will be rapturous!). Either way, what is important is that the Scottish people and the Scottish media will judge the efforts of their representatives in Kuala Lumpur purely in terms of results. No matter how many personal best performances are registered and positive personal developments take place, if the medal count is less than 20, with fewer than six gold, then the athletes and their coaches can expect a hard time from the Scottish media. Drysdale (1994), commenting on Scotland's track and field team's performance in the 1994 Commonwealth Games, wrote that '... a valid rationale would contend that one solitary success is a paltry return on the estimated £75 000 invested to send the 39-strong team to Canada'. Such a sentiment was expressed widely in 1994, and no amount of education of the general public or the media by National Governing Bodies of Sport, National Coaches and Scottish Sports Council will change their orientation and attitude after the 1998 Games.

Winning and success

At the elite end of competitive sport there is a public perception that effective coaching is simply another term for successful coaching, and success is mostly equated with winning – medals, knockout competitions and leagues. However, being successful does not always have to mean finishing in first place. For instance, the first three football teams in the Scottish Premier League qualify for European competition in the following season, and the coach of each would undoubtedly be regarded as successful. Similarly, had Scotland qualified for the second round of the World Cup in France then the players and coaches would have been hailed as heroes. Winning, or being successful, *does* mean gaining a positive outcome, which brings tangible rewards, but it is outside the direct control of the coach concerned. The coaching process is characterized by the coach's attempts to control the variables influencing performance. This means that the coach will be able to exert some control over the performance of the athletes, but not necessarily how their performance will rate in comparison to others. In addition, the coach has to operate within the matrix of recruitment, facilities, finance and support services (and of course, knowledge and experience). Nevertheless, most coaches do attempt to attend to all aspects of the coaching process, and this may explain why sport psychology is now playing an ever-increasing role in the preparation of elite athletes for national and international competition in a wide variety of sports. Of course, it has to be recognized that sport psychologists are only one element in the coaching process and that they do not have any greater control over winning than coaches. Their ever-increasing involvement does, however, point to the fact that those who hire their services believe that psychological preparation is an essential element in the coaching process, and that sport psychology can help athletes to become more successful – why else would they want a sport psychologist in the first place?

To become more successful is to invite comparison with a previously established standard, and can only be registered in an appreciable improvement of some kind. To improve is to do things better than ever before, albeit in a particular context, and that means something(s) must have changed. To 'change things for the better' is a more challenging statement than 'to improve', and tends to focus the mind on more objective criteria. These criteria are particularly relevant if success is the raison d'être for employing a coach in the first place – which, in professional sport, it usually is.

So, what would coaches change in order to improve performance or bring about success? What *could* they change? In professional sports, the short answer to both of these questions is 'the athletes'. In football, for instance, each season sees a large movement of players from one team to another. (In this sense, change usually means replacement.) For some, the reason for transfer is for their club to make money, but often it is because they are no longer wanted by their coach. It is of particular interest to count the number of players who are sold each season to another club in the same league, for if they are no longer regarded as good enough for one club, how can they be good enough for another in the same league? Admittedly this question is too simplistic, for it takes no cognizance of different tactics and strategies employed by different coaches across different teams, nor of players at different stages in their careers. Changing the playing staff, as the only change in a professional set-up, could also be regarded as a simplistic approach, particularly when the coach in question has previously been sacked from a club in the same league. An analysis of the English Premiership and the Scottish Premier League in any one season would quickly reveal several coaches/managers who, during their career, have been employed by as many as four different clubs in the same league.

There are many other aspects of the coaching process that can be changed. In terms of external management of resources, additional finance can mean access to competitions, a better training environment or a larger support personnel. Indirect aspects of the process, as well as of the planning and monitoring procedures, can be improved, and the coaches' direct intervention can also be changed. This might be the detail of training matters, techniques or tactics, or the way in which performers are treated by the coaches. Changing the athletes' overall lifestyle, including activities and specific performance-related behaviours, is also an important part of improving the process. Therefore, changing athletes could also mean keeping the same athletes but changing the way they do things. For instance, many elite athletes in Scotland have, in the past 5 years or so, changed their eating patterns and habits. This has been brought about largely through the increasing influence of sports science and the education that has come with it. Most elite athletes are now quite knowledgeable about what and when to eat and drink, although my experience with them suggests that there is still a long way to go in this respect. A major problem is the fact that greater knowledge does not in itself necessarily result in a change in behaviour, and many nutritionists and dieticians have still to appreciate fully the fact that eating and drinking are largely psychological rather than solely nutritional behaviours. In other words, we eat and drink what we *like* to eat and drink, and do so in accordance with long established habits. To change such habits requires insight into human behaviour and how it is motivated.

This is where such matters become complicated, because psychologists have never reached agreement about the sources of human motivation. Some believe it is intrinsic to human nature. For instance, psychoanalysts (see Freud, 1933) believe the wellspring of human motivation lies in our libidinal instincts and energies and that, through such psychological mechanisms as displacement, regression and repression, all human behaviour can be accounted for in these terms. Among those who reject this theory are those who call themselves humanists, for they believe that human behaviour is not controlled by an internal energy system or, for that matter, by any system, internal or external. Their theoretical stance revolves around the belief that human beings are free agents in this world and that they choose to do what they do, when they want to do it, and are under the control of nothing and nobody but themselves (Sage, 1980).

This debate could well occupy the remainder of this chapter, for there are several other types of psychology, but this is not its purpose. The important point is that the methods adopted in attempting to change a person's behaviour should be consistent with the theoretical stance adopted, and will differ from theory to theory. For what it is worth, my own stance is that of radical behavioural psychology and, as such, I believe that all forms of human behaviour (above reflexive movement) are shaped by their consequences. This means that human beings are motivated by the contingencies of reinforcement, positive and negative, that operate in their lives. For present purposes, it means that coaches, providing they understand the effects of their own behaviour on others, can change the motivation of the athletes in their charge. The swimming coaches Gambril and Bay (1985: 23) appeared to believe this when they stated that: 'There is a way to motivate every person, there is a way to inspire every swimmer. Finding this way is the key to the art of coaching.'

Changing for success

Perhaps a useful starting point for discovering the way to change the behaviour of elite athletes is to study what they like about training or practice sessions, and what they look for in an 'effective' coach. If this is known with some certainty, then it makes sense to use the information to induce a positively reinforcing training environment in which athletes feel they want to work longer and with greater commitment and quality. Rushall (1995: 0.1) claimed to have completed such a study for, as the basic thesis of his book, he stated that: 'There is a group of overt and covert behaviours that are common to sporting champions irrespective of sex, nationality, or activity. We now know how champions think and behave in the social aspects of the sport setting, at training, prior to and in competitions, what experiences are rewarding to them and how sport is considered relative to other activities.' Moreover, he claimed that his checklist of behaviours was stable over time, for he had researched the behaviour of 155 champions and record-holders over a 20-year period and found that 'there are no new items that differentiate old-previous champions from today's champions. The basic core of behaviours and thoughts that it takes to be a champion are as valid today as they were 15 years ago' (Rushall, 1995: 13.3). It seems sensible, therefore, to examine the results of this research with a view to finding out which of these behaviours and thoughts can be promoted directly by coaches. Before doing so, however, it must be acknowledged that in order to promote any particular behavioural change in any one of their athletes it might be necessary for the coaches to modify (a euphemism for 'change') their own behaviour first. In many sports the stereotypical coach would be described as more rather than less authoritarian and, by definition, resistant to change, at least in interpersonal style and attitude. My experience of football, rugby and swimming has provided many examples of this, and these sports are not alone. Interestingly, the presence of such coaches begs the question of whether these sports attract this type of personality to their coaching ranks in the first place, or whether those who aspire to coach these sports believe they have to behave in this way in order to be seen as credible. If the coaches were former athletes in the sport and were coached in this manner themselves, then it would hardly be surprising if they behaved similarly. This raises the further question of whether an examination of coaching styles and their different, predictable effects upon the behaviour of athletes is a sufficient part of the coach education programmes for these sports.

From the 100 items identified by Rushall (1995) as being representative of the predilections of champion athletes, 10 have been identified as particularly relevant because they are under the direct control of the coach. It is contended here that if coaches can make all 10 happen on a regular basis, then they will go a long way towards motivating their athletes positively and thereby raising the probability of changing their behaviour for the better. These 10 items are presented in Figure 4.1.

Each of the 10 items presented in Figure 4.1 raises several questions for coaches. For instance, why are champion athletes motivated positively by them? How different are they from what coaches do already? How much extra work do they necessarily involve? Are they relevant for either less able or less experienced athletes? These questions are important, for if coaches do not have answers to them then they are unlikely to attempt to implement any of the behaviours involved in any meaningful way, or even to recognize that they already characterize their coaching practice. For this reason, each of the 10 items will now be considered in detail.

Excellent coaching sessions:

1   Are planned and published in advance of the session.
2   Start and end on time.
3   Keep athletes busy the whole time.
4   Promote competition between friends.
5   Include a lot of variety.
6   Include behaviours required in competitions.
7   Involve each athlete in goal-setting.
8   Generate as much feedback to each athlete as possible.
9   Are evaluated as soon afterwards as possible.
10 Encourage interested family and friends to make a positive contribution.

Figure 4.1 Characteristics of excellent coaching sessions

Excellent coaching sessions are planned and published in advance

All coaching sessions should be planned well in advance, and preferably as part of an overall plan rather than an isolated event. Any coaches who are still deciding what they are going to ask their athletes to do while travelling to the coaching venue are bound to be less effective than they might otherwise have been. This is because they can give little or no consideration to anything other than the basic content of the session, and the importance of doing more than this is borne out by the fact that the first six items in Figure 4.1 are all dependent on planning. If athletes do not know what their coach has in store for them, then they are likely to hold their personal resources back in case a 'maximum' effort is required in a particular activity later in the session.

In addition to identifying the content of any coaching session, the coach should consider how long each activity is to last, the organization and objectives (criteria for performance and criteria for success) of each activity, where the feedback to each athlete is to come from and when, and the coaching style most suited to achieving the objectives. More importantly, making all this known to the athletes in advance empowers them to set personal goals for each activity and plan the management of their physical and mental resources. A coach who has planned well should have no qualms about letting his athletes know in advance what is expected of them. Therefore, there is no reason why the day's programme (and preferably a whole week's programme) should not be posted on a notice board (perhaps in the changing room) before the athletes arrive for each session. It is also important, however, to acknowledge that a degree of contingency planning is required because of injury, player availability, weather, and the progress made in previous sessions. Competition programmes may also change with short notice. Nevertheless, informing athletes of the coach's intentions is a key factor in developing their sense of self-management.

Excellent coaching sessions start and end on time

This is a very basic requirement, but it is surprising how often it is offended in practice. Many coaching sessions in a wide variety of sports fail to start and end on time, and seldom is this caused by any contingency outside the coach's control. The first requirement is for coaches to organize their time such that they are ready some time before the appointed hour, and this readiness should be visible to the athletes. This allows the coach to organize any equipment and personnel required to assist with the session. From a psychological point of view, the athletes quickly appreciate that their coach is punctual and well organized, both of which indicate that he or she cares about the impending session. It also means that the coach can reasonably ask the athletes to arrive with sufficient flexibility so as to be ready to start work at the appointed time.

Having arrived early and set up everything that is necessary, the coach should begin the session exactly on time, even if the 'star' athlete(s) has still to appear. Nothing is more galling to those who *have* made the effort to arrive early than to be kept waiting for one or two latecomers, regardless of their importance. I have witnessed this event on numerous occasions in more than a dozen rugby clubs over a 25-year time span (human behaviour of this kind is not altered by the passing of time!). It takes no more than two promptly started sessions to communicate to everyone concerned that the coach means business. In professional clubs, athletes can be (and often are) fined if they are not ready on time, so it is less of a problem than in amateur clubs. However, while a punitive system such as fines for misbehaviour of this kind is usually effective, something else must happen if the athletes concerned are to change their behaviour permanently. The acid test is to remove the punishment (the fines) and study the behaviour in question as a consequence. If athletes start to arrive later and even miss the start of a session because the system of fines has been suspended, then it becomes obvious that the behaviour has not changed, but merely been suppressed. This highlights a common misunderstanding in trying to change a behaviour in another person, and it is manifested in the differences between what behavioural psychologists refer to as 'punishment' on the one hand and 'extinction' on the other. Both are known as behaviour modification techniques, and though punishment is intended to eradicate a behaviour from a person's repertoire it is, nevertheless, quite different from extinction. (For detailed explanations and discussion of these important concepts see Leslie, 1996.)

In behavioural modification terms, the undesired behaviour in question is weakened by the presentation of a punisher (an aversive stimulus or event) following the behaviour. The closer in time the presentation, the more effective the punishment is likely to be. The ideal is within 30 seconds of the undesired behaviour occurring. Moreover, the punishment should be delivered immediately after *every* instance of the undesired behaviour, as occasional punishment is not nearly as effective, and is even less so when it is delayed in time. More importantly, perhaps, the person administering the punishment should remain calm when doing so, as anger and frustration may inadvertently either reinforce the undesired behaviour positively or alter the consistency of the intensity of the punishment. Martin and Pears

(1992) explained how punishment should never be administered in a humiliating or degrading manner if it is to be effective.

However, punishment (or the threat of punishment) does not always bring about the intended effects, as is evidenced in the behaviour of many a 'star' athlete. In football, for instance, the names of players such as George Best, Vinnie Jones and Paul Gascoigne spring to mind. These players were disciplined on several occasions for breaches of football regulations but whatever the sanction they received it appeared not to bring about the desired change in behaviour for which, presumably, it was intended; other reinforces in their lives were obviously far more powerful. Players will also weigh up the severity of the punishment against the benefits of the undesired behaviour, and may decide that the latter outweigh the former. This is certainly the case with on-field disciplinary punishments. In 'extinction', a behaviour is weakened as a result of occurring without being reinforced. This is extremely difficult to do in practice, because it means ignoring the undesired behaviour while at the same time waiting to reinforce positively any behaviour that approximates that which is desired. For example, in trying to persuade athletes to arrive in time for the beginning of a coaching session, it would mean paying no attention whatsoever to anyone who was late, but praising and thanking those who were ready for the start of the session. This would have to apply to all other athletes present as well as to the coach. In professional terms, it would mean having a monetary bonus scheme in place for all those who arrive early (paid on an intermittent time schedule), and no sanctions at all for anyone who turns up late. This highlights what is arguably the most challenging aspect of trying to change the behaviour of anybody. The great majority of coaches (and teachers, officials and even parents) are quick to punish undesirable behaviour in a multitude of different ways, but slow (if at all) to reward the desired behaviour they want to see instead. All too often, behaviour is punished without the recipient ever being told what to replace it with. Thus, expressions such as 'don't do that', 'stop that' and 'do that again and you'll be ... (punished in some way)' are commonplace, but seldom is the alternative, acceptable behaviour spelled out immediately following. Furthermore, it is extremely difficult not to reinforce undesirable behaviour negatively, particularly when the person concerned has a long history of doing so, and suddenly to be invited to ignore the unwanted behaviour rather than punish it has proved to be beyond the capabilities of many. One other complication is the fact that, in administering the punishment, a form of attention is being given to the culprit concerned, and this can be interpreted as a form of positive reinforcement – in lay terms, the recipient gains notoriety, and it would not be the first time that athletes have courted the sanctions imposed by officials in their sports in order to enhance their reputation as a 'bad boy'.

Ending a coaching session on time is equally important. Many coaches have been tempted to keep a session going for longer than anticipated when the quality of work being produced is high. However, to do so is to ignore the strong possibility that several of the athletes concerned have arranged appointments straight after the stipulated end of the session. Elite athletes are typically very good managers of their own time. Consequently they expect others to be so, and especially their coach. If the session is described in advance as a 2-hour session, beginning at 7.00 pm and ending at 9.00 pm, then that is precisely what elite athletes expect. They will organize other events in their lives around these times. More importantly, they will plan to give all that they can to the 2 hours, but no longer. If they are asked to work beyond 9.00 pm or, worse, the coach is unaware that 9.00 pm has come and gone and shows no sign of ending the session, then their motivation will decrease rapidly and so will the quality of their work. Good time management is a relatively simple skill for coaches to develop, but it pays huge dividends in terms of effectiveness.

Excellent coaching sessions keep athletes busy the whole time

Elite athletes have a large capacity for hard work, and they like to make maximum use of the time available. Except for appropriate recovery periods, they prefer to be kept busy for the duration of the session. Thus, it makes sense for coaches to capitalize on the productivity of their athletes by not wasting time. A consequence of this is that the athletes will perceive the value of the session as being high, and their motivation for it will increase accordingly. This can only be achieved through detailed planning in advance.

Organizational matters can sometimes interfere with the flow of a coaching session and appear to waste time. Successive practices may need large amounts of different equipment set out in particular, strategic places around the practice environment. If the coach is fully occupied in observing the athletes at work, as should be the case, then who is to set out the equipment for the next practice? If the coach does it, then the athletes are kept waiting and, though this might lead the coach to think the session is busy because he or she is working hard, nobody else will think so. The athletes will see the coach as disorganized for failing to make appropriate arrangements, and their motivation for the session will decrease as a result. This is where the coach can encourage injured athletes in attendance, as well as interested friends and family members, to make a positive contribution. It is important to realize, however, that not all athletes will be making an equal contribution to the exercise at any given time, nor will they be receiving equal amounts of attention. This will depend on the focus of the drill, and the athletes' specialisms.

Excellent coaching sessions promote competition between friends

When the 1997 British Lions were practising one day during their tour of South Africa, the intensity of a practice scrummaging session was so great that scuffles broke out on more than one occasion between the two sets of forwards. The coaches were quick to intervene but it was largely of their own making, for they had been demanding such intensity from the beginning. They knew, from previous experience, what was going to be required of their first choice pack when they faced the Springboks in the forthcoming three Test matches.

This level of 'competition between friends' is obviously an extreme example, and must not be taken out of context. That is to say, it occurred during a particularly tough coaching session for one of the most physical, confrontational games ever devised; it was prompted by poor scrummaging that had led to a defeat in the previous match; it was in preparation to play the then world champions on their home soil in front of a hostile crowd; it was in response to the South African media which had written them off with taunts such as 'pussycats' rather than 'lions'; and it was fuelled by unexpected and surprising combinations of players in both packs. One of these was the probable pack for the first Test that no one, least of all the players themselves, had predicted in advance. Nevertheless, it was hailed by the coaches involved as the turning point for what turned out to be a highly successful tour, for the Lions won two of the three Tests against South Africa and were feted on their return home.

Elite athletes do like to compete against each other during training or preparation sessions, but it must be kept in perspective. While the reason for any coaching session must be to prepare athletes to compete, competing against each other should never become the raison d'être for any coaching session. Competition is much more likely to be used for specific competition rehearsal and for the evaluation of training targets. However, it should also be viewed as an opportunity in some sports for athletes to air their pent up competitive frustrations – to let off steam. As such, it is probably most effective if it occurs every fourth or fifth normal training, or practice session.

Interesting examples can be provided from my experience with the British Swim Team during a training camp in Florida, some 4 months prior to the 1992 Olympics in Barcelona. The team had travelled to Florida in search of warm weather training outdoors and, as a form of light relief from the daily diet of hard training, two competitions were organized on different days. Everyone was invited to take part in the first, and only one out of 24 swimmers declined. On the whistle, everyone had to swim 100 m (without a dive to start – they could begin at either end of the pool) with the knowledge that the second whistle would sound after 80 s. On that second whistle they had to swim another 100 m, knowing that the third whistle would sound after 79 s, the fourth after 78 s, and so on. If any swimmers were still swimming the previous 100 m when the whistle was blown to start the next, they were obliged to drop out. Thus, the challenge was to be the last swimmer(s) left in the water and to swim as many 100 m distances as possible with 1 s less time for each. It turned out to be a quite incredible event, enjoyed by all who took part, with the two eventual winners completing 22 consecutive 100 m swims before the clock beat them both during the 58 s leg. Not surprisingly, both were male 400 m freestyle specialists, but it was a female medley swimmer who finished third.

The second event was organized 4 days after the first and involved the whole team being divided into four mixed teams, each of six swimmers. The programme comprised a series of relay races across the width (25 m) of a pool, involving all four strokes used in competition and in different combinations. Points were awarded to each team that finished the race legitimately, and the winning team was the one with the most points at the end. Again the event proved to be highly enjoyable, although it had to be suspended at one point because some of the swimmers were so competitive they were cheating in their desire to win!

These two competitions were designed to provide enjoyable relief from the 'slog' of normal training. They were also intended to raise the feeling of team spirit while, at the same time, achieving a high level of intensive work. Furthermore, they were no threat to anyone's status or reputation, because the swimmers were never asked to compete over their preferred race distance and stroke. These principles should be borne in mind when incorporating competition into any coaching session for elite athletes. However, it should be noted that many sports have activities within their normal training regimes that involve interaction between players and in which an opportunity exists for performers to test themselves against others.

Competition can be against fellow athletes, against some standard of performance established by other elite athletes or against previous personal best performances. Elite athletes are, by definition, goal-directed, and the most basic goals are those set for each task during a coaching session. No performance in practice is done without the intention to achieve a self-set goal, and nor should it be. When the practice performance has been completed, its standard of performance is assessed against the goal set for it. By doing this, the benefits of every practice are maximized, and this is designed to ensure the highest rate of improvement possible. Elite athletes do not need to wait to be told what they should be aiming for in practice, and they will turn the most co-operative activity possible into some form of competitive exercise and set themselves a goal to achieve in it. However, there is evidence to show that some elite athletes often work at a higher intensity than that sought by the coach. In some cases, this may even lead to overtraining. One of the main reasons why research into goal-setting and its effects on performance is so difficult to conduct is because it is virtually impossible to establish a 'no goals' control group with athletes of any standard, as Weinberg *et al.* (1990) demonstrated. It is out of the question with elite athletes.

Excellent coaching sessions include a lot of variety

Repetitive work eventually becomes boring, and that applies to beginners as much as it does to elite athletes. The only difference is that beginners will become bored much more quickly. Elite athletes like variety, but with three qualifications. First, all activities must be understood to be relevant to the requirements of competition. For instance, tasks which do not train the energy systems required for competition will not be appreciated, for they will be perceived as invalid. Secondly, while different activities are welcomed, they should produce similar performance effects in keeping with the overall aims and objectives for the macro-cycle being undertaken. Troup (1990) provided examples of how swimmers can experience many different training elements, all of which produce consistent levels of effort and energy expenditure in the body. Thirdly, as with any training programme, those different activities should be evaluated periodically, both individually and collectively, in light of any improvement in performance by the athletes concerned. If improvement has taken place, then the variety in training activities will be judged as having been worthwhile, although it will be difficult to establish that the variety has contributed significantly to the improvement. In many games and sports, the variety of techniques involved and the phase of the game lend themselves to variety in designing training sessions.

Excellent coaching sessions include behaviours required in competitions

This item introduces the principle of specificity, which was described in detail by Rushall (1985: 40), who indicated that 'task repetitions should be as physiologically, psychologically and biomechanically similar to the sport performance criteria as is possible'.

This is a controversial statement, as evidenced by the wide-ranging discussions concerning motor behaviour and motor skill development, but it is not unusual in the coaching practice of many games and racket sports. For instance, the merits or otherwise of Schema Theory (Schimdt, 1975) and the more recent Dynamical Systems approach (Kamm *et al.*, 1994) have fully occupied those researching these areas of concern for some time now, and the debates show few signs of lessening. (They are discussed in some depth in Chapter 6 of this book.) Nevertheless, it seems logical to practise those behaviours required in competition on a regular basis, and efforts to simulate the demands of competition can be seen in most sports. For instance, the use of a scrummage machine and body protection suits to allow full contact is commonplace now in virtually every rugby club in the country, and the full version of rugby in coaching sessions, without any modifications, appears to be gaining in appeal. Having said this, however, a lack of specificity is noticeable in some training programmes with regard to competition behaviour. For instance, members of the British Swim Team (1990–1992) would regularly complete training sessions of anything between 3000 and 10 000 m, depending on their event. At every training camp the pool was 50 m in length, which meant the swimmers were completing between 59 and 199 turns each session. (These figures would be doubled for sessions in their home club, as most had to train in 25 m pools.) In a long distance microcycle, the swimmers would complete two training sessions each day for six consecutive days before 'resting' with a single session on the seventh day. This meant completing 13 sessions per week, which produced an approximate range of turns (in a 50 m pool) of between 750 and 2500. Even the lowest figure in this range is a huge number, for some things are being practised and reinforced at every single turn. Through simple observation, it became obvious that what was often being practised was slow turning with sloppy technique, the very antithesis of what is required in a competition. When added to the fact that the only dive during these sessions was to enter the water at the beginning, and that it too was executed (not surprisingly) with nothing like the technique required for competitive races, it is not difficult to appreciate that these fundamentally important aspects of race requirements were often being neglected. Of course, the swimmers would be asked to practise racing starts and turns during the 'taper phase' of their preparation, but not with sufficient frequency to overcome the effects of long-term practice in training and thereby ensure maximum effectiveness. In top class swimming, when swimmers are rested and fully fit, the two phases of any race (with the possible exception of the long distance events) that produce the greatest variability in time, both within and between individual swimmers, are the start and the turns. The actual swimming speeds and number of strokes taken to complete all but the final length for each elite swimmer show little variability. This is why swimming a personal best by

0.5 s over 200 m would represent a huge improvement for any of them. While acting as timekeeper for four sprint swimmers at a British training camp in Cyprus (in preparation for the 1991 European Swimming Championships to be held in Athens 1 week later), variations in time were recorded, over eight separate attempts, ranging from 0.25 to 0.4 s to complete a distance of 15 m from a racing dive start. This could have been due to a number of reasons, though lack of recent practice and lack of consistent and appropriate thought content featured prominently. Moreover, the swimmers themselves knew as soon as they stopped whether they had produced a fast start or not. Obviously a time recorded by hand, as opposed to electronic timing, is going to be less than 100 per cent reliable, but not by as much as 0.4 s. Remembering that Adrian Moorhouse won his Olympic gold medal in Seoul for the 100 m breaststroke by 0.01 s, it becomes clear that a variability of 40 times that figure in the first 15 m of a race is simply unacceptable. Moreover, this will be made considerably worse by neglecting the turns in a swim race, which the swimmers themselves acknowledge can be solely responsible for separating the winner from the losers, especially in short course (25 m pool) championships.

The reason offered by the swim coaches concerned for not practising racing starts and turns more often was that time spent swimming was more profitable. From ensuing conversations, it was quite clear that those coaches believed physiological training to be the major determinant of successful performances, though they never agreed among themselves as to the amount or type of training required to produce winning performances despite any appeal to the principle of individualizing programmes. It is argued here that preparation for competition swimming should reflect much more of the behaviour required for racing than it does at present, and that applies even to physiological training – as Mahoney (1995) so ably demonstrated in his work with a seasoned sprint swimmer.

Excellent coaching sessions involve each athlete in goal-setting

Goal-setting in this sense could mean either setting goals for certain aspects of the coaching session itself or, through discussion, for the next competition. Obviously, the two are not unrelated. Much has been written about goal-setting in the sports psychology literature over the past 25 years, and it is probably one of the top three subject matters in terms of time and attention devoted to it. Debates about the merits of product, or outcome goals as opposed to process or performance goals, have been recorded in several books (for example, Kremer and Scully, 1994; Cox, 1994), and research into their efficacy has been conducted by too many to mention here (see Locke and Latham, 1985 and Beggs, 1991 for summaries). For present purposes, three points are worth recording:

1. The behaviour of elite athletes in sporting contexts is always goal-directed, which means that they will set goals for themselves for just about everything they do, whether it be for training sessions or for competitions. Thus any coach who attempts to set goals for an elite athlete, regardless of the situation, is bound to come into conflict, sooner or later, with that athlete's self-set goals. This is one important reason

why goals should always be negotiated between coach and athlete, and this process cannot be started too early in an athlete's career. It is the coach's responsibility to ensure that the goals agreed upon are realistic for an athlete's current capacities, developmental stage and preparation because, left entirely to their own devices, many athletes will set outcome goals that are either beyond their capabilities or so beneath them that success is ensured. Neither will help to produce top class performances.

2. Negotiating a goal for oneself is pointless if the means of achieving it are not identified at the same time. This is probably the most neglected feature of goal-setting at all levels of sport, and is the main reason why adherence (particularly to long-term goals) is a problem for many athletes. Moreover, it is the steps that lead to goal achievement in training and competitions that should be the focus of attention, and not the goal itself. Anything less will produce a less than optimal performance. Goal-setting will provide significant psychological benefits for the athlete, but the identification of goals is also a vital part of the coach's planning procedures.

3. The idea of involving each athlete in goal-setting introduces the principle of individuality which, broadly stated, means that coaching sessions should be structured around each athlete's individual needs and capacities. Any session in which all athletes are given the same programme (or, even worse, the same goal – this *does* happen!), although easy to administer and supervise, is bound to be inappropriate for some. It is important to recognize that coaching practice in relation to team sport and individual sport practice management is different (and difficult), although there is no excuse for undifferentiated goal-setting.

Excellent coaching sessions generate as much feedback to each athlete as possible

Feedback provides information about our interaction with the world through our visual, auditory, tactile/kinaesthetic, olfactory and gustatory sense modalities, and this information is usually matched against our prior learning and experience before being interpreted as either positive or negative. (The exception to this process is an interaction that produces instant pain – such as spilling boiling water onto a hand – which causes a reflex reaction that is not processed by any cognitive mechanism.) The consequences of our behaviour can only be made known to us through feedback of one kind or another, and it is the reinforcing properties of these consequences, together with their interrelationships with the stimuli provided by the occasion upon which the behaviour occurs, that shape it in some way. Behaviourists refer to this as the 'contingencies of reinforcement', a detailed discussion of which was provided by Skinner (1969).

Feedback comes from two major sources. Primary feedback comes from everything we think, feel, say, hear and do, and has some level of consequence for us. We are not always aware of these consequences and, even when we are, it does not follow that we are necessarily capable of changing our behaviour in order to change the consequences, however desirable the latter may be. Much depends on the strength of the reinforcement previously received from the established responses to the stimuli in question.

Secondary feedback comes mainly from other people's reactions to what we say and do (which are their only means of accessing our thoughts and feelings). Thus, coaches are a major source of secondary feedback in that they comment on their athletes' performances and often demonstrate, in a number of ways, what they want them to do.

In sport, feedback provides information and reinforcement about performance and results. Feedback about both is intrinsic to the task, and therefore primary in nature. However, many athletes are poor at using such information, and often want their coach to interpret and evaluate their performances for them. They frequently evaluate their performances solely in terms of results, which explains why many good performances are dismissed when the results are not to their liking. Coaches provide secondary feedback and reinforcement through their evaluations of performance. In today's technological world, they often do so through video recordings, which allow them to replay parts of a performance in slow motion and even frame-by-frame in order to highlight successful aspects of performance or technical shortcomings. Moreover, they can do this many times over whenever the need arises.

Verbal feedback
This is a vitally important issue in any consideration of effective coaching, and one that was dealt with by Cox (1991). Its importance has not waned since then and never will, simply because it comes from the main source of secondary feedback for most athletes – their coach. Verbal feedback can take several different forms, each of which reinforces athletes in a predictable fashion. As Cox pointed out, a coach need only ask himself four questions in order to test the effectiveness of his own verbal feedback (1991: 22):

1. Are the majority of feedback statements I make to my athletes *value* statements? That is, do I say such things as 'well done', 'good shot', 'that's great', more than any other type of statement?
2. When I give *corrective* feedback, such as 'you failed to keep your wrist cocked' or 'your feet were in the wrong position', is it usually phrased negatively, as are these examples, rather than positively?
3. When coaching more than one athlete at a time, do I usually give feedback to an individual so that others can hear what I am saying?
4. Do I usually give feedback to my athletes whilst they are actually working and practising?

If the answer to each of these four questions is 'yes', then the coach needs to reconsider typical verbal behaviour of this type for the following reasons. First, if the feedback is mainly value-laden then it is imprecise. What does 'good shot' or 'that's great' actually mean? Do these kinds of statements tell the athlete concerned what precisely he has done well and, more importantly, does it raise the probability of being able to reproduce that part of the performance that the coach is obviously pleased with? Of course not, and while feedback of this kind can motivate athletes initially, it soon loses its effect and eventually may become mildly irritating. Secondly, if feedback that contains information (corrective feedback) is negative, then it is likely to make the majority of recipients anxious to please. This, in turn, can lead to increased tension in the skeletal muscles, which rarely helps any athlete to perform effectively. Thirdly, these problems are likely to be exacerbated if negative feedback is given such that others can hear and, finally, it is more likely that verbal feedback will prove to be a source of distraction, rather than encouragement, if it is given during performances. This is one very good reason why football coaches should reconsider their behaviour in the dugout during matches, in addition to the efficacy of the communication itself.

Cox went on to claim that (1991: 23):

> In general, the negative effects are worse for beginners than for experienced athletes. But for all athletes it is better to...
>
> 1. Give praise (value-laden feedback) only when athletes understand clearly the reasons for it.
> 2. Phrase corrective feedback in the positive, such as 'try to do this' rather than 'don't do that'.
> 3. Impart criticism privately so that athletes do not suffer the added embarrassment of having their 'weaknesses' exposed to others.
> 4. Give feedback immediately after performance, rather than during it or sometime after it has been completed.

For coaches who are concerned enough about these matters to do something to improve them, I have devised a means of checking on the quality of interactions they have with their athletes. This can be seen in Figure 4.2. The important point to note about this checklist is that it has to be given to the athletes, who then respond anonymously to it. Thus, not only do coaches have to be concerned about these matters but they also have to be brave, because they risk receiving a lot of negative feedback about their own performance. Imagine how a coach will feel if his athletes respond mostly to the 'never' box and only seldom to the 'always' one. On a similar note, I recall conducting a Nominal Group Technique (NGT) evaluation (see O'Neil, 1981) of a professional football club in Scotland and producing over 30 suggestions from the players for improving the running of the club, all of which were phased positively and constructively. A few seconds after handing the list to the manager, I was told in no uncertain terms that I should not have done the exercise as the manager perceived it as usurping his authority. Needless to say, his style of managing and coaching could only be described as strictly authoritarian, and there would have been little room in his club for most of the ideas presented in this chapter.

Two other points about generating feedback during coaching sessions are worth making here. The first is to encourage coaches to give more thought to the nature and design of practices adopted for improving skill levels, and for one simple reason: motivation is increased when athletes are engaged in practices that provide as much primary feedback as possible through their design, and thereby reduce the need for secondary feedback from the coach. Identifying the criteria for performance in any practice is usually done efficiently by coaches, but identifying the criteria for success is less so. All too often, coaches reserve providing feedback about whether athletes have been successful in a practice for themselves. Even with only one athlete to coach this can be problematic, but with a group it is nigh on impossible to do to maximum effect.

For practising athletes (regardless of your sport)

1.   How are you usually greeted (if at all) by your coach when you arrive for training?

....

2.   Does your coach use your Christian name when talking to you?

☐   ☐   ☐

Always   Sometimes   Never

3.   Does your coach tell you what kind of session has been planned for you before you warm up?

☐   ☐   ☐

Always   Sometimes   Never

4.   Does your coach (help you to) set goals for your training sessions?

☐   ☐   ☐

Always   Sometimes   Never

5.   Does your coach congratulate you when you train hard?

☐   ☐   ☐

Always   Sometimes   Never

6.   Does your coach criticize your training/competitive performances *constructively*?

☐   ☐   ☐

Always   Sometimes   Never

7.   If your coach tells you off for something, is it done privately?

☐   ☐   ☐

Always   Sometimes   Never

8.   Does your coach talk to you *individually* about your progress?

☐   ☐   ☐

Always   Sometimes   Never

9.   Does your coach say goodbye to you at the end of training sessions?

☐   ☐   ☐

Always   Sometimes   Never

10.   Does your coach ask you to tell him/her what you like and what you don't like about his/her training sessions?

☐   ☐   ☐

Always   Sometimes   Never

Figure 4.2 A checklist for interactions between coach and athlete

The second point refers to the source of secondary feedback. Many Governing Bodies of sport, probably through their coach education programmes, encourage the belief that only the coach can offer meaningful assessments of performance. Although this is a generalization, it may lead to feedback from one athlete to another being regarded as unimportant and, in some cases, actually stifled. This issue was addressed by Mosston and Ashworth (1986), who identified a spectrum of teaching styles that can be adopted directly by coaches. Most coaches adopt a style that Mosston and Ashworth would have identified as a mix of Style A, the command style, and Style B, which they termed the practice style. In both styles, it is the coaches who provide all the secondary feedback in accordance with their own criteria for performance. Mosston and Ashworth highlighted the assets and liabilities of these styles, and the biggest liability was the fact that one teacher/coach cannot provide appropriate feedback to more than one learner/athlete at any one moment in time. Thus, if all athletes in a group are engaged in the same practice as each other, then only some will receive feedback contingent upon their performance; for others it will inevitably be delayed. This liability provided the rationale for the shift to Style C, the reciprocal style, in which athletes are paired and one acts as a surrogate coach to a partner, the performer. Roles are reversed after a number of trials, and the effectiveness of this arrangement is supported by research conducted by Rushall (1982, 1991a), who claimed that athletes generally provide feedback to other athletes more effectively than coaches do. Rushall later (1995: 0.3) argued that 'coaching programmes should emphasize an expected role of athletes as providing fellow athletes with positive and constructive suggestions and discussions about performance ... By doing that, performance will progress because of the increased amount of task-oriented feedback.'

Part of the explanation for why athletes assisting fellow athletes in this way is effective is the fact that the surrogate coach is constantly rehearsing the criteria for performance and articulating each one of them in feedback statements. As a consequence, surrogates become acutely aware of what is required for performance and, when it is their turn to perform, these criteria provide a sharp focus for their concentration throughout the practice.

In conclusion, then, it is worth emphasizing that no change in performance of any kind will ever take place without feedback. Feedback is the one essential element in behavioural change and, as such, should be given the most careful consideration by all coaches whenever and wherever they interact with their athletes. Even the most innocent and generalized comment, perhaps made in jest, is likely to be dwelt upon sooner or later by one athlete, to the point of producing a decrement in performance. The contingencies of reinforcement produced by coaches' verbal feedback probably rank alongside the nature and quality of work that they ask their athletes to do as the most important of all. As such, all coaches are recommended to increase their awareness of what they say to their athletes, how and when they say it and the reactions that it produces. Carrying a voice recorder occasionally during a coaching session is one good way of doing this, and a videotaped recording is even better because all the 'body language' of the coach and the physical responses of the athletes to any remarks can be studied retrospectively in detail and at length.

Excellent coaching sessions are evaluated as soon afterwards as possible

Elite athletes use information gained from coaching sessions and competitions to plan for the next. They evaluate their own performances on every occasion, regardless of whether it is in training or competition. Thus for coaches not to evaluate performances (including their own) would be tantamount to folly, for their athletes would expect them to. Indeed, if any coaching session or competition was not prefaced by the coach providing a detailed evaluation of performances in the previous session or competition, then the athletes concerned would question the degree of continuity in the programme. The moment this happened, the motivation of the athletes would be affected adversely and 'coaching effectiveness' reduced accordingly.

When a session or competition has been completed, the coach should ask two questions. First, which aspects of performance were performed to a high level and therefore need only be maintained rather than changed? Secondly, which aspects of performance need to be changed in order to improve? Subsequent coaching sessions should be focused on changing these aspects in order to bring about an improvement in the next competition. Of course, these evaluations are added in an incremental fashion to previous evaluations, and the coach should be careful not to react hastily to variability in performance. The coach will also need to distinguish short-term preparation from longer-term improvements.

This may sound like basic common sense, but it is surprising how often post-competition coaching sessions do not aim to improve those aspects of performance that need it the most. For elite athletes this is a recipe for frustration, and they will quickly become disenchanted with such sessions.

After the initial warm up, a suitable arrangement for an excellent coaching session based on the psychological principles of primary and recency effects (essentially, these state that what is practised first and last in any sequence are remembered best of all) is to begin with practice of aspects of performance that are already of a high standard and continue this for 20 per cent of the time available. This should be followed with specific practice of those aspects of performance that need to be improved the most, for 60 per cent of the time available, through a variety of activities that are alternated and returned to more than once (the principle of distributed practice). The final 20 per cent of the session should be completed by returning to practice of aspects of performance that were performed excellently the last time out, and which were practised in the first 20 per cent of the session. This arrangement will go a long way towards both improving performance and maintaining high levels of motivation, though it must, of course, take into consideration other important principles such as energy systems and progressive overload.

Excellent training sessions encourage interested family and friends to make a positive contribution

Elite athletes welcome attention from family members and friends to their sporting activities, and they are encouraged when these important others provide positive support. Coaches can do a lot to develop this type of support by, for instance, inviting family and friends to watch coaching sessions, making special arrangements for them to spectate at competitions and, whenever possible, talking to them and making them feel welcome. If it is financially possible, an occasional social evening involving friends and family is always welcomed, and helps foster a sense of belonging to the group by creating the feeling that the coach and any assistants actually care about the athletes as people as well as about their athletic performances.

As mentioned earlier, elite athletes like to be kept busy the whole time, which means that ideally someone else has to set out any equipment needed for successive practices. This provides a golden opportunity for the coach to invite family members and friends not only to attend, but also to help out. Most will do so willingly, for they like to feel involved and it gives them a sense of worth. Nevertheless, this must be interpreted as a principle, and will not be achieved easily on all occasions. Athletes in training camps, in traditional professional clubs and in some forms of training sessions might not feel comfortable with the presence of the friends of other athletes.

Summary

Ten characteristics of coaching have been described, each of which has been identified by elite competitors as contributing to their perception of effectiveness in the coach. Taken together, they constitute an approach that will lead to more satisfied, happier, more focused and motivated athletes. This psychological state helps to facilitate the degree of training and co-operation required to be successful. None of the principles is, of itself, a guarantee of success. Effectiveness has been interpreted throughout as the satisfaction of the elite athlete, and a more receptive athlete. It is a reasonable assumption that the conditions associated with these principles will be more likely to lead to the quality of coaching process required for success. However, there are many other aspects of the coaching process and many other contributory factors to successful performance. Nevertheless, the 10 items identified here will help the coach to organize and bring a sense of purpose to the discipline and sports-specific knowledge, skills and experience required. These points are primarily concerned with the direct intervention aspects of the coaching process.

These 10 items, which amount to characteristics of excellent coaching sessions, can be incorporated into a plan of action that coaches can use as part of every coaching session for which they are responsible. Such a plan is illustrated in Figure 4.3, and helps both in the planning stage and when evaluating the session afterwards. It is contended here that if coaches can honestly say they consider all 10 characteristics on a regular basis, then their athletes will come to regard them as excellent coaches. Of course, this is assuming that they have intimate, detailed and firsthand knowledge of their sport before even considering these 10 points. Indeed, it is highly unlikely that, without such knowledge, they would ever begin to consider the points, for novice coaches (which is what they would be) often seek to gain credibility through demonstrating their technical knowledge and seldom give consideration to other criteria.

Aims	Action Taken
1 To plan and publish the programme in advance of each training session	
2 To start and end on time	
3 To keep athletes busy the whole time	
4 To promote competition between friends	
5 To include a lot of variety	
6 To include behaviours required in competition	
7 To involve each athlete in goal-setting	
8 To generate as much feedback to each and every athlete as possible	
9 To evaluate each training session as soon afterwards as possible	
10 To encourage interested parents to make a positive contribution	

Figure 4.3 Towards excellent coaching sessions

Of course, it is still possible that, after doing all that is recommended in this chapter, coaches may notice that the athletes appear to be 'flat' in the sense that their training effort is poor and their motivation apparently low. Athletes get tired and they become ill, neither of which is necessarily anything to do with the coaches concerned, although they may be responsible for over-training, which can lead to both. With the help of the British Swim Team medical doctor, I devised one way of monitoring the overall physical and psychological health of the swimmers for precisely these purposes and a version of it can be seen in Figure 4.4. This particular version is for outdoor team games such as football, rugby and hockey, but is easily modified to suit the needs and demands of any sport.

Figure 4.4 is called an 'early warning response sheet' (EWRS) because it is meant to provide an early warning that something is not all that it should be with a particular athlete. The criterion for the latter is five or more ticks in the right-hand column (in practice, even four ticks should usually be followed-up with an enquiry as to whether everything is all right). For athletes who are training every day, this sheet is administered every 48 hours, at the same time of day.

A slightly different version of Figure 4.4 was first used with the British Swim Team in 1991 at a training camp in the South of France, and to great effect. On two occasions apparent problems were identified and dealt with quickly, one by the medical team doctor and the other by myself as team psychologist. The first concerned a female swimmer who, it was later diag-nosed, had contracted a viral illness, and the second concerned a case of

Name . . . .   ***Date*** . . . .

Please tick the box that best represents how you have been feeling and reacting during the past few days. Please respond truthfully. False answers will render useless any help and advice given to you.

	Better than Normal	Normal	Worse than Normal
1 General Health			
2 General Fitness			
3 General Appetite and Digestion			
4 General Effort in Training			
5 Quality of Sleep			
6 Stamina			
7 Acceleration Over First 20 Metres			
8 Feelings Towards Others (In General)			
9 All-Round Muscular Strength			
10 Flexibility (Ability to Stretch)			
	Less than Normal	Normal	More than Normal
11 Feeling Irritable			
12 Time Taken to Recover Between Training Sessions			
13 Stiffness or Soreness from Training			
14 Minor Internal Aches and Pains			
15 Frequency of Arguments			
16 Feeling Bored			
	More than Normal	Normal	Less than Normal
17 Time Taken to Recover During Training Sessions			
18 Feeling Happy and Cheerful			
19 Enthusiasm for Training			
20 Enthusiasm for Playing Matches			

Figure 4.4 Early Warning Response Sheet

what could only be termed semi-starvation. This involved a 1.95 m (6'5") tall young man who was full of admiration for what the team nutritionist had done. The nutritionist had liaised with the hotel management in advance of the camp, and established menus for each day based on the nutritional needs of the swimmers. The only problem was that the food was not to the athlete's liking and, as a consequence, he had been spending a considerable amount of money in a local supermarket in a futile (as it turned out) attempt to make up for what he wasn't eating in the hotel. In the process he had become socially withdrawn and homesick, and had little enthusiasm for the hard work he was meant to be doing twice a day in the pool. Even though he was somewhat embarrassed by the attention his responses to the EWRS had drawn, he agreed to my suggestion that we approach the team manager to see if anything could be done about the situation. This we did together, but not before identifying the types of meal he would enjoy. After explaining the problem to the hotel manager he agreed to provide the meals requested, and the young man in question was delighted and much relieved. Two days later, his next EWRS showed five ticks in the left-hand column and the remainder in the middle rather than the eight ticks in the right-hand column that had been recorded previously. A simple solution to a simple problem but one which, had it been left to fester, could have developed into major proportions and possibly even caused the individual concerned to consider whether he wanted to continue in international swimming. Similar cases, though perhaps not quite as dramatic, have been identified in other sports in which I have used the EWRS, and it has proved to be extremely useful. As a consequence, it is recommended as an aid to coaches in their efforts to become as effective as possible.

To become a truly effective coach can take a lifetime of endeavour, and it requires a very high degree of professionalism in all aspects of the role. This is why coaching has a professional structure with formal qualifications; why Governing Bodies of Sport exist and have full-time representatives who meet regularly to discuss the best ways forward; why coaches typically belong to an Association that meets annually (at least) in order to discuss the latest developments in its field; and why coaching has its own monitoring system for technical and ethical standards. It is a highly professional concern, and it is hoped that this chapter can make one small but significant contribution to this concern.

References

Beggs, W. D. A. (1991). Goal-setting in sport. In *Stress and Performance in Sport* (J. G. Jones and L. Hardy, eds), pp. 135–70. Academic Press.

Cox, R. L. (1991). Motivation and goal-setting. In *Sports Psychology: A Self-Help Guide* (S. Bull, ed.), pp. 6–30. Crowood Press.

Cox, R. H. (1994). *Sport Psychology: Concepts and Applications*. Brown Communications.

Drysdale, N. (1994). Golden dreams end in cinders. *Scotland on Sunday*. Glasgow, 28 August.

Freud, S. (1933). *New Introductory Lectures on Psychoanalysis*. Norton.

Gambril, D. and Bay, A. (1985). Motivation. *Swimming World*, **26(7),** 23–4.

Kamm, K., Thelen, E. and Jenson, J. (1994). A dynamical systems approach to motor development. In *Movement Science*, pp. 11–23. APTA.

Kremer, J. M. D. and Scully, D. (1994). *Psychology in Sport*. Taylor and Francis.

Leslie, J. C. (1996). *Principles of Behavioural Analysis* (3rd edn). Harwood Academic Publishers.

Locke, E. A. and Latham, G. P. (1985). The application of goal-setting to sports. *J. Sport Psychol*, **7**, 205–22.

Mahoney, C. A. (1995). Psychological interventions with an elite swimming squad: Processes and products. Unpublished Ph.D. thesis. The Queen's University of Belfast.

Martin, G. L. and Pears, J. J. (1992). *Behaviour Modification : What It Is and How To Do It* (4th edn). Prentice-Hall International Editions.

Mosston, M. and Ashworth, S. (1986). *Teaching Physical Education*. Merrill Publishing Company.

O'Neil, M. J. (1981). Nominal group technique: An evaluation data collection process. *Evaluation Newsletter*, **5(2)**, 44–60.

Rushall, B. S. (1982). What coaches do – behavioural evidence on coaching effectiveness. In *Psychology of Sport and Motor Behaviour: Research and Practice* (L. Wankel and R. B. Wilberg, eds), pp. 185–202. University of Alberta.

Rushall, B. S. (1985a). Several principles of modern coaching. *Sports Coach*, **8(3)**, 40–44.

Rushall, B. S. (1991a). Motivation and goal-setting. In *Better Coaching* (F. S. Pyke, ed), pp. 151–74. Australian Coaching Council.

Rushall, B. S. (1995). *Think and Act like a Champion*. Sports Science Associates.

Sage, G. M. (1980). Humanism and performance. In *Sport Psychology: An Analysis of Athletic Behaviour* (W. F. Straub, ed.), pp. 215–30. Mouvement Publications.

Schmidt, R. A. (1975). A schema theory of discrete motor learning. *Psychol. Rev.*, **82**, 225–60.

Skinner, B. F. (1969). *Contingencies of Reinforcement: A Theoretical Analysis*. Appleton-Century-Crofts.

Troup, J. P. (ed.) (1990). *International Centre for Aquatic Research Annual Studies*. International Centre for Aquatic Research 1989–90, Colorado Springs. US Swimming Press.

Weinberg, R. S., Bruya, D. and Jackson, A. (1990). Goal-setting and competition: A reaction to Hall and Byrne. *J. Sport Exer. Psychol.*, **12**, 92–7.

5

Applied physiology in sports coaching

Andrew Maile

- The role of the coach in planning physical preparation programmes
- The key principles to be considered in planning preparation programmes
- An enhanced appreciation of the role of specific training
- The provision of anaerobic energy for performance
- The provision of aerobic energy for performance
- How coaches can improve energy provision
- Important elements associated with the development and delay of fatigue
- The use and value of physiological assessment for the coach

Introduction

The pursuit of excellence in sports performance depends on a large number of interrelated and interdependent elements. Consequently, the absence of appropriate attention to any one of these elements makes progress difficult. As a result, priorities have to be established and detailed planning carried out in a variety of contributory sub-disciplines in order to design an appropriate performance plan. The objectives of such a plan have to be clear and unambiguous, and linked to an overall performance development strategy. The plan needs to be clearly understood and accepted by everyone – managers, administrators, coaches, athletes and support personnel – and, finally, defined tightly enough so as to establish performance indicators that can be used to effectively monitor progress. Sport sciences have a self-evident part to play in improving sports performance. Important features of the coaching process, such as devising training schedules, monitoring performance, establishing technique or preparation for competition, are informed by such knowledge. Within the context of performance planning, the Sports Council (1993: 12) has considered that:

> Sports Science has been recognized as a key ingredient in assisting those with talent, commitment and interest to reach their potential... The theory of Sports Science should be integrated with practice to address relevant problems.

It is important therefore to ensure that appropriate physiological principles are incorporated into coaching practice. In these circumstances, the performance plan should indicate the nature and scale of the involvement of any sports science assistance needed to complement the work of the coaches. In addition, it is essential that the manner in which sports science input is to be incorporated into coaching practice should be identified.

The role of the coach

In many circumstances coaches operate with a group of athletes without the benefit of specialist support personnel. However, preparing these individuals for competition in elite sport increasingly involves the coach, the athlete and one of a number of sports scientists. Each needs to appreciate the significance and complementary nature of one another's roles if performance is to be effectively enhanced. Coaches need to have sufficient knowledge and understanding of the principles of applied physiology, and how to use these principles in a planned and systematic manner, in order to recognize and address all of the relevant training issues. In elite sport, the coach may require access to a sports physiologist to assist with this process for, as Dick (1986: 5) has reminded us:

> Coaches working at this level will need to be familiar with the vital contribution the sport scientist, sports medicine practitioner and nutritionist can make. Without such understanding, they will be unable to make valued judgements as to the role each has to play in a programme co-ordinated by the coach.

Co-operation between sports scientists and athletes is best co-ordinated by the coach. It is the coach who will assimilate information, analyse the effectiveness of the programme, construct specific training sessions and co-ordinate and supervise these. Such an approach will maximize the training effect of time spent in preparation, and is acknowledged as important for a successful sporting performance (Scottish Sports Council, 1998).

Although a variety of sports science disciplines will impact upon sports performance and the coaching process, this chapter will focus specifically on the physiological aspects of performance planning and consider appropriate principles that should be incorporated into coaching practice.

Appropriate knowledge and help is currently available to guide the coach's thinking on the most efficient strategy for the physiological preparation of athletes. Guidelines have been established which, if adhered to, may prevent time being wasted. With a number of areas being of special importance to high performance athletes, including lifestyle and medical management as well as physical conditioning, it is vital that the coach understands the value of each facet and can identify and draw on relevant expertise to ensure an effective training programme (Sports Council, 1991). At the elite performance level, the coach becomes not only facilitator and mentor but a manager of resources as well.

The efficient use of time, when applied to physiological preparation, should leave the coach with more time to attend to the other important aspects of performance. It should be noted here that the physiological preparation of an athlete is only one part of the jigsaw that makes up the complete picture of a successful performance. However, despite the importance of this particular part of the total picture, it cannot and should not be viewed in isolation. Attendance by the coach to the following set of

principles will go a long way in guiding the application of appropriate training procedures.

In order for the coach to efficiently utilize the time that is available, the
following steps must be attended to. First, the coach needs to analyse the
sport with which he or she is associated, in terms of overall movement
patterns. This will include technical considerations and time on task. There
must be some recognition of the intensity, frequency and duration of exercise
associated with successful performance. Secondly, this information needs to
be translated into sports-specific conditioning components. This translation
will form the basis upon which work associated with training methods and
systems will be designed. Thirdly, the organization, design and prescription
of relevant training methods and systems needs to consider the major conditioning principles, particularly those associated with progressive overload
and specificity of training. The application of these principles in a planned
progressive manner, in my experience, is the key not only to increased
physiological preparation but also to enhanced motivation and confirmation
of the coaching relationship.

Analysis such as this is more likely to occur in those sports that tend to be
dominated by the physiological condition of the performer; for example,
athletics and swimming. In those sports more dependent on technique,
skill or 'team' organization, this type of analysis will provide important specific, position and event requirements that will need to be considered. It is in
this important area of event, sport and game analysis that the coach is able to
co-ordinate specific technical knowledge and the principles associated with
the planning of efficiently designed training programmes.

The present technological capability associated with digital video and
interactive analysis through the developing field of notational analysis provides objective data for the coach to review technical, strategic and physiological demands placed on performers. Whilst coaches may not be in a
position to undertake such analysis themselves, the sports scientist can be
used to provide reports following prior discussion and planning such that
analysis provides clear data on which the coach can make informed decisions within the planning process.

One of the roles of the coach is to plan, lead, design or manage physiological preparation in such a way that potentially isolated physical preparation is applied in context. The analysis of specific movement patterns will
help determine an understanding of the integration of the energy processes
involved. Thus, a particular aspect of the coach's role is to appreciate,
develop and enhance the specificity of energy integration, for without such
integration the athlete may succumb to fatigue at an earlier stage in performance. This may be manifested by a loss of concentration and a subsequent
reduction in the quality of technical performance caused by a loss of timing
associated with less effective muscular stimulation and co-ordination.

For coaches to undertake the increasing sophistication of tasks expected
in the twenty-first century, their knowledge and understanding of physiological principles and practices needs to be constantly updated. This will
enable coaches to become increasingly involved not only in planning
more sports-specific programmes, but also in expanding their analytical capabilities of what these planned programmes should deliver. In this way, the
ability to organize, communicate and plan for performance enhancement will

be considerably developed. This chapter will address the physiological basis of effective and efficient energy integration for sports performance, and the implications of this for coaching practice. In so doing, it seeks to assist in the provision of knowledge and understanding that coaches can draw on and subsequently apply in order to improve their practice and enhance the coaching process. Specifically, this chapter will consider aspects of physiological planning, such that excessive and inappropriate training is not pursued. There will be a need to consider elements associated with effective and efficient energy provision, specificity of training, aspects of fatigue, effective recovery, and the monitoring and evaluation of planned programmes. It is the knowledge and understanding associated with the integration of these considerations that will determine a well-structured progressive plan designed to provide performers with the necessary physiological adaptation to compete successfully.

The game plan

A knowledgeable coach, in terms of specific training and its application, would wish to plan training peaks to coincide with important events, tournaments, championships or selection trials that occur during a year's programme. Cross and Lyle (1996: 34) have highlighted the need for planning when they note that 'good practice does not consist of episodic attention to variables but forms part of a systematic process'. Bompa (1994: 233) confirms this in stating that 'long term planning is one of the characteristics and requirements of modern training. A well organized and planned training program over a long period of time greatly increases the efficiency of the preparation for major future competitions.'

It is in the context of this systematic planning process that the coach needs to consider the contribution and design of physiological preparation. In order to do this, a number of training principles must be built into the programme. These will help to determine:

- The duration of exercise needed (how much?)
- The appropriate relative intensity of exercise (how hard?)
- The frequency or density of training (how often?)

These elements need careful consideration, and should be integrated into the coaching process in order to provide the best possible service to athletes. Knowledge to date should enable coaches to recognize that the first development of physiological preparation should be to increase the *extent* of training – that is, to increase the time spent on a particular session. In this regard, little and often is better than longer and harder, which can leave the athlete overtired and which will require more extensive recovery periods. The relative *intensity* of these sessions should be gradually and cautiously built up as specific adaptations begin to occur. It is always good practice to develop sessions progressively, with planned increases in the intensity of work. Subjecting athletes to sudden large increases in intensity can cause stiffness, soreness and demotivation, whilst at the same time running the risk of injury (Appell, 1992). Frequency or *density* of training is dependent on the athletes' lifestyles, commitment, facilities available, training objectives and contact with their coach. A further consideration is necessary; one that demonstrates the inter-relatedness of performance variables. Organized high performance training means that coaches need to recognize the need to implement appropriate nutrition strategies in order to fuel the energy systems and components under stress in the training programme (Williams and Devlin, 1995; Hargreaves, 1995; Maughan *et al.*, 1997). If coaches, through lack of planning or understanding, increase intensity or density of training prior to increasing its extent, or increase density prior to intensity, they will not maximize efficiently the training time at their disposal. Indeed, they may even propagate injury or demotivation amongst their athletes prior to or during a season's performance (Bompa, 1994; Fry *et al.*, 1991). Certainly, failing to apply training considerations such as these may significantly affect the peaking process when it occurs later in the season.

There may still be a belief amongst athletes and coaches in many sports that 'no pain means no gain', and that it does not really matter when this pain is inflicted in relation to competition. Whilst some fitness benefits associated with intense exercise may accrue from such a philosophy, whether the athlete will be able to give of their best in competition soon after is another question. In such cases, athletes may wish to ask the coach who holds to such a philosophy why they become injured, cramped or heavy-limbed at worst, whilst at best their sharpness seems to be impaired (Appell, 1992). As Cross and Lyle (1996: 40) have noted:

> More and harder is not always better ... the perception of overtraining lies with the attention to the performer's response to training loads that can only come from a processional approach to coaching.

As a result, a guiding principle for all planning is that the programme of physiological preparation should develop from general to specific requirements, and be coupled with the development of training duration towards and including specific intensity requirements. In addition, appropriate frequency of training needs to be both maintained and developed. The coach must allow adequate rest and regeneration within such progression. This process should enable athletes to become event or match fit immediately prior to competition. The progressive balance of work can be seen through the general demands of training associated with pre-season planning, whilst the gradual movement towards specific demands is encapsulated within the planned progression of training leading up to, and immediately prior to, the start of the competitive period. This process is particularly appropriate when considering physiological preparation for all the major games, whether field or court.

In this regard, training sessions should incorporate elements of warming up to enhance body temperature, increase the catalytic effect of enzymes and reduce muscular viscosity. High intensity speed work should follow, with adequate recovery time between repetitions and sets to allow continual energy resynthesis via the creatine phosphate (CrP) and adenylate kinase shuttle systems. Subsequent stimulation of the aerobic metabolism will promote enhanced energy provision by the facilitation of nicotinamide adenine dinucleotide (NAD) and lactate dehydrogenase (LDH) shuttle systems, coupled with effective stimulation of the appropriate fuel source. Glycogen stores may then be both enhanced and spared for subsequent activity.

Finally, the anaerobic lactate metabolism should be stimulated via intensity of work and/or reduced recovery periods to stimulate lactate clearance, shuttling, buffering and subsequent toleration. Particular lactate characteristics are stimulated specifically by the relative intensity of training and time on task. These considerations have to be applied carefully by the coach. Cessation of a hard, demanding session should incorporate an active recovery to promote replenishment of energy stores and removal of metabolic waste and elevated hormonal concentrations. This general appraisal will need adjustment to specific sporting contexts, which some see as the key element in the coach's facility for co-ordinating physiological preparation.

The increased professionalization of sport, and the rewards available to athletes, have led to increased pressure to intensify training. In order to make informed judgements about physiological demands in training, the performance coach needs to pay particular attention to a number of aspects of training; namely specificity, integrated energy provision, the development of fatigue and effective recovery. Without this attention the planning process will be less systematic and less effective, possibly leading to demotivation, unnecessary injury, lack of physiological adaptation and poor performance. The present state of coaching knowledge appears to indicate that this is a matter of some concern in a large number of sports, including those with a professional orientation. The exceptions to this statement include swimming, athletics, cycling and rowing, due to the more central part that physiological preparation plays in successful performance in these sports. Rugby Union has also recently benefited from knowledge gained from rugby league in this respect. The advent therefore of enhanced professional attitudes in sport holds a distinct challenge for the coaching process as it is presently understood by a large number of practising coaches who wish to develop performance. The lack of sophistication of coaching practice in a number of sports, particularly in some professional team sports, suggests that the physiological adaptation required in training is sometimes approached less systematically than it might be. However, while this may reflect a lack of awareness of the appropriate principles by the coach, it may also be because physical condition is, in some sports, only one of a number of determining factors in performance. This chapter now goes on to examine in greater detail the key principles of physiological preparation identified above.

Specificity: the key

With the increasingly prevalent application of science to sport and exercise, advances in research techniques have permitted direct investigation into specific muscular training adaptations (Green, 1992; Shephard, 1992). In addition, the design of training programmes based on sound physiological principles requires an understanding of the acute and chronic metabolic and biochemical responses to exercise and how these are modified by repeated exposures over time. Achieving a match between a training stimulus and the actual demands of the competitive performance is a difficult task. However, specificity of training is important if improvement in athlete performance and adaptation to competition stress is to be most effective. A key objective for the coach, therefore, is to achieve this specificity through the design and content of an appropriate training programme. This is particularly important for programmes in which there is a need to maintain specific movement patterns despite the necessary addition of weighted or drag resistance. The use of weighted jackets for speed, speed endurance and power training provides a good example here, as they allow relatively unhindered and specific court and field movements. This utilizes specific muscular overload, yet enables the appropriate recruitment of muscle fibres to occur with the correct sequence and timing associated with the technical demands of the sport in question. Incorporating the specificity of muscular activity into training requires an appreciation of muscle function in order that a particular fitness component and/or combination of components, for example, in a gymnastic manoeuvre, can be developed for a particular sport. It is important to realize that, irrespective of whether muscles are working to develop tension or power, the muscular structure of individual fibres incorporating the myofibrillar protein complex operate in the same way in all the voluntary muscle groups. The implication for coaches is that they must select a specific mode and design of resistance training to suit the required physiological development.

The ultimate effect of nervous stimulation and subsequent protein regulatory activity is that actin sites in the muscle fibres are exposed, allowing crossbridge formation and the resultant generation of force (Macdougall *et al.*, 1991). With all voluntary muscle operating in this way in sporting techniques, the effective sequencing of fibre stimulation co-ordinated by the necessary timing of central nervous system stimulation will enable the correct force to be applied to the implement, body weight, racket or ball. At low force levels, the slow twitch fibres (type I) are recruited first, followed by fast twitch type IIa and fast twitch type IIb fibres as the force of contraction required exceeds certain thresholds. The high threshold IIb units are not recruited until the force required is greater than 90 per cent of the maximum (Sale, 1992). Therefore, where specific power and speed is required to be developed, a certain amount of the athlete's training should involve fast twitch fibre and the recruitment of a higher number of motor units at increased firing rates in order to achieve the required force. Green (1992) suggests that skeletal muscles exhibit a wide diversity in mechanical function, and that the fundamental basis for diversity resides in the muscle cell itself at the level of the various excitation, contraction and energy producing processes. If all variations of the three myofibrillar-controlling proteins are considered, the potential for diverse composition, structure and function between fibres is staggering. The present view is that the diversity in composition between fibres can provide a continuum in mechanical function, at least with regard to dynamic activities. As a consequence of this, it is imperative that physiological preparation and planning incorporates the necessity for specificity associated with both training and assessment procedures. If this does not occur, the development and application of power, which is the hallmark of successfully prepared athletes in most sports, will be much less effective.

Implicit in all discussion associated with the need to increase power is the crucial role of co-ordination. This is demonstrated in the static generation of force, such as in holding a gymnastic movement, or in the front row of a rugby scrum. It is also important in the dynamic isotonic force exhibited in the timing of a well-executed cricket or golf shot, soccer or rugby pass. As all sporting techniques have as their basis an identical structure of muscular composition, which is innervated by the same processes in the nervous system, what distinguishes one technique from another is the amount, sequence and timing of muscle fibre stimulation. When this is applied to a game situation, the athlete exhibits skill in either the completion of an appropriate movement sequence or the selection of the correct movement appropriate to the sporting context. This is a question of effective decision making by the athlete, incorporating past experience, existing technical competence and perceptual capacity.

The generation of strength by a muscle which underlies the generation of power only occurs under maximal activating conditions in which the excitation of the muscle is sufficient to ensure maximum cross-bridge interaction in the myofibrils, muscle fibres and appropriate muscles. On the other hand, activity that emphasizes the generation of maximal speed at low force levels depends on different factors. Here, the emphasis is not on increasing the number of myofibrillar protein interactions, but rather on the rate at which these interactions can occur (Green, 1986). This rate depends on the muscle's ability both to translate high-frequency impulse excitation through the various excitation processes with minimal time delay and to associate and dissociate the actin and myosin as they repeatedly rotate through successive cross-bridge cycles. A primary determinant of this type of behaviour is the rate at which adenosine triphosphate (ATP) can be hydrolysed and the energy released. Thus, the sports-specific differences exhibited by a variety of sportsmen and women hinge on the co-ordination, timing, sequencing and control of a range of identical muscles and muscle fibres. The coach must take account of this in the design and prescription of appropriate training.

The implications for coaching practice are that the design of resistance training should incorporate conditioning for muscular strength and the specificity of speed development if power is required. The combination of speed and strength will produce a more powerful athlete who may need to use plyometric training. This will enhance inherent muscular characteristics of stored energy and elasticity coupled with the physiological adaptation of an increased myofibrillar protein density. The specific co-ordination of this process must be reflected in the specific training patterns of movement and the extent of muscular overload. The use of weights in jumping activity, weighted belts and jackets in court and field games, elastics in gymnastics and tyres in sprinting are all examples of mechanisms that enable the coach to design specific programmes and implement the principles necessary to achieve physiological adaptation in a sports-specific context.

Sports performance in activities that involve varying degrees of velocity and force depend on a combination of the cross-sectional area of the muscle and the rate at which ATP hydrolysis and energy release can occur. In order to fuel these contractions, the turnover of ATP must increase 1000-fold, particularly in relation to sprint activities (Newsholme, 1993). Because ATP is in very low concentration in the muscle and decreases only minimally even in the most intense voluntary contraction, there must be tightly controlled mechanisms that continually regenerate ATP as the contractions occur. It is the integration of these mechanisms into the training programme that is so important in the physiological preparation of the competitive athlete.

The implication here for the design of the training programme is that coaches need to include sufficient rest and regeneration for their athletes when demanding intense training activity from them. High quality, intense stimulation must be accompanied by adequate rest and regeneration between bouts of exercise. This is the rationale for interval training, which is used to maximize physiological adaptation from specific training stimuli. In my experience with a range of athletes, the concept of incorporating sufficient rest and regeneration is difficult to grasp for both coach and athlete alike. Whilst this may be a particularly British trait in some sports, it is not characteristic of those who habitually exhibit high quality performance in international competition.

In relation to the metabolic considerations that are essential for high intensity exercise, the muscle type that possesses the metabolism to meet these demands is that of the Type II variety, or the fast twitch fibres of skeletal muscle. Not only do these fibres have the metabolic characteristics that high intensity activity requires, but they are superior in a number of neuromuscular and morphological factors that are considered advantageous for elite performance in intense activity. Type IIb fibres are considered to be utilized most during the initiation of intense activity because of the high forces needed to overcome the inertia of body weight. In order to support continued intense activity, Type IIa fibres remain stimulated to generate forces at high speeds and attempt to maintain maximal activity when central and peripheral fatigue becomes a factor. The principal difference between Type IIa and IIb fibres is that the Type IIa fibres have a much higher resistance to fatigue. This implication for the coach is that specific intensity of work needs to be included in any training programme, otherwise physiological stimulation will not be applied to the correct muscle fibre type.

Further consideration must be given to the fact that ATP for energy is produced not only from the breakdown of creatine phosphate, but also by the process of glycolysis (Jacobs, 1986; Newsholme, 1993) during the first few seconds of any intense activity, and predominantly by glycolysis if the intense activity is maintained. The rate of glycolysis increases rapidly during intense activity, blood lactate accumulates and blood pH falls. Reduced rates of glycolysis, reduced times to fatigue and a reduction in isometric tension have all been demonstrated with a decline in intramuscular pH (Parkhouse and McKenzie, 1984). As a result of the greater resistance of Type IIa fibres to fatigue, it seems likely that athletes will rely most on these fibres if speed endurance is required. Therefore, intense activity, although it may last for less than 10 s, will still place a significant physiological demand upon the ability of the skeletal muscle to buffer H+ accumulation, assessed by the drop in blood pH level. This will certainly be the case in intense exercise lasting in excess of 10 s.

The coach needs to appreciate the physiological basis of this process, for in this understanding lies the framework for the effective design of training programmes intended to accommodate the specific work/rest ratios of a particular sport. In understanding this process, it has to be acknowledged that boundaries separating the various categories of activity are not precisely defined and that the key to specific adaptation lies in the integration of all energy provision. With progressive training, physiological adaptation will require frequent re-adjustment in order to maximize the physiological parameters. Physiological systems do adapt to both an acute bout of exercise and a planned programme that emphasizes a particular metabolic energy provider. As a consequence one cannot say with any certainty that, at a particular intensity of work, one energy system changes to another. However, it is possible for the coach to manipulate a change in emphasis between the different energy systems through changing the intensity, frequency and duration of training.

Energy for performance

Anaerobic mechanisms

With creatine phosphate being extremely limited in its ability to regenerate large amounts of ATP, other metabolic pathways must predominate beyond the first few seconds of intense exercise if ATP levels are to remain high (Sjodin, 1992). The resynthesis of ATP through anaerobic glycolysis involves the breakdown of muscle glycogen to lactic acid. Although substantial amounts of ATP can be regenerated from this energy pathway, it is not possible for contraction to continue for prolonged periods through anaerobic glycolytic processes (Sjodin, 1992). The large acidosis resulting from lactic acid accumulation and/or the rapid rate of glycogen depletion will ultimately result in a reduction in work intensity.

However, the role of anaerobic glycolysis in multiple and single bouts of intense performance is crucial, being supported as it is by the systems dependent on creatine and adenylate kinase. It has been suggested that the decline in performance in this type of activity is as a direct result of the increased proportion of ATP that needs to be resynthesized by glycolysis when stores of creatine phosphate become low (Hirvonen *et al.*, 1987). Fatigue results, as the supply of ATP is insufficient to meet demand. This would apply equally to any repetitive high intensity activity that has a duration longer than 5–7 s. Not only may a deterioration in high intensity performance take place when stores of creatine phosphate approach depletion, but this may be exacerbated by the glycolytic rate declining because of a fall in blood pH inhibiting PFK and the glycolytic rate limiting enzyme phosphofructokinase (Gaitanos *et al.*, 1993).

This has implications for training programmes. Research suggests that, to elicit adaptations to the anaerobic glycolytic pathway, exercise should be performed at the highest order of intensity (Jacobs *et al.*, 1987). As part of a periodized plan, training of this type will facilitate adaptations to increase the rate of ATP resynthesis attained and maintained by anaerobic glycolysis (Sahlin, 1992). Adaptations specific to high training intensity may include an increased buffering capacity (Parkhouse and McKenzie, 1984) or an increased concentration of PFK (Nevill *et al.*, 1989; Brooks *et al.*, 1993). The former will enhance the ability of the musculature to tolerate a greater production of H+ ions, and the latter will enhance the ability of glycolysis to meet the resulting additional requirements for ATP.

In order to facilitate ATP production via anaerobic glycolysis, coaches need to plan for intensive forms of training associated with anaerobic tolerance. Whilst it is difficult to generalize, athletes who are mature and experienced will generally be required to operate in a band of intensity commensurate with 85–95 per cent of their maximum heart rate in order to achieve this objective. This can only be achieved by taking part in intense training with limited recovery. Having already suggested that rest and regeneration are important, coaches should approach this area with care. This type of work should be based on previous well-planned training that has developed the athlete's adaptation to aerobic or local muscular endurance. From this base, the athlete will gradually be able to tolerate the demands of an intense session, albeit only for short periods in the first instance. As tolerance improves, so too can the frequency of the training stimuli within a particular training session that seek to challenge this particular pathway. High intensity training sessions should not be carried out back to back because glycogen stores, the fuel for anaerobic high intensity work, can take in excess of 24 hours to be replenished. The manipulation of interval training is a classic training method that can be organized to suit this objective.

Long-term adaptation to anaerobic, sprint-type training has also been shown to produce a glycogen sparing effect, resulting in maintenance of muscle glycogen concentrations (Boobis *et al.*, 1983). In addition, it has been noted that glycogen synthesis activity increases after anaerobic training. This adaptation serves to increase the synthesis of glycogen from glucose, thus increasing the concentration of stored muscle glycogen. The anaerobically induced adaptations in glycogen storage and the glycolysis mechanism are of great importance in multi-sprint, intermittent sports such as all the major field games. Enzyme activity will, in part, determine the rate and efficiency of an individual's ability to replenish depleted stores of fuel following maximal, short duration exercise. Increased glycogen stores will therefore permit the maintenance of supramaximal workloads for longer periods of time, thus permitting a player to sustain high intensity activity for longer periods. Increases in glycolytic enzyme activity will serve to enhance the efficiency of ATP production and shorten recovery time between bouts of high intensity activity. Therefore without an effective and efficient recovery and replenishment system, the athlete's ability to perform repeated sprints is limited, thus affecting competitive performance (Spriet, 1995). As has already been stated, the energy systems responsible for ATP production are integrated, and emphasis will shift according to intensity, frequency and duration of exercise. Despite this an energy continuum does exist, and the principles of time on task and intensity may provide the coach with a useful indication of the emphasis being placed on a particular pathway.

Aerobic mechanisms

The integration of aerobic and anaerobic systems is demonstrated in the athletes' capacity to utilize an appropriate percentage of their individual oxygen uptake capability. This is particularly pertinent for those sports that depend on large muscle groups, such as swimming, cycling, athletics, rowing and cross-country skiing. These activities greatly increase the overall metabolic demand, and lead to a significant change in the functions of the respiratory and cardiovascular systems. The factors responsible for increased VO_2 max have been identified and occur as either adaptations in the oxygen delivery system or in the mechanism of oxidative metabolism itself. Fuel utilization is also an important factor in aerobic activity Costill and Hargreaves, 1992; Maughan, 1992). Therefore, providing an enhanced oxygen delivery system is an important adaptation to aerobic exercise. However, in order for this to be of any benefit to the individual, the capacity of the muscle to utilize the extra oxygen also has to be increased. As a result, appropriate aerobic training induces changes in mitochondrial function that improve the muscle fibres' capacity to produce ATP via aerobic metabolism. As a consequence of such aerobic exercise, muscle fibre mitochondrial density is increased via an enhanced size and number of mitochondria. The value of this adaptation is that it reduces the diffusion distance between the blood capillaries and the mitochondria, hence facilitating oxygen delivery (Wagner, 1991). It also provides an increase in the area of the sites where oxidative metabolism can occur. Underlying this increased capacity to generate ATP via oxidative metabolism is a rise in the levels of activity of the mitochondrial enzymes responsible for these processes.

In general, aerobic performance exercise is of a low to moderate intensity lasting up to 2 hours and beyond. Therefore, a sustainable energy source for the duration is vital for physical and mental wellbeing. The only available fuel substrate that is in abundant enough supply to sustain prolonged exercise is stored fat, with muscle glycogen storage providing an energy source for only approximately 7 minutes of work at higher levels of intensity (Sjodin, 1992). Consequently, there is an adaptive response in aerobic metabolism and a shift towards a greater reliance on free fatty acid as a source of energy for extended periods of exercise (Maughan, 1992; Wilmore and Costill, 1994). This is facilitated by enzymatic adaptation, which serves to enhance the activation, transport and oxidation of fat, thus increasing the efficiency of ATP production via lipid metabolism. It appears probable that the shift towards a greater reliance on fat is a result of the increase in the individual's capacity to oxidize fatty acid acting in synergy with the increased rate of fatty acid mobilization (Abernethy *et al.*, 1990).

These particular fat metabolism adaptations are of great importance in duration and multi-sprint sports. In the latter, despite activity being characterized as intermittent and regularly changing in intensity, low to moderate intensity activity during the major games is relatively continuous. Utilizing fat as an energy source not only produces a higher energy yield per unit than glycogen, but it also depletes negligibly in relation to its abundant storage level, thus sustaining exercise for a longer period of time. Fat metabolism will help to protect depletion of the valuable glycogen stores, thus saving energy for activities of high intensity and short duration (Saltin, 1973). Increasing free fatty acid metabolism and the oxidation of free fatty acid produces citrate, which consequently inhibits anaerobic glycolysis via PFK inhibition. This glycogen sparing effect (Maughan, 1992) also decreases the production of lactic acid, which has the potential to limit and even decrease performance. This particular adaptation, along with the increased removal and clearance of lactic acid via increased capillary and mitochondrial density, accounts for the aerobically induced increase in lactate threshold. This can be defined as the band of work intensity, associated with an individual's lactate profile, above which lactate production becomes significantly elevated.

The implication for the coach is that aerobic training, at an appropriate intensity in the order of approximately 70 per cent of the maximum heart rate for the experienced performer, will improve lactate turnover and clearance. As a result, athletes will be able either to do more work at this intensity or to handle higher intensities before succumbing to fatigue. This adaptation of aerobic metabolism has the facility to push back the boundary of an individual's lactate threshold (Spurway, 1992). Consequently, regular monitoring and evaluation will enable the coach to plan a continually adjusted overload, in terms of intensity, in order to maintain a challenge to the aerobic mechanisms.

In addition to producing adaptations that promote aerobic energy production, aerobic exercise also produces adaptations that benefit the anaerobic energy system. Enhanced capillary density via aerobic adaptation not only assists in oxygen delivery for oxidative metabolism, but also assists in recovery from short bouts of high intensity exercise. During the rest and recovery periods of low to moderate activity, continual mitochondrial respiration assists in the resynthesis of creatine phosphate, and a large blood flow helps to remove any wastes such as lactate and hydrogen ion by-products which may inhibit ATP production if they are allowed to accumulate. The more quickly this recovery from exercise is achieved, the sooner an athlete can repeat any high intensity sprint activity that may be demanded. An active recovery from training or performance will promote this situation. Consequently, coaches would be well advised to build this into their programmes.

How can coaches improve energy provision?
This section examines the physiological training principles for the anaerobic alactic, anaerobic lactate and aerobic energy systems. The anaerobic alactic pathway, which is fuelled by creatine phosphate, operates on an approximate 1 : 5 work : rest ratio. One bout of very high intensity work lasting less than 10 s should be accompanied by a rest interval of at least five times the length of the work period (Armstrong and Welsman, 1997). Note that, while the work period is very intense activity of very short duration, the rest period can also be of an active nature, but should be at a very low intensity. Active rest promotes recovery by incorporation of the creatine phosphate shuttle in which isosyme creatine kinase promotes the resynthesis of creatine phosphate from mitochondrial ATP production (Sjodin, 1992). This is particularly characteristic of recovery which incorporates low-level sub-maximal intensities.

The essential principle that should guide this type of work is the provision of adequate rest and recovery, and coaches will need to build this into their programme. If specific speed is a key consideration within this programme, each training session should incorporate this element following an adequate warm up. The intensity of activity should be maximal, lasting between 5 and 10 s. Recovery should be five times the length of the activity. Specific speed development requires frequent stimulation in order to achieve adequate adaptation. Repeated speed work organized in sets, with at least five repetitions in each set, will need to be accommodated such that other elements of the programme are not neglected. Little and often is the key, thus allowing full recovery between high intensity bursts of activity. This may necessitate 5–10 minute recovery periods between sets. In my experience, this may require explaining to the athletes who, unless they feel tired, may consider that they are not training hard enough. Therefore, quality as opposed to quantity is the essential understanding to facilitate successful training of this system.

To avoid deterioration in the quality of repetitive intense training, the additional utilization of the adenylate kinase system is likely to be called upon – particularly if sufficient recovery time has not been allowed. The more exhausted the CrP stores become around the muscular contractile apparatus, and the higher the local concentrations of adenosine diphosphate (ADP) and Pi (inorganic phosphate) become, so the more the adenylate kinase system is stimulated. This may result in the continued breakdown of adenosine diphosphate to adenosine monophosphate (AMP) as the demand for ATP is maintained. Subsequent breakdown of AMP could lead to a loss from the adenine nucleotide pool. The long-term effects of attempting to maintain ATP levels may be an increased susceptibility to overtraining syndrome, or at least the inability to reach a physiological peak for competition. As a result, coaching practice must include the necessary rest and regeneration previously indicated when repetitive quality training is required.

The anaerobic lactic glycolytic pathway operates on an approximate 1 : 2 work : rest ratio (Armstrong and Welsman, 1997). Note that the work period is intense and quality orientated, whilst the rest period should be of a low-level active nature. Exercise intensity corresponding to 70–80 per cent maximum heart rate in experienced athletes will increase lactate and H+ ion concentration such that a small increase in intensity will cause a large increase in anaerobic glycolysis, presently defined as the 'lactate threshold' (Spurway, 1992). At work intensities below this figure, the integrative nature of the lactate shuttle keeps the damaging products of glycolytic activity in check as the muscular capability for lactate clearance is stimulated (Brooks, 1986). At exercise intensities above 80 per cent maximum heart rate, the production of AMP is increased as ADP is further reduced in the bid to provide sufficient ATP in order to maintain exercise intensity. Simultaneously, a gradual increase of the AMP breakdown products inosine monophosphate (IMP) and ammonia can be observed intramuscularly. At this intensity only minor increases are observed, indicating that the adenylate pathway is capable of shuttling these breakdown products back to the adenine nucleotide pool (Sjodin, 1992). However, with further increases in intensity in excess of 100 per cent max VO_2 and up to maximum heart rate, plasma levels of breakdown products increase exponentially. This may result in a net loss from the adenine nucleotide pool, with a subsequent impact on the athlete's capacity for recovery.

To maintain a high intensity of 80 per cent maximum heart rate and beyond for extended periods during a training session, recoveries should be long enough to return muscles to their pre-exercise state (Bangsbo, 1994). However, work periods lasting 5–30 s with 0.5–5 min recoveries have been recommended in order to facilitate adaptations of the glycolytic pathway (Bangsbo, 1994). Clearly, a compromise has to be reached between returning the musculature to its pre-exercise state and maintaining a certain level of physiological and psychological readiness. Therefore, the necessity to maintain very high work rates means that strategies should be undertaken to facilitate recovery and hence offset fatigue in subsequent exercise bouts. Low intensity recovery exercise may present just such a strategy, and be a valuable tool for both coach and athlete to use. Jacobs *et al.* (1987) have noted that exercise which raises blood lactate concentrations can reduce subsequent performance; consequently, post-exercise stimulation of creatine, lactate and adenylate shuttle systems during recovery exercise is essential to maintain both the volume and frequency of an intense training stimulus.

The key principles in developing the anaerobic glycolytic energy source revolve around continuous high intensity activity at 85–95 per cent maximum heart rate for up to 30 s, with at least twice this period as low-level active rest. When the athlete fails to accomplish the work set in the time allowed, the session should be terminated. With muscle glycogen being the fuel source for this activity, at least 24 hours must elapse before such a session is repeated. It would certainly not be wise to hold such a session within 48 hours of competition, due to the degradation of the fuel source that would be most needed for the high intensity work of the competition. Three such sessions, equally spaced within the week and located in the overall training plan such that the athlete has already achieved aerobic adaptation, would enable the intensity of the work to be accommodated and lactate tolerance to be enhanced. Lactate tolerance training is demanding, and the athlete must be well prepared for it in order to diminish the detrimental effects that can occur. These effects include stiff and sore muscles, demotivation and the risk of injury. As a result, coaches need to exhibit care and sensitivity in the design and planning of such sessions and in their communication and feedback to the athlete.

The aerobic system operates on a 1 : 1 work : rest ratio. One bout of work lasting in excess of 3 minutes should be accompanied by a similar rest period. This time period is necessary in order to ensure that 'steady state' activity is developed. Note that the work period is concerned with quantity and extension of work rather than quality. Time on task and relative intensity of exercise are the two considerations that determine the contribution of aerobic energy provision to any particular sporting context. Inevitably there is a progression of anaerobiosis as more and more muscle fibres reach a situation in which perfusion is insufficient to match metabolic demand (Shephard, 1992). This progression lies within a relative intensity of exercise normally of 70–80 per cent maximum heart rate, but must be qualified by genetic individuality and trained metabolic efficiency. Endurance capacity can be increased as a result of training by increasing the time an exercise task can be sustained, or by increasing the work rate that can be sustained for a given time (Maughan, 1992). Key considerations associated with central and peripheral adaptation, coupled with an adjusted fuel balance, underlie this increase in endurance capacity. The adaptation is enhanced by the co-enzyme NAD shuttling across the mitochondrial membrane, facilitating production of ATP. The contribution of glycolysis terminating in lactate to the overall energy output will remain negligible whilst the relative intensity allows lactate dehydrogenase (LDH-H) to assist in lactate clearance (Spurway, 1992). The enzyme LDH-H is responsible for driving the reconversion of lactate back through aerobic metabolism. Whilst lactate production occurs at all levels of work intensity, provided the intensity is such that LDH-H is stimulated to facilitate lactate clearance, lactate build up will be negligible. Hence the lactate shuttle is an important mechanism for the maintenance of aerobic activity.

The reason for establishing these training guidelines is the need to maximize the training stimulus and the amount of work that an athlete can do in the training period. The coach should now be aware of the work/rest ratios applicable to his or her specific conditioning requirements. In effect, a well designed conditioning programme has one 'goal'; that is, to improve the efficient and effective production of energy so that athletes can accommodate the challenging metabolic demands placed on them by their sport. In my experience, the athletes' awareness of being prepared specifically for the demands of competition has a psychological as well as a physiological benefit. It is imperative, therefore, in terms of physiological training and adaptation, that coaches understand how effective energy is produced in their particular sporting context. They can then apply the appropriate training stimulus coupled with an effective recovery strategy such that fatigue, overuse injuries, staleness and demotivation are avoided.

Feeling tired and need a rest?

The muscular fatigue associated with physical performance manifests itself in the loss of perceptual and decision making capability, together with a loss of timing and the application of muscular force. The coach should recognize that the smooth, effective and efficient movement exhibited by a well-trained, technically proficient athlete reduces the onset of muscular fatigue. This is accomplished by using only the critical generation of muscular force required to accomplish the task in question. It is apparent, therefore, that training the muscle will help to delay the onset of fatigue. This is especially relevant when training incorporates overload, and is specific to the muscle groups and patterns of movement required (Green, 1992; Powers and Howley, 1994). This reinforces the need for muscular training to be as sports-specific as possible.

Coaches will benefit from an awareness of the potential causes of fatigue. This will result in an informed approach being taken in managing recovery during the training process. Numerous excitation–contraction processes occur within the muscle, which may or may not be limited by the particular energy system being challenged. Consequently, the onset and progression of fatigue can be due to both central and peripheral disturbances (Gandevra, 1992; Sahlin, 1992). During intense activity, these include the ability of the muscle fibres to maintain regulation of Na^+ and K^+ in order to ensure the transmission of action potentials at maximum speed (McKenna, 1992). The ability of the sarcoplasmic reticulum to release and sequester Ca^{2+} ions may be inhibited by protons (Allen *et al.*, 1992) and, since sarcoplasmic reticulum function is of particular importance for the rapid contractions and relaxations during intense activity, the need for muscle fibres (especially Type IIa) to possess an adequate buffering capacity and ion regulation becomes critical (Sahlin, 1992).

Particular attention has been paid to the role of metabolic end products in the inhibition of the cross-bridge cycle, and in the capacity of the muscle to resynthesize ATP sufficiently to meet demands to maintain muscle contractions (Sahlin and Ren, 1989). A decline in pH could induce fatigue at a number of sites, and pH could act directly upon myosin ATPase and ATP hydrolysis due to end product inhibition by the direct action of H^+ ions. H^+ ions could decrease the sensitivity of Troponin C to Ca^{2+} ions by competitive inhibition, and the accumulation of H^+ ions in the sarcoplasmic reticulum could affect the release and uptake of Ca^{2+} ions (Allen *et al.*, 1992). A decline in pH has been shown to inhibit phosphofructokinose and, thus, glycolytic rate (Newsholme and Leech, 1983). However, it is likely that, in addition to the inhibition of PFK by low pH, other mechanisms may be responsible for the reduction of glycolytic rate. These may include the accumulation of citrate and changes in Ca^2+ concentration (Bangsbo, 1994), coupled with glycogen depletion (Costill and Hargreaves, 1992). The apparent reduction in glycolytic rate in repeated high intensity exercise has implications for the type of training that may be undertaken to increase glycolytic power and, consequently, those fitness components that depend on this energy source. These include local muscular endurance, which will be sports-specific, and speed endurance.

The complexity of the physiological processes responsible for energy provision, subsequent delay in fatigue, effective technique and the possibility of overtraining should inform coaches of the necessity to consider appropriate rest and regeneration in their work with athletes. It is important that the coach remembers that one of the outcomes of effective planning is a reduction in the physiological fatigue that can accompany a poorly prepared athlete, not to mention the avoidance of muscular damage.

The demands placed on athletes, if not carefully monitored and controlled, may lead to staleness coupled with a stiff and sore musculature. This is particularly the case when the athlete is asked, or expected, to do too much too soon. The difficulty of planning sufficient rest and recovery periods into the training programme is complicated in certain sports such as association football and rugby by their onerous and dynamic competitive schedule. In addition, issues to do with selection or trials may not have been incorporated into the overall plan and, as a result, exacerbate the problems of planning, particularly when these are unforeseen. However, research into the recovery process over the past 10 years has identified factors that will, if given careful consideration, improve performance by:

- Maximizing the training process through the benefits of short duration intense activity.
- Maximizing the training process in terms of the amount and quality of work undertaken.
- Maximizing the competitive performance of athletes, particularly in tournament play
- Improving the advice available to athletes and coaches about the recovery of fluid and energy loss during intense competition.

A number of the physiological principles identified earlier illustrated the need for coaches to be increasingly aware of the value of recovery as an essential part of performance planning. These included the development of sports-specific speed work, the rationale underlying interval training, the ability to withstand frequent tournament play and the dietary ingredients necessary for full recovery from intense competition. A further factor concerns the removal of metabolic waste products and the replenishment of the raw material that is the basis of energy production (Williams and Devlin, 1995). Research suggests that enhancing glycogen storage can be achieved by tapering training and increasing carbohydrate intake to 70 per cent of the total energy intake (Sherman *et al.*, 1981). It is possible that some of the feelings of tiredness associated with the training process are related, in part, to lowered glycogen reserves (Costill *et al.*, 1988). As a result, pre-exercise meals should consist primarily of carbohydrate, and be ingested 3–4 hours prior to competition or training. This should ensure easy digestion and the normalization of blood glucose and insulin levels prior to exercise (Costill and Hargreaves, 1992). During intense exercise, athletes need to ingest between two-thirds and one litre of a 6–10 per cent carbohydrate solution in order to maintain adequate carbohydrate for the latter stages of prolonged exercise. At the cessation of intense exercise, at least 24 hours are required for complete restoration of muscle glycogen stores as a result of the rate of post-exercise muscle glycogen resynthesis. The rate of resynthesis is faster if carbohydrate is ingested shortly after exercise rather than delaying carbohydrate intake. A final point that should be considered is that high intensity exercise, which can produce muscle damage and soreness, stimulates the presence of inflammatory cells, which possess a large capacity for glucose oxidation. Within damaged muscle, this probably results in less glucose being available for glycogen-depleted muscle cells (Appell, 1992). Therefore, athletes and coaches should be aware of the potential need for increased dietary carbohydrate following intense prolonged exercise that produces muscle damage and soreness.

The practical implications of these guidelines will be demonstrated in the coach's weekly packaging of intensive training in preparation for competition, or the amount of intense training in the planned programme of preparation for an identified event. It is essential that, in designing training, the frequency of high intensity sessions allows enough recovery time for athletes to train and perform with a full fuel tank. There is considerable research to suggest that active recovery promotes the enhanced removal of blood lactate faster than passive rest (Brooks, 1986; Gupta *et al.*, 1996). As demonstrated earlier, this can be attributed to the greater turnover and metabolic clearance rate of lactate during moderate exercise. Active rest of low and moderate intensity is therefore important after high intensity work in order to ensure that lactate is removed and subsequent performances are not adversely affected (Signorile *et al.*, 1993; Ahmaidi *et al.*, 1996). The removal of blood lactate allows a continued efflux of muscle lactate and H+ ions, hence playing an important role in the regulation of intramuscular pH and the recovery from fatigue. It has previously been stated that lactate retards the rate of glycolysis by inhibiting the activity of lactate dehydrogenase and phosphofructokinase (Spriet, 1995). Therefore, the removal of lactate after exercise is crucial for continued performance. A variety of exercise intensities have been suggested to enhance the removal of blood lactate and alleviate the decline in subsequent exercise performance (Bangsbo and Saltin, 1993; Bell *et al.*, 1997). With appropriate training, it has been shown that the changes that occur in muscle with regard to the proportion of LDH-H enzyme, the capillary density and the ability to shuttle H+ ions will enhance the oxidative capacity of the slow twitch fibres and thus the removal of lactate during non-dynamic low intensity activity. For the coach this is an important consideration. Bompa (1994) recommends light, relaxing activity during recovery, and confirms that subsequent performance is dependent on adequate rest. This enables the athlete to arrive at competition having benefited from the most appropriate balance of training stimulus and recuperation. If enough rest is written into the programme, sessions can be planned to maximum effect and the quality and quantity of each training stimulus selected for its specificity to the relevant energy system. Consequently, time spent on training will reap positive and lasting benefits.

Test results show the value of assessment

The use of physiological test results as a means of establishing selection criteria or the erroneous use of them immediately preceding competition leaves the competitor with little faith in the process of formal monitoring, and can have a detrimental impact on the ability of the athlete to perform well. Quite simply, physiological assessment should not be used in this way but as a means of objectively assessing the progress of both the athlete and the preparation plan. As such, it should provide information for analysis and subsequent action by both coach and athlete. In order to achieve this, assessment needs to be built into the training plan at regular and appropriate intervals. In this way it will assist the design and regulation of a well-structured and meaningful programme. The assessment mechanisms will require the involvement of the coach and athlete and, possibly, additional support from an appropriate sport scientist. This team has to consider why and when assessment is to be carried out, and the most appropriate form of assessment to be used. Laboratory assessment can provide effective measurement of energy production but, due to the limitations of laboratory equipment, it may not be specifically related to the movement patterns involved in the actual sporting context. As a consequence, it may be more appropriate to consider field measures that provide evidence of specific movement patterns, albeit at the potential expense of laboratory objectivity. Ideally, assessment should be focused on physiological parameters that are most relevant and most informative about the sport. In order to achieve the most beneficial results, three principles need to be considered. First, all those involved in the process must be aware of the benefits that can accrue from a well-structured, monitored and regulated programme. Secondly, the athlete and coach should be conversant with the procedures involved and thirdly, the sport scientist should be able to link specific assessment procedures to the sport in question. The results from such tests used will be reliable, valid and relevant. Analysing and interpreting the results needs to be a process in which the coach is involved with the sport scientist. The coach is then responsible for the appropriate modifications to the overall training plan. Quite clearly, this information provides feedback for both coach and athlete; for the coach the effectiveness of the programme can be monitored, and for the athlete it can provide an objective view of the current state of preparation and assist in boosting confidence. A final common point for consideration is the educative information provided to both coach and athlete by a well-planned assessment procedure. Involvement in testing physiological variables is an opportunity for the coach to improve knowledge of applied physiological principles, for the athlete to take home 'ownership' of the training process, and for the sport scientist to improve the capacity to translate data into meaningful and relevant sports specific information and advice.

The systematic assessment of an athlete's physiological performance is not therefore simply a means of collating relatively sophisticated data. It does not merely provide the athlete and the coach with scientific data to reinforce the outcomes of already known adaptations. If interpreted appropriately by the sports scientist and applied correctly by the coach, the resultant data can be used to effect optimal training and thus improve performance. The coaching process requires sub-processes of planning, monitoring and regulation. For this reason, a judicious balance of field and laboratory testing can provide the coach with the data to improve the physiological components associated with performance preparation.

Summary

This chapter has considered the role of the coach in relation to the physiological preparation of athletes preparing for competition. This role is quite clearly associated with bridging the gap between appropriate physiological knowledge and the understanding and application of this in a specific sports context. For this reason, it is apparent that coaches need to have an enhanced appreciation of the principles identified in each of the sections in this chapter. An important skill for the coach is the management and manipulation of the intensity, frequency and duration of exercise associated with physiological preparation for their particular sport. Effective energy provision will result from the implementation of integrated and effective work/rest ratios, which delay the onset of fatigue, facilitate effective recovery and, perhaps more importantly, eradicate the potential problems associated with overtraining. The 'shuttling systems' of creatine kinase, adenylate kinase, nicotinamide adenine dinucleotide and lactate dehydrogenase need to be stimulated by the organization, design and prescription of relevant training methods. The integrated application of the principles outlined in this chapter in a planned, progressive and regulated manner is the basis of specific performance preparation. However, it must be acknowledged that the diversity of structure and function between different muscle fibres provides a continuum of force production in dynamic activities. Training effectiveness will therefore be improved by a better understanding of metabolic limitations supported by physiological assessment, which means that training can be made more specific. This will result in a more appropriate integration of the relevant systems, which is necessary to help the athlete to address the specific metabolic challenges associated with their sport. There is little doubt about the centrality of the physiological components of performance. More specific physiological preparation will allow the coach to make a significant – some might say *the* significant – contribution to the training process that forms such a substantive part of the coaching process.

References

Abernethy, P. J., Thayer, R. and Taylor, A. W. (1990). Acute and chronic responses of skeletal muscle to endurance and sprint exercise: A review. *Sports Med.*, **10(6)**, 365–89.

Ahmaidi, S., Granier, P., Taoutaou, Z. *et al.* (1996). Effects of active recovery on plasma lactate and anaerobic power following repeated intensive exercise. *Med. Sci. Sport Exer.*, **28(4)**, 450–6.

Allen, D. G., Westerblad, H., Lee, J. A. and Lannergren, J. (1992). Role of excitation–contraction coupling in muscle fatigue. *Sports Med.*, **13(2)**, 116–26.

Appell, D. G. (1992). Exercise muscle damage and fatigue. *Sports Med.*, **13(2)**, 108–15.

Armstrong, N. and Welsman, J. (1997) *Young People and Physical Activity*. Oxford University Press.

Bangsbo, J. and Saltin, B. (1993). Recovery of muscle from exercise, its importance for subsequent performance. In *Intermittent High Intensity Exercise, Preparation Stresses and Damage Limitation* (D. A. D. Macleod, R. J. Maughan, C. Williams *et al.*, eds), pp. 49–70. EFN Spon.

Bangsbo, J. (1994). The physiology of soccer – with special reference to high intensity exercise. *Acta Physiol. Scand.*, **51**(Suppl. 619).

Bell, G. J., Syndmiller, G. D., Davis, D. S. *et al.* (1997). Relationship between aerobic fitness and metabolic recovery from intermittent exercise in endurance athletes. *Can. J. Appl. Physiol.*, **22(1)**, 78–85.

Bompa, T. O. (1994). *Theory and Methodology of Training: The Key to Athletic Performance* (3rd edn). Kendal Hunt.

Boobis, L. H., Williams, C. and Wootton, S. A. (1983). Influence of sprint training on muscle metabolism during brief maximal exercise in man. *J. Physiol.*, **342**, 36–7.

Brooks, G. A. (1986). The lactate shuttle during exercise and recovery. *Med. Sci. Sport Exer.*, **18**, 360–8.

Brooks, G. A., Melvil, M. E., Gaitanos, G. and Williams, C. (1993). Metabolic responses to sprint training. In *Intermittent High Intensity Exercise, Preparation, Stresses and Damage Limitation* (D. A. D. Macleod, R. J. Maughan, C. Williams *et al.*, eds), pp. 33–48. EFN Spon.

Costill, D. L., Flynn, M. G., Kirwan, J. P. *et al.* (1988). Effects of repeated days of intensified training on muscle glycogen and swimming performance. *Med. Sci. Sport Exer.*, **20**, 249–54.

Costill, D. L. and Hargreaves, M. (1992). Carbohydrate nutrition and fatigue. *Sports Med.*, **13(2)**, 86–92.

Cross, N. and Lyle, J. (1996). Overtraining and the coaching process: implications for the management of coaching practice. *Scot. J. Physical Ed.*, **24(3)**, 28–43.

Dick, F. W. (1986). Coaching: the way ahead. *Coaching Focus*, **3**, 3–6.

Fry, R., Morton, A. R. and Keast, D. (1991). Overtraining in athletes: an update. *Sports Med.*, **12(1)**, 32–65.

Gaitanos, G. C., Williams, C., Boobis, L. H. and Brooks, S. (1993). Human muscle metabolism during intermittent maximal exercise. *J. Appl. Physiol.*, **75(2)**, 712–19.

Gandevra, S. C. (1992). Some central and peripheral factors affecting human motor neuronal output in neuromuscular fatigue. *Sports Med.*, **13(2)**, 93–8.

Green, H. J. (1986). Muscle power: fibre type recruitment, metabolism and fatigue. In *Human Muscle Power* (N. L. Jones, N. McCartney and A. J. McComas, eds), pp. 65–81. Human Kinetics.

Green, H. J. (1992). Myofribrillar composition and mechanical function in mammalian skeletal muscle. *Sport Sci. Rev.*, **1**, 43–64.

Gupta, S., Goswani, A., Sadhuklan, A. K. *et al.* (1996). Comparative study of lactate removal in short-term message of extremities, active recovery and a passive recovery period after supramaximal exercise sessions. *Int. J. Sports Med.*, **17(2)**, 106–10.

Hargreaves, M. (ed.) (1995). *Exercise Metabolism*. Human Kinetics.

Hirvonen, J., Rehunen, S., Rusko, H. *et al.* (1987). Breakdown of high energy phosphate compounds and lactate accumulation during short supramaximal exercise. *Eur. J. Appl. Physiol.*, **56**, 253–9.

Jacobs, I. (1986). Blood lactate: implications for training and sport performance. *Sports Med.* **3(1)**, 10–25.

Jacobs, I., Esbjornsson, M., Sylven, C. *et al.* (1987). Sprint training effects on muscle myoglobin, enzymes, fibre types and blood lactate. *Med. Sci. Sport Exer.*, **19(4)**, 368–74.

Macdougall, J. D., Wenger, H. A. and Green, H. J. (1991). *Physiological Testing of the High Performance Athlete*. Human Kinetics.

Maughan, R. (1992). Aerobic function. *Sport Sci. Rev.*, **1**, 28–42.

Maughan, R., Greeson, M. and Greenhaff, P. L. (1997). *Biochemistry of Exercise and Training*. Oxford University Press.

McKenna, M. J. (1992). The role of ionic processes in muscular fatigue during intense exercise. *Sports Med.*, **13(2)**, 134–45.

Nevill, M. E., Boobis, L. H., Brooks, S. *et al.* (1989). Effect of training on muscle metabolism during treadmill sprinting. *J. Appl. Physiol.*, **67**, 2376–82.

Newsholme, E. A. (1993). Application of knowledge of metabolic integration to the problem of metabolic limitations in sprints, middle distance and marathon running. In *Principles of Exercise Biochemistry* (J. R. Poortmans, ed.), pp. 230–247. Karger.

Newsholme, E. A. and Leech, A. R. (1983). *Biochemistry for the Medical Sciences.* John Wiley and Sons.

Parkhouse, W. S. and McKenzie, D. C. (1984). Possible contribution of skeletal muscle buffer to enhanced anaerobic performance: A brief review. *Med. Sci. Sport Exer.*, **16**, 328–38.

Powers, S. K. and Howley, E. T. (1994). *Exercise Physiology: Theory and Application to Fitness and Performance.* Brown and Benchmark.

Sahlin, K. (1992). Metabolic factors in fatigue. *Sports Med.*, **13(2),** 99–107.

Sahlin, K. and Ren, J. (1989). Relationships of contraction capacity to metabolic changes during recovery from a fatiguing contraction. *J. Appl. Physiol.*, **67**, 648–54.

Sale, D. G. (1992). Neural adaptation to strength training. In *Strength and Power in Sport* (P. V. Komi, ed.), pp. 249–65. Blackwell Scientific.

Saltin, B. (1973). Metabolic fundamentals in exercise. *Med. Sci. Sports*, **5(2),** 137–46.

Scottish Sports Council (1998). *Sport 21: Nothing Left to Chance.* SSC.

Shephard, R. J. (1992). Exercise physiology and performance in sport. *Sport Sci. Rev.*, **1**, 1–12.

Sherman, W. M., Costill, D. L., Fink, W. J. *et al.* (1981). The effect of exercise and diet manipulation on muscle glycogen and its subsequent utilization during performance. *Int. J. Sports Med.*, **2**, 114–18.

Signorile, J. F., Ingalls, C. and Tremblay, L. M. (1993). The effects of active and passive recovery on short-term, high intensity power output. *Can. J. Appl. Physiol.*, **18(1),** 31–42.

Sjodin, B. (1992). Anaerobic function. *Sport Sci. Rev.*, **1**, 13–27.

Sports Council (1991). *Coaching Matters: A Review of Coaching and Coach Education in the UK.* Sports Council.

Sports Council (1993). *Sport in the Nineties: New Horizons.* Sports Council.

Spriet, L. L. (1995). Anaerobic metabolism during high intensity exercise. In *Exercise Metabolism* (M. Hargreaves, ed.), pp. 1–40. Human Kinetics.

Spurway, N. C. (1992). Aerobic exercise, anaerobic exercise and the lactate threshold. *Br. Med. Bull.*, **18(3),** 569–91.

Wagner, P. D. (1991). Central and peripheral aspects of oxygen transport and adaptations to exercise. *Sports Med.*, **11(33),** 133–42.

Wilmore, J. H. and Costill, D. L. (1994). *Physiology of Sport and Exercise.* Human Kinetics.

Williams, C. and Devlin J. T. (1995). *Foods, Nutrition and Sports Performance.* EFN Spon.

6

Skill learning principles: implications for coaching practice

Malcolm Fairweather

- The operational definitions of skill and skill learning
- A discussion of the theoretical issues in skill learning
- Implications of skill learning research for practice structure and organization
- Implications of skill learning research for feedback provision
- Recent changes in skill learning theory: Dynamical Systems theory
- Implications of skill learning research for sports coaching

Introduction

Coaches are faced with multidimensional challenges that continually evolve at both the theoretical and practical levels (Lyle, 1996). In addition, the underpinning knowledge base that supports the coach within the coaching process is also comprised of multidimensional and eclectic fields. This knowledge base constantly evolves in response to research activity and coaches' experiences, which means that the progressive coach must strive to keep in touch with important changes in theory and practice across many areas. Some expert coaches recognize the implications of changing theoretical notions very quickly, and it is their astute application of this knowledge that will ultimately affect future coaching practice. Therefore, an important task for the authors contributing to this book is to present a comprehensive picture of recent changes in applied practical knowledge that, to date, may not have been accessible to all coaches. Given this task, the specific goal of this chapter will be to offer practical knowledge and insight from the skill learning area that can be incorporated within coaching practice. Of course, skill learning as a distinct area represents only one dimension of the coaching process. However, from a viewpoint of applied coaching practice, it is perhaps one of the most influential and practical knowledge areas.

There are many factors that facilitate or inhibit skill learning. A primary responsibility for the coach who wishes to facilitate skill learning is to understand the concepts involved. Following an understanding of these concepts, coaches may then recognize the various facilitating and inhibiting effects that the coaching environment can have upon skill learning activities. Fortunately, little time is required to secure an understanding of the term 'skill learning'. However, a lifetime may be required before an appropriate understanding of the many factors that influence skill learning is achieved and translated into practice. Some expert coaches appear to develop an intuitive grasp of such factors, and display this understanding within their coaching behaviour. Nevertheless, despite this evidence of good practice, present research suggests that at times neither intuition nor experience may provide the most accurate or appropriate pathways when attempting to improve skill.

Over the past 70 years, skill learning researchers have produced a number of theoretical perspectives from which skill can be appraised. Throughout this period, researchers have continually adapted their theoretical notions in line with the findings of related empirical investigations (see, for example, Schmidt, 1991; Magill, 1998). This research effort has produced a mass of applied information as well as more fundamental and basic theoretical information. Unfortunately, within the coaching literature there is often a notable absence of many of the findings gleaned from this research. As a result many coaches, perhaps the majority, remain ignorant of the implications and applications of this research effort. Thus, the availability of practical information may remain limited to scholars who investigate skill learning issues in depth. The transmission and dissemination of findings may well be the responsibility of both academics and coach educators. What is clear is that, despite the problems, it is vitally important that students and coaches are continually informed of new knowledge. This chapter will provide a starting point for a developing awareness in the skill learning area.

Of course, it is well beyond the scope of the present chapter to divulge all the skill learning research information that is relevant to the coaching process. Instead, the information presented will focus on selected theory and research content, whilst still attending to applied research findings and practical examples. In particular, the content will focus on instructional and practice issues that require identification and understanding by both the coach and athlete. The goal of developing independence and understanding within the athlete will be promoted throughout the chapter. In addition, the requirement for the athlete to present effort in processing information during practice activities will also be viewed as critical.

In recent years, skill learning research has produced some intriguing counterintuitive data that question the very essence of our traditional instructional behaviour. The purpose of this chapter is therefore to provide insight into this research knowledge and to evaluate the effectiveness of skill learning activities within the coaching process. The terms 'skill' and 'learning' will be considered briefly and individually prior to discussing both topics within a framework of skill learning theory. This framework will be used to appraise the efficacy and explanatory power of both past and present research investigating skill learning phenomena. Following this theoretical discussion, coaching implications will be identified and practical solutions will be suggested for a number of skills and for individuals who present different performance levels. These solutions are based upon recent research observations, and will at times be supported by personal coaching experience.

Skill

Magill (1998:7) defines skill as 'a task that has a specific goal to achieve'. Within sports environments skill requires a movement (motor) component, and Magill considers this movement component when defining a motor skill as 'a skill that requires voluntary body and/or limb movement to achieve the goal'. In addition to this intentional nature of skilled behaviour, Higgins (1991) considers expert motor skill behaviour as consistently successful despite changing environmental factors. Inherent within both Magill's and Higgins' definitions of skilled behaviour is the view that skilled behaviour requires voluntary action at either the body or limb level. In order to perform voluntary action(s) comprising a skill, many abilities may be required. The term 'ability' in this sense refers to a general characteristic or trait that may be fundamental to the performance of a number of motor skills (for example, strength). Abilities can be enhanced with training, and prowess in certain key ability areas may enhance skilled performance. It should be noted that the term 'ability' is often confused with skill and that, because abilities can be affected positively by training, skill can also be enhanced. More specifically, this enhancement will be more likely if the trained abilities are important in the performance of the required skill activity.

There are a number of different forms of skill, including: fine (small muscles) and gross (large muscles); discrete (requiring a distinct movement) and continuous (repetitive movement); and open (variable environmental conditions) and closed (consistent environmental conditions). The modern perspective of skilled behaviour is that both the skill's characteristics and the environmental conditions pertaining to the skill must be closely considered when designing training programmes, creating the practice environment, providing instruction and, finally, appraising the efficacy of coaching behaviour. Consistency in skilled behaviour despite altered environmental conditions (as suggested by Higgins, 1991) clearly differentiates skill levels. If environmental pressure is increased, then this pressure can have a detrimental effect upon even the most rudimentary of skills. For example, kicking a ball becomes a far more difficult task as the supporting surface underfoot becomes less stable, or when the time available to perform the kicking action is reduced. Skilful individuals display consistent behaviour despite such potentially interfering conditions. These individuals recognize problems quickly, and possess appropriate movement solutions to solve a multitude of skill problems (Abernethy *et al.*, 1994).

Within open skill environments (involving changing environmental conditions and externally paced tasks; for example, tennis serve returns), skilled behaviour may require problem-solving at the cognitive level in addition to an appropriate display of physical behaviour. There are at least two levels of activity within such circumstances – a recognition level (often associated with cognitive control functions) and a movement level (again often associated with cognitive functions, although more recently recognized as a multidimensional activity). The time taken to develop the movement component of a skill is dependent upon the functioning of a number of systems (Clarke, 1995). In walking, for example, each system involved in the task could be recognized as an ability area, and so only when the many critical systems for the walking task are sufficiently developed will the skilled behaviour emerge. The transitory nature of skilled behaviour at the environmental level is clearly highlighted when babies present difficulty in coping with novel terrains and obstacles. In addition, energy systems at the physiological level, and the consumption of food, may radically influence the display of walking behaviour.

Transferring the discussion from walking at a basic level to race walking, it is obvious that the pattern of movement that is presented in race walking is not only related to the locomotive element of the task, but also to the rules governing this event. The function of the coach from a skill development perspective is to recognize the various problems posed by critical systems involved in the skill. The coach also needs to recognize the extra problems posed by the skill environment, and the rules governing the skilled behaviour. Addressing all of these problems in a systematic fashion is the essence of programme planning, preparation and implementation. Recognition of the abilities required to perform a skill is a first step that the coach must take when helping athletes to solve movement problems. The training programme must be sympathetic to the athlete's skill requirements in a particular sporting domain and, in addition, training activities should enable the athlete to display active problem-solving behaviour in order to seek task solutions (Newell and McDonald, 1992). Active involvement in the development of skill by the athlete will be reinforced within this chapter.

Following an understanding of the term 'skill', a further step is to recognize the appropriate responses by the coach for dealing with different skills, different individuals and, finally, the different environments in which skills are performed. A major factor that differentiates effective from ineffective coaching is the understanding and awareness that coaches have of the components of skill learning, and the issues involved in translating this into practice. Recent research activity in skill learning has reinforced the interdisciplinary nature of the factors that influence skill. However, little of this research has been applied to work conducted within natural coaching environments. The research information included within this chapter is designed to facilitate the understanding of skill learning principles required by coaches.

Skill learning

Skill learning is the process of behavioural change that results in a relatively stable and resistant skilled behaviour. Schmidt (1991) defines skill learning in terms of relative permanency. The relative permanency principle means that performance should be observed on several occasions prior to considering the effectiveness of any coaching activity and/or athlete behaviour. Practice performance viewed in isolation is considered by skill learning scholars to be a relatively poor indicator of permanency (for a detailed discussion see Salmoni *et al.*, 1984). This means that practice performance behaviour (known as skill acquisition behaviour) may not be predictive of later behaviour (known as skill retention behaviour), or of the ability to perform within novel environments (known as skill transfer behaviour). Once this skill learning perspective is understood by both the coach and athlete, then both parties may appraise their individual and interactive behaviours from many different levels. The coach has a natural viewing advantage over and above the teacher in this area as, in performance coaching, the coach is typically in constant interaction with the athlete, and skill changes can be perceived beyond isolated events. Furthermore, the coach will also be in a position to monitor competition behaviour.

The various factors that affect the development of retention and transfer behaviour are critical in an understanding of the skill learning process, and a major role of skill learning research has been to identify these key factors. The important research issues that have influenced this search for key skill learning variables will be outlined. Many of these issues provide insight for coaching practice and the coach–athlete interaction in general. First, a historical perspective of skill learning theory will be outlined in the following appraisal of theoretical perspectives. Thereafter, attention will be drawn to the appropriateness of specific coaching practices, given recent advances in theoretical and empirical skill learning research.

Theoretical issues

Research in skill learning from the 1970s to the present date has been heavily influenced by two motor (movement) learning theories, both based upon information-processing models of skilled behaviour (see Schmidt, 1975, for a review). Adam's (1971) closed-loop theory and Schmidt's (1975) schema theory stimulated enormous amounts of research activity through the 1970s and 1980s. Information-processing theories focused upon the internal activity of the central nervous system and hypothetical processing models of skilled behaviour. More recently, however, information-processing theories in general have been challenged by a new perspective in skill learning research called the dynamical systems theory (Thelen, 1992). The following discussion will outline each of these theories, and will identify the implications that each theory presents for coaching practice.

Adam's closed-loop theory

Adam's closed-loop theory of motor learning stimulated early research into the role of feedback in skill learning. The theory assumed two forms of internal representation; a long-term memory system called the memory trace, which initiates actions, and a further sensory system called the perceptual trace. The notion of a perceptual trace is fundamental to closed-loop theory. Its role is to assess ongoing movement behaviour and, if required, alter movement in response to the available external and internal feedback information. This perceptual trace activity is viewed as critical to producing accurate responses. With practice and knowledge of results (KR), the suggestion is that the perceptual trace strengthens as comparisons of the task outcome are actively compared with intrinsic feedback received during the performance of the task. Providing external feedback information (known as augmented feedback) in addition to any task outcome-related external feedback reinforces discrepancies between the actual movement and the preferred response. With practice and the guiding role of augmented feedback, the perceptual trace should become stronger, enhancing the like-lihood of more accurate responses in the future. Adam's closed-loop theory suggested that errors in practice would degrade the perceptual trace. This view therefore reinforced the importance of error-free practice, characterized by frequent reinforcement in the form of augmented feedback.

From a coaching perspective, this would mean that an athlete in the early stage of practice should ideally practise skills under conditions of constant feedback and with minimal error. Therefore, free exploration within practice attempts would not be encouraged by the closed-loop approach to practice. Instead, early guidance from the coach would be reinforced until the athlete displayed relatively error-free behaviour, indicating perceptual trace devel-opment. Research findings from investigations into closed-loop theory emphasized augmented feedback in the form of knowledge of results, and assessed only practice activity behaviour when evaluating learning. The con-clusions drawn from such research suggested that augmented feedback should be presented frequently and immediately.

Problems with the closed-loop theory were soon recognized. In particular, Adam's theory failed to account for the performance of fast-moving motor skills, where the perceptual trace would be unable to affect an action due to time constraints. In addition, closed-loop theory failed to explain why prac-tising different variations of a skill during the same practice session produced greater practice error, yet improved performance capability in retention assessment or in the transfer to novel movements (for example, Shea and Kohl, 1990). Furthermore, the motor skills employed in the examination of closed-loop theory involved restricted limb movements utilizing unidimen-sional limb positioning tasks. These skills do not reflect the difficulty posed by applied sports skills, and the efficacy of transferring the results of such closed-loop investigations is therefore questionable.

The credibility of any skill learning theory for coaches must include the transferability of experimental observations to sports-specific environments. Given the limited nature of closed-loop investigations, the multidimen-sional characteristics of sports skills displayed by sports performers remain unaccounted for by research examining this theory. A further problem in research investigating closed-loop theory was that many conclusions were based solely upon practice period behaviour. A review paper by Salmoni *et al.* (1984) examined this issue, and presented a strong case suggesting that practice performance is not the best predictor of subsequent skill behaviour.

Adam's theory proposed that feedback should be provided in a manner that reinforces the strength of the perceptual trace. However, when assessing feedback frequency effects (that is, how often we present feedback) and feedback delay effects (the number of practice trials prior to feedback avail-ability), the role of feedback on acquisition performance versus retention performance appears to be very different. In many ways Adam's theory underpinned a commonly observed coaching practice in which one task is practised consistently over many trials. Within such practice conditions, aug-mented feedback from the coach may be presented frequently, at least until a relatively consistent form of practice success is achieved. Later research evi-dence arising from Schmidt's (1975) schema theory is critical of this form of coaching behaviour and of other closed-loop theory suggestions.

Schema theory

Advances in the information-processing theoretical progression were signified by Schmidt's (1975) schema theory, which closely followed Adam's closed-loop theory. Underpinning schema theory is the notion of generalized motor programmes (GMP). Generalized motor programmes are fundamental to the schema perspective and are thought to produce skilled movements sharing specific invariant features, such as the relative timing and organization of limb parts in co-ordination. An example of a generalized motor programme in action would be a GMP for walking which produces walking behaviour. The relative timing component within walking is displayed by the sequential organization of movement in the thigh, shank and foot. These limb parts perform their respective movements, taking up a constant proportion of time (relative time) during one complete step-cycle in walking regardless of walking speed. This means that, when walking is speeded up or slowed down, the individual limb parts take up the same proportion of time within the overall timing pattern of walking. Schema theory suggests that, because the parameters of speed and force are free to vary when walking, then the walking movement can vary in speed and stride length.

However, as speed is increased to a critical level, walking is clearly discontinued from a relative timing perspective and is replaced by jogging. Jogging is therefore a different mode of gait than walking, and can be characterized by a new relative timing of limb part co-ordination. Therefore, according to the generalized motor programme explanation, a new programme is activated to produce the behaviour (a jogging programme). To control the parameters influencing the functioning of a GMP, Schmidt suggested two forms of schema; the recall schema and the recognition schema. Schema are common to information-processing models and, at the fundamental level, are abstract rule-based mechanisms.

The role of the recall schema is to specify parameters for the appropriate operation of a GMP, given task conditions. These specifications are thought to be based upon previously learned relationships between initial environmental conditions/body conditions, previous response specifications and previous outcomes. Following the initiation of a movement, the recognition schema analyses the sensory consequences of movement along with the environmental outcome. This task analysis is then compared with previous experiences of the skill. During the production of slow-moving tasks, parameters may be varied during the task. However, in fast-moving skills, parameters may only be altered following movement production prior to a new attempt at the skill (Schmidt, 1975). Schema theory therefore overcame one of Adam's major problems by explaining the potential control mechanisms involved during fast-moving skills.

For many years, schema theory has received the greatest amount of research attention in skill learning. This research interest has been achieved despite strong criticism of schema theory, including a general lack of clarity in explaining the emergence of novel movements in human behaviour that would presumably require the capacity of new GMPs. Despite this criticism, information-processing research designs and schema theory have underpinned many motor learning researchers' activities over the past 25 years. In particular, researchers have investigated schema theory predictions under a variety of feedback and practice conditions (e.g. Swinnen, 1990; Landin *et al.*, 1993).

Schema theory and variable practice

An important prediction arising from schema theory is that variable practice should significantly alter the specification process available when processing the parameters for motor programmes. This should be superior to constant practice conditions in developing the effectiveness of the recall and recognition schema. Schmidt's variability-of-practice hypothesis critically questioned the idea of the repetitive 'perfect' practice experience promoted by earlier closed-loop theory research and, in doing so, also suggested that errors were essential for skill learning to occur. In coaching terms, this means that the developing athlete should be encouraged to vary the parameters of a specific skilled movement – such as a push pass in hockey or a free kick in soccer – during practice sessions.

The expected increase in errors that may be observed during practice, from a schema perspective, acts as an investment towards future skill production via the development of stronger schema mechanisms. The role of both the coach and the athlete during variable practice activity, therefore, is to recognize the cause of error yet not dwell upon the skill output. Research investigating Schmidt's variability-of-practice hypothesis suggests that variable practice activity can enhance skill learning (e.g. Landin *et al.*, 1993) and skill transfer (e.g. Shea and Kohl, 1990). These experimental data are contradictory and relatively damaging to Adam's closed-loop theory of skill learning. For example, in basketball free-throw shooting, Landin and colleagues found that constant practice from the free-throw line was not as beneficial to learning free-throw shooting in novices when compared to variable free-throw practice from around the key.

Practice schedules and contextual interference

Research suggests that practice organization is critical to the development of skill. A practice phenomenon known as the contextual interference effect provides significant insight into the organization of practice activities. Originally observed by Battig (1979) in verbal learning research, the contextual interference effect suggests that practising various skills in a random manner will typically reduce practice performance, especially when compared to more repetitive practice schedules that provide less variety. However, despite random skill practice presenting clear practice decrement, retention and transfer performance typically show marked benefit, presumably as a result of the effects of random skill practice organization.

Low contextual interference conditions are present when one task is performed repeatedly. For example, blocked practice of a skill involves practising the same skill repeatedly, and this practice behaviour presents a low form of contextual interference. An example of this form of contextual interference on the golf driving range would be to hit 50 shots in succession with a driver. High contextual interference conditions, on the other hand, involve practising several different skills within a discontinuous random practice framework. An example of a random practice schedule would include practising a variety of golf shots in succession (for example, driver, 5-iron, wedge, putter). Motor learning research has shown benefits for skill transfer when practising in high contextual interference conditions (e.g. Lee and Magill, 1983; Goode and Magill, 1986). However, similar to the 'variability of practice' research, high contextual interference has a dampening effect upon the practice behaviour prior to the potential learning benefits within retention or transfer conditions being observed. The coach must therefore consider the effects of increased practice error upon athletes' motivation and self-confidence when employing contextual interference within the practice schedule.

At present, skill learning research suggests that skill practice organization, even at the earliest stages of skill development, should include some form of random behaviour. In soccer, for example, this random behaviour may require changes to parameter modifications such that speed and force are altered systematically during practice. The length, the angle and the speed of a pass could be altered under fairly constant environmental conditions. A further contextual interference step would then be to alter practice conditions by providing increasing variability in the environment. Thereafter, the sequence of skills may be varied. The contextual interference effect implies organizing practice so that the soccer passing skills are increasingly per-formed in a random order. Where possible, this order should reflect passages of play and movement sequences that naturally occur in the game. The goal of these progressive activities would be to provide practice conditions that provide optimal transfer to the competitive environment. The ultimate trans-fer development given these passing activities would be for a player to demonstrate novel yet appropriate passing behaviour in a game situation.

The role of the coach within such practice progressions is to help the athlete to recognize that a greater number of errors will occur given more complex practice conditions and, most importantly, to explain why this is of benefit. If athletes know why such practice conditions are being implemen-ted, and they also concurrently possess a basic understanding of potential skill retention and skill transfer benefits (that seem to be facilitated by skill production or processing errors), then the commonly held negative view of errors held by coaches and athletes alike may require change. In particular, in open skill activities the athlete should be encouraged to be active in processing information during practice activities. Processing links between practice activities and competition activities may be further established by the assessment and comparison of elite video footage. The proposed active involvement of both coach and athlete that is expressed here needs to be approached in a very positive and sympathetic fashion in which errors are viewed in a knowledgeable and insightful fashion. The main problem observed with this approach is that athletes can be impatient, and personal experience suggests that patience is essential when using these strategies. A further problem that can arise in team sports is whether or not practice behaviour is viewed as critical to team selection. Few team players will wish to demonstrate errors in practice if they perceive that they are a selec-tion criterion. As a result of this extra pressure players may revert to more conservative actions during practice and thereby display less exploratory behaviour, thus possibly limiting their future progress.

Feedback research and schema theory
When analysing coach/athlete interaction in relation to feedback, the way that both parties view the use of feedback information also appears to be

critical for effective skill learning (for a review, see Magill, 1994). Cognitive engagement in the use of augmented feedback by the athlete seems essential, for example, when relationships must be established between internal mechanisms and external outcome (Lee *et al.*, 1994). Research investigating the availability of augmented feedback suggests that by increasing augmented feedback, the requirement for cognitive effort is lessened. Reducing the availability of augmented feedback facilitates internal processing during non-feedback trials, and is thought to promote skill retention and transfer (Winstein and Schmidt, 1990). High frequency augmented feedback, on the other hand, may limit the necessary processing of internal sensory systems. Furthermore, the ability to relate this information to naturally occurring environmental feedback would then also be limited. Instead, the athlete may respond directly to the augmented information and bypass critical internal processing mechanisms.

Analysis of the research literature investigating feedback effects upon motor skill learning over the past 10 years reveals important information for the coach. A brief appraisal of this literature shows that both the characteristics of the learner and those of the motor skill should be considered. For the development of fairly simple skills where a level of success can be achieved quickly by the performer, research suggests that the provision of high frequency feedback restricts skill learning (e.g. Nicholson and Schmidt, 1991). Furthermore, this research suggests that performers tend to respond to high frequency augmented feedback in a variable manner, altering their responses from trial to trial (e.g. Lai and Shea, 1998).

Within a recent review of augmented feedback research, Magill (1994) clearly suggested that the characteristics of a skill and the learner are critical factors that affect the augmented feedback and skill learning interaction. A summary of Magill's review is that the effects of augmented feedback in skill learning are now regarded as a much more complex issue than the notion that feedback is necessary and more is better. The interaction of internal mechanisms and supplemental guidance (or augmented feedback) is not a simple issue. In fact, for some motor tasks such as anticipation timing skills (e.g. cricket batting, or service returns in tennis), laboratory-based tasks suggest that additional augmented feedback in the form of timing error (representative of the disparity between racket and ball at the point of serve return) provides no distinct advantage to learning over and above naturally occurring task-intrinsic feedback (e.g. Magill *et al.*, 1991). Task-intrinsic feedback in this case represents the naturally occurring feedback that is presented within the working environment. Magill therefore states that the accuracy of statements suggesting that augmented feedback is essential for all skill learning activities has been brought into question by recent motor learning research.

Proteau and Cournoyer (1990) suggest that augmented feedback is stored as part of the memory structure for a particular skill. This view increases the ability to explain positive skill retention effects when augmented feedback in practice is made less available. The reliance upon augmented feedback seems to become less necessary when the memory representation of a skill has been formed by the activity of independent processing mechanisms by the athlete. Providing immediate and frequent augmented feedback during practice conditions can therefore act negatively by developing a memory structure that depends upon the coach's augmented information for success. Delaying feedback, on the other hand, stimulates the development of more independent processing mechanisms and the advanced understanding of the important relationships between varied outcome and internal sensory factors (Anderson *et al.*, 1994).

To facilitate independence and stimulate active processing by performers, research suggests that estimating errors and the cause of errors following practice trials will help skill retention and transfer (Swinnen, 1990). Delaying feedback may encourage the athlete to react to internal sensory feedback mechanisms and, through active cognition, may reinforce the connections between perception and action. The interesting nature of recent feedback experiments is that, if practice data alone were assessed, then the conclusions from these data sets would be reversed.

Less frequent augmented feedback during practice may benefit learning by strengthening the response to sensory detection mechanisms such as vision and proprioception. More frequent feedback appears to guide practice performance. However, this guidance seems to distract attention from important sources of sensory information by replacing the role of this information during practice. Practice conditions that minimize the development of sensory mechanisms may also minimize learning and independence in the learner. By delaying augmented feedback the learner is allowed some time to interact with his/her response, and this interaction seems critical for optimal learning to occur.

As suggested, motor learning researchers throughout the 1980s and 1990s have changed the way that they assess learning. Retention tests present a more insightful and longer-term view of the effects of practice by examining the relative permanency of practice behaviour. An example of this retention perspective would involve assessing badminton serve performance during a series of daily practice sessions under coach feedback conditions (acquisition), and then reassessing serving performance, say, 2 days later, at a weekend competition (retention) when coach feedback was less available. Retention assessments may provide some insight to the relative independence factor and, as such, to the effects of this particular aspect of coaching practice. Performing under novel task conditions, no matter how slight, requires the transferability of memory and skill behaviour. To avoid limiting transfer behaviour, skill practice should be directed at developing independent and sophisticated processing mechanisms under the athlete's control. The role of the athlete in developing such mechanisms given augmented feedback research findings should be an active one. The athlete must be aware of the many reasons for errors occurring in practice, and learn to understand and accept that practice without error may be insufficient to stimulate further development.

Recent motor skill research has shown that the performance level of the athlete and the complexity of the motor skill are important factors when considering the provision of feedback information (e.g. Guadagnoli *et al.*, 1996; Wulf *et al.*, 1998). Low skill-level performers may require high frequency feedback in order to grasp a basic problem-solving behaviour. The complexity of the sports skill should also be considered prior to employing reduced frequency or delayed feedback practice conditions. A criticism of the motor skill literature is that research has predominantly investigated simple laboratory skills that are low in terms of dimensionality. The three-dimensional problems faced by sports performers may require greater feedback reinforcement, at least at the early stages of skill development. For example, augmented feedback from the coach (or some external mechanism) appears essential in the learning of skills where objects or limb parts disappear beyond visual control (e.g. tennis serving). There are of course many situations within sports environments where implements move beyond visual control, such as in golf and tennis. Acknowledging the previous research discussion, the relative frequency and delay in providing augmented feedback should be closely considered. In the early stages, young, developing athletes may require an abundance of information in order to develop an understanding of the relationships between task goals, intrinsic feedback and freely available extrinsic feedback. As this understanding establishes itself, the principles provided by more basic motor learning research may be acknowledged, and the athlete may then gradually be weaned off high frequency or immediate augmented feedback practice conditions so that more independent self-detection mechanisms may mature. The interaction of augmented feedback and the amount of independence required should therefore be taken into consideration by both coach and athlete in designing and implementing practice sessions.

Feedback and practice summary
The processing mechanisms identified by schema theory clearly influence both feedback provision and practice behaviour. In summary, the frequency and timing of augmented feedback should be carefully considered along with the characteristics of the athlete and the sports skills involved. A long-term goal should be to develop relative independence in information processing within the athlete. Augmented feedback information may eventually be delayed to allow athletes time to process and access relevant information by themselves. Contrary practice would involve providing augmented feedback constantly during practice, perhaps resulting in dependency behaviour by the athlete, which is not clearly observable in practice behaviour. However, this dependence may be more easily observed in competition behaviour. If competition behaviour constantly drops below practice levels, then consider the feedback and practice conditions that prevailed prior to competition. This can be carried out within the overall appraisal process that follows competitions. Of course, there are many other factors that can influence competition performance, and these processing factors are but one aspect.

Both the coach and athlete, however, must develop an understanding of practice and competition errors. An important factor in the athletes' progress is that they are encouraged to understand their own errors and, perhaps just as importantly, others' errors. By so doing, the coach may facilitate the development of active processing abilities. There is a danger that coaches will make the mistake of merely judging their coaching success in practice outcome terms and not in processing terms. In physiological terms, coaches often plan training activities that are designed to limit performance ability in the training phase. Following this phase, rest is incorporated within the programme to optimize competition potential. Training theories follow a compensation principle which suggests that, as a result of progressive training, athletes will demonstrate improvement only some time after the training activity is completed. This planning and awareness of training effects is perhaps analogous to the discussion of skill development at the informa-tion-processing level.

Dynamical systems theory

A major problem for GMP advocates is that, once a successful GMP has been developed, why should behaviour (particularly at the highest level of sport) display inconsistencies? A classic example in recent years is the problem experienced by the golfer Ian Baker-Finch. Once a consistent world leader in the game, his performance became variable and ultimately disastrous in terms of his world ranking. A GMP account might have some difficulty in explaining this slump purely in information-processing terms. If the indivi-dual has obviously shown ability in the past to operate the various golfing programmes required at the elite level, then why would such error arise if physically no observable difference may be observed? Some answers to this question may rest in other domains, such as sports psychology. However, even if the motor programmes are in good order, the body itself can act as a constraint and thereby limit skilled performance. In recent years a more holistic and, to some extent, more physical theory of skill learning has emerged. This theory is known as the dynamical systems theory (Kugler *et al.*, 1980).

The dynamical systems theory of skill learning presents a very different perspective to the information-processing theories presented thus far. The concept of motor programmes is eliminated. Less concern is directed to neurophysiological mechanisms; instead, the human being and the environ-ment are considered inseparable and are studied interactively from the per-spective of non-linear dynamics. Newell (1986) suggests that skilled behaviour emerges from a system that is enveloped by constraints. Constraints are observed in the human being, the environment and the skill itself. An example of an organismic constraint would be body composi-tion; of an environmental constraint, gravity; and of a task constraint, the rules affecting behaviour. Fundamental to Newell's perspective of constraints is that they present a holistic and interactive effect upon the system. This effect is therefore multidimensional and so, for the coach, this perspective recognizes the complexity of the skilled performance and provides potential insight into the many variables operating within skill development beyond the employment of information-processing analogies.

In nature, non-linear systems display system change that may not be predicted in linear terms. This means that a system such as wind may alter its behaviour radically despite apparently small perturbations (disturbances), including humidity. Extending this perspective to human behaviour, and the walking example employed during the earlier motor programme discussion, may help to exemplify theoretical differences. The change from walking behaviour to jogging behaviour in motor programme terms is accounted for by moving from one form of motor programme control to another. However, in terms of dynamical systems, as one increases the speed para-meter in walking, the body reacts to changes in energy consumption. The mechanical result of this linear change in the speed parameter is the non-linear emergence of a new movement pattern. This change in movement co-ordination is known as self-organization (Werbos, 1994), and is governed by factors such as gravity, energy, the physical structure of limbs and the environmental surface. The extent of the movement change is predicted by the continuous alteration of only one variable, i.e. speed. However, the discontinuous result is the change from walking to jogging. From the dynamical systems perspective, many more factors are soon involved in the discussion than simply the top-down control of a motor programme. Changes in behaviour exemplified in Ian Baker-Finch's golf game may therefore also be considered at multiple levels, especially if the behaviour displayed by the individual is problematic or requires intervention.

Researchers working from an information-processing perspective and those from a dynamical systems perspective ask very different questions of skilled behaviour. In coaching terms, the refreshingly holistic nature of the dynamical systems perspective offers a theoretical approach which has the potential to offer critical insights into movement problems and reinforces the need to consider movement solutions at many levels. Dynamical systems researchers are at present asking questions that seek to explain behaviour without the requirement for hypothetical information-processing mechanisms. An example of this is the approach to co-ordination that is evaluated by treating co-ordinative behaviour as the interaction of the self-organizing properties of limb and body structures, given various stable environmental rules that govern all organisms (for further clarification, see Turvey, 1990).

Stability and transitions in behaviour are emphasized in studies by dynamical systems researchers. By employing the mathematical principles that govern non-linear dynamics, researchers have explored movement behaviour from new angles. Preferred states (attractor states) are thought to represent stability in a movement system. However, these states are somewhat fragile given the behaviour of variables known as control parameters (Abraham *et al.*, 1992). The walking example may help explain this idea further. If the relatively stable state of walking behaviour is perturbed via the control parameter of speed, then increased speed can, at a critical point, send the system into a very brief transition state, known as a phase transition. Phase transitions predict the emergence of new behaviours. Then, as self-organization occurs, the new behaviour that quickly emerges is jogging. In this way, and for this particular skill, there is no need to store motor programmes. The interactive effects of the limb structures, energy release and gravity predict the new stable attractor state.

Coaching practice, therefore, should be attempting to create environmental conditions that promote the development of strong, stable attractor states. These stable states may be developed by providing a variety of perturbances such as variations in task demands, environmental conditions and opponent pressure in practice behaviour so that the physical and perceptual systems become relatively resistant under competitive pressure. In the early stages of skill development, relatively novel behaviour could also be perturbed in many ways until this fragile behaviour also remained stable under many more conditions. Think back to the earlier example involving kicking a ball. When the support surface presented by muddy conditions provides less purchase, individuals with stronger postural muscles, lower centres of gravity and better studs may well display less variable balance behaviour and, hence, more consistent kicking behaviour than individuals who possess relative weaknesses in any of these areas.

Changing skilled behaviour may therefore be viewed in a number of ways, such as facilitating the emergence of a stable attractor state or perturbing a stable attractor state towards a new stable state. An example of the latter would involve changing an individual's preferred running pattern. To do this effectively may take a very long time, and would require an understanding of the constraints that influence running development. In addition, there is a phenomenon observed in non-linear dynamics whereby under certain conditions previous and relatively stronger attractor states may re-emerge. This means that the individual who wishes progressively to alter a stable movement may well be entering a long-term problem-solving process, particularly if the movement has already been strongly stabilized and is of the gross motor skill variety. A golfing example is that of Nick Faldo, who spent a number of years reorganizing his golf swing in the belief that better, more consistent competition behaviour lay ahead as a result of appropriate long-term practice behaviour.

A personal example of the problems that may result from the re-emergence of stable attractor states involved changing the running mechanics of one of Scotland's leading international rugby players. The individual concerned demonstrated fairly rapid improvement in body mechanics in training. However, to witness these changes in the pressure of international match conditions took over 1 year. The benefits to the player were reduced injury, an increased pace and a greater change of pace and direction. The difficulty of transferring these changes to a more complex environment is that old movements (from a dynamical systems perspective) are relatively stronger than the new desired patterns. At present the work continues, and further advantages are being strived for. This example, and that of Nick Faldo, emphasizes the importance of patience, insight and self-belief when attempting to change complex skill behaviour.

Skill learning research and implications for coaching

A number of significant changes in skill learning theory have been emphasized. Knowledge and awareness of these changes bring significant insight into the coaching environment. A common thread reinforced throughout the chapter is the requirement for athlete independence at a number of levels. Information-processing research suggests that, for athlete autonomy to be achieved, practice activities should accentuate the development of independent and adaptive processing mechanisms. The role of the coach is to recognize these important implications for coaching practice, and then evaluate current coaching practice and assessment to bring it into line with the radical changes in theory presented in this chapter.

The dynamical systems theory suggests that there are many factors beyond the development of internal processing mechanisms that require further consideration in skill learning. These factors include the transitory nature of skill and the likelihood that skill development will present non-linear patterns of improvement. This chapter has attempted to introduce the reader to the most basic of these issues, and further reading in this area of skill learning research is highly recommended.

Perhaps one of the most important implications for coaching that requires further investigation at this time is the role of assessment within coaching accreditation procedures. If assessment procedures ignore skill retention and transfer issues and focus solely on methods that accentuate acquisition success, disparity seems likely to emerge between skill learning theory and current coaching practice. The skill learning process is important to both the participation coach (a teacher of skill) and the performance coach (a manager of skill development). Both forms of coach must understand the factors that influence skill learning. This is particularly true when considering that skill demands upon athletes competing in international environments are continually increasing. To match and exceed these demands, the principle of non-linear progress must be recognized. To facilitate coaches in their quest for skill development, researchers must therefore strive toward ecological validity in their work. Essentially, this suggestion supports longitudinal study of skill development within relevant environmental conditions. In addition, this research should identify how the various systems that contribute to skill learning affect the learning process. Research in skill learning examining changes in applied skill movement with practice (e.g. Anderson and Sidaway, 1994) presents a step in this direction.

References

Adams, J. (1971). A closed-loop theory of motor learning. *J. Motor Behav.*, **3**, 111–49.

Abernethy, B., Burgess-Limerick, R. and Parks, S. (1994). Contrasting approaches to the study of motor expertise. *Quest*, **46**, 186–98.

Abraham, F. D., Abraham, R. H. and Shaw, C. D. (1992). Basic principles of dynamical systems. In *Analysis of Dynamic Psychological Systems: 1, Basic Approaches to General Systems, Dynamic Systems and Cybernetics* (R. L. Levine and H. E. Fitzgerald, eds), pp. 35–143. Plenum Press.

Anderson, D. A., Magill, R. A. and Sekiya, H. (1994). A reconsideration of the trials–delay of knowledge of results paradigm in motor skill learning. *Res. Q. Exer. Sport*, **65(4)**, 286–90.

Anderson, D. A. and Sidaway, B. (1994). Co-ordination changes associated with practice of a soccer kick. *Res. Q. Exer. Sport*, **65(2)**, 93–9.

Battig, W. F. (1979). The flexibility of humans in memory. In *Levels of Processing in Human Memory* (L. S. Cermak and F. I. M. Craik, eds), pp. 23–44. Erlbaum.

Clark, J. E. (1995). On becoming skillful: patterns and constraints. *Res. Q. Exer. Sport*, **66(3)**, 173–83.

Goode, S. and Magill, R.A. (1986). Contextual interference in learning three badminton serves. *Res. Q. Exer. Sport*, **57(4)**, 308–14.

Guadagnoli, M. A., Dornier, L. A. and Tandy, R. D. (1996). Optimal length for summary knowledge of results: the influence of task-related experience and complexity. *Res. Q. Exer. Sport*, **67(4)**, 239–48.

Higgins, S. (1991). Motor skill acquisition. *Physical Ther.*, **71**, 123–39.

Kugler, P. N., Kelso, J. A. S. and Turvey, M. T. (1980). On the concept of co-ordinative structures as dissipative structures: 1. Theoretical lines of convergence. In *Tutorials in Motor Behaviour* (G. E. Stelmach and J. Requin, eds), pp. 3–47. North-Holland.

Lai, Q. and Shea, C. H. (1998). Generalized motor program (GMP) learning: effects of reduced frequency of knowledge of results and practice variability. *J. Motor Behav.*, **28**, 233–40.

Landin, D. K., Hebert, E. P. and Fairweather, M. (1993). The effects of variable practice on the performance of a basketball skill. *Res. Q. Exer. Sport*, **64(2)**, 232–7.

Lee, T. D. and Magill, R. A. (1983). The locus of contextual interference in motor skill acquisition. *J. Exp. Psychol. Learning Memory Cognition*, **9**, 730–46.

Lee, T. D., Swinnen, S. P. and Serrien, D. J. (1994). Cognitive effort and motor learning. *Quest*, **46**, 328–44.

Lyle, J. (1996). A conceptual appreciation of the sports coaching process. *Scot. Cent. Res. Papers Sport Leisure Soc.*, **1(1)**, 15–37.

Magill, R. A. (1994). The influence of augmented feedback on skill learning depends on characteristics of the skill and the learner. *Quest*, **46**, 314–27.

Magill, R. A. (1998). *Motor Learning Concepts and Applications* (5th edn). McGraw-Hill.

Magill, R. A., Chamberlin, C. J. and Hall, K. G. (1991). Verbal knowledge of results as redundant information for learning an anticipation timing skill. *Hum. Move. Sci.*, **10**, 485–507.

Newell, K. M. (1986). Constraints on the development of co-ordination. In *Motor Development in Children: Aspects of Co-ordination and Control* (M. G. Wade and H. T. A. Whiting, eds), pp. 341–60. Martinus Nijhoff.

Newell, K. M. and McDonald, P. V. (1992). Practice: a search for task solutions. In *Enhancing Performance in Sport: New Concepts and Developments* (American Academy of Physical Education, The Academy Papers 25), pp. 51–9. Human Kinetics.

Nicholson, D. E. and Schmidt, R. A. (1991). Scheduling information feedback to enhance training effectiveness. *Proceedings of the Human Factors Society 35th Annual Meeting, Santa Monica*, pp. 1400–3. Human Factors Society.

Proteau, L. and Cournoyer, L. (1990). Vision of the stylus in a manual aiming task: the effects of practice. *Q. J. Exp. Psychol.*, **42B**, 811–28.

Salmoni, A. W., Schmidt, R. A. and Walter, C. B. (1984). Knowledge of results and motor learning: a review and critical appraisal. *Psychol. Bull.*, **95**, 355–86.

Schmidt, R. A. (1975). A schema theory of discrete motor learning. *Psychol. Rev.*, **82**, 225–60.

Schmidt, R. A. (1991). *Motor Learning and Performance: From Principles to Practice*. Human Kinetics.

Shea, C. H. and Kohl, R. M. (1990). Specificity and variability of practice. *Res. Q. Exer. Sport*, **61(2)**, 169–77.

Swinnen, S. P. (1990). Interpolated activities during the knowledge of results delay and post-knowledge of results interval: effects of performance and learning. *J. Exp. Psychol: Learning Memory Cognition*, **16**, 692–705.

Thelen, E. (1992). Development as a dynamic system. *Curr. Dir. Psychol. Sci.*, **1**, 189–93.

Turvey, M. T. (1990). Co-ordination. *Am. Psychol.*, **45(8)**, 938–53.

Werbos, P. J. (1994). Self-organization: re-examining the basics and an alternative to the Big Bang. In *Origins: Brain and Self Organization* (K. Pribram, ed.), pp. 16–52. Erlbaum.

Winstein, C. J. and Schmidt, R. A. (1990). Reduced frequency of knowledge of results enhances motor skill learning. *J. Exp. Psychol.: Learning Memory Cognition*, **16**, 677–91.

Wulf, G., Shea, C. H. and Matschiner, S. (1998). Frequent feedback enhances complex motor skill learning. *J. Motor Behav.*, **30**, 180–92.

7

Biomechanics and its application to coaching practice

Simon Coleman

- The understanding and application of Newton's laws of motion to coaching
- The different areas of sports biomechanics
- Measurement techniques in qualitative and quantitative sports biomechanics
- Links between biomechanics and other sports sciences
- Biomechanical analysis of sports techniques
- Fault identification and correction using biomechanics
- Problems and limitations of sports biomechanics for the sports coach
- Future predictions in the use of biomechanics in sports coaching

Introduction

In the fifteenth century, Leonardo da Vinci wrote:

> Mechanical science is the noblest and above all other, the most useful, seeing that by means of it, all animated bodies which have movement perform all their actions

(Ariel and Amherst, 1979). However, it was not until Isaac Newton published his *Principia* in 1687 that a full and correct understanding of the laws of motion was gained. These laws remain the foundation for all human movement and, despite being superseded at quantum and astronomical levels by the laws of Heisenberg and Einstein, provide the fundamental relationships between forces and motion during everyday life.

Newton's three laws of motion (and the law of gravitation) are critical to an understanding of sports performance, and it is therefore appropriate to describe them at this early stage and to illustrate them with examples from sport.

The first law states:

> Every body continues in its state of rest, or of uniform motion in a right (straight) line, unless it is compelled to change that state by forces impressed upon it

(Cohen and Westfall, 1995). This means that an object (or the human body) will stay at rest, or continue moving in a straight line at constant speed, unless acted upon by an unbalanced force. For example, a ball will stay at rest until hit or kicked, and will then keep moving in a straight line unless a force (gravity, air resistance or lift) acts upon it to curve the flight. It is worthwhile noting that this means that objects will continue in their motion without an external force to drive them (although a driving force may be needed to overcome gravity or friction, which are slowing them down).

The second of Newton's laws states:

> The change of motion is proportional to the motive force impressed; and is made in the direction of the right (straight) line in which that force is impressed

(Cohen and Westfall, 1995). This is often translated as force = mass × acceleration, where acceleration is defined as a change in motion and mass the amount of matter in an object. This implies that the greater the required change in motion of an object, the greater the force that has to be applied. For example, a tennis player wishing to hit a fast serve must apply greater forces than required to hit a slow serve. The force must also be in the correct direction, as any object will change its movement in the direction of the force. Thus, the muscle forces required to move limbs must be applied in the correct directions, otherwise incorrect or unintended actions will result.

Finally, Newton's third law states:

> For every action there is always opposed an equal reaction; or, the mutual actions of two bodies upon each other are always equal, and directed to contrary parts

(Cohen and Westfall, 1995). This law is well known by non-scientists, but its comprehension is often incomplete. There must be two bodies involved (although not necessarily in contact), the forces on the two bodies must be opposite in direction but equal in size and occur at the same time, and there must be no 'ownership' of the forces. For example, a small rugby player in collision with a larger moving one will experience exactly the same size of force as the other (although in the opposite direction). It is Newton's second law that explains why the smaller player is knocked backwards (he or she has less mass, and so the same size force causes a greater acceleration).

It should be noted that these laws apply to all forces normally experienced by the human body, whether they are muscular forces, 'lift' forces, air resistance or contact forces. The important aspect is that Newton's laws of motion relate the forces to the ensuing motion.

The science of biomechanics is the application of these mechanics to the human body and sporting implements, and studies the forces on (and caused by) the human body and the subsequent results of those forces. Sports performance is at the heart of the coaching process. It is the transformation of sports performance that is the essential and defining element of the process. Clearly, an understanding and awareness of the application of biomechanical principles to sports performance is an important part of the coach's technical repertoire. This chapter will describe biomechanics and biomechanical methods of analysis, move on to the application of biomechanics within the coaching process and, finally, suggest future directions for biomechanics research and application in coaching. Sporting examples are used wherever possible, with particular reference to those sports in which the author has some expertise.

Kinetics and kinematics

Kinetics is the direct study of the forces on or by the human body, and usually requires the use of force transducers to convert the forces into measurable signals. This is relatively simple for external forces created by the human body or other objects, and devices such as force platforms, force pedals and dynamometers are often used to give insights into the forces of human motion. However, forces created within the human body (usually by muscles) are more difficult to measure. The direct measurement of these forces would require surgical intervention to attach force transducers to muscles (or more usually tendons). Whilst this is a recognized procedure in animal studies, only one group has attempted to carry this out on humans by attaching a buckle transducer to a subject's calcaneal (Achilles) tendon (Komi *et al.*, 1987; Komi, 1990). There are obvious ethical considerations for this type of work – let alone the difficulty of finding volunteers for the research!

Kinematics is the measurement of the changes in motion caused by both internal and external forces. This field of study does not seek to measure the forces, but simply to record accurate position and time information about the human body's motion in space. From these two variables, other measurements such as velocity and acceleration can be calculated. The collection of the position–time data is relatively easy, usually requiring the use of one or more cameras to record the movement of the body. Procedures for the recording of this type of information are well established, and do not present a major problem for the sports biomechanist (Challis *et al.*, 1997).

If internal forces are required, it is possible to employ inverse dynamics. This method uses the kinematic data with anthropometric measures (such as limb masses and moments of inertia) to calculate joint torques (turning forces) and forces. However, it is only possible to calculate net joint torques and forces (the difference between all torques and forces applied), and so the contributions of individual muscles are very difficult to ascertain. There have been recent studies (Baltzopoulos and Iossifidou, 1998) in which inverse dynamics combined with computer modelling has been used to try to quantify muscle forces, but these studies are limited to very simple movements, such as knee extension in one plane. Another difficulty with inverse dynamics arises due to the problems of measurement errors. The kinematic data utilized will always contain errors due to digitization or recording limitations (particularly in accelerations), and anthropometric variables are usually calculated from standardized tables. The combination of these errors, along with uncertainties in joint centre positions (unless multiple X-rays are used), can make the calculation of muscle forces hazardous and, in the worst case, incorrect (Challis, 1997). Fortunately for the sports biomechanist and the coach, there is much useful information to be gained from simple kinematic analysis, such as limb paths, movement patterns and displacements, velocities and accelerations of joints and body segments.

Finally, there is the technique of forward dynamics. This uses mathematical modelling (often with a microcomputer) and kinetic data to produce simulated movements of the body. The input data for the models usually consists of anthropometric parameters and the initial position of the body, from which subsequent positions can be calculated. Muscle forces can also be incorporated to examine the effects of voluntary movements. However, forward dynamics has several limitations. First, it is limited to (mathematically) simple actions such as gymnastics or diving. This is due to the mathematics becoming indeterminate or unsolvable for more complex actions (particularly those involving opponents, tactics or external objects). Secondly, it requires the use of a powerful computer to solve the equations. Finally, there is often a lack of realism due to the simplifications required to make the mathematics manageable. None the less, the forward dynamics method has been used to gain useful insights into sporting techniques, three examples of which will be given here. Yeadon *et al.* (1990) and Yeadon (1998) modelled airborne gymnastic techniques in order to examine different methods of twisting during somersaults. By examining the trading of angular momentum around the three principal axes of the body (twist, somersault and tilt), he found that gymnasts used different methods to create the required twisting movements. He then modified the actions to create new methods for twisting, and it was possible to teach these to gymnasts who had never previously used these techniques. Alexander (1991) simulated three different methods of throwing (pushing, underarm and overhand), and found that there were optimal time delays between extension of the different joints. If the distal segments were moved too early, the proximal segments had not reached maximum speed, but if they were moved too late, then the proximal segments were already slowing down. Alexander gave different time values depending on the mass of the object being thrown, and applied this to shot putting, bowling and softball pitching. Finally, Bobbert and Van Ingen Schenau (1988) studied the timing of lower limb movements in vertical jumping. By using a forward dynamics model, they found that maximal performance was reached if muscles were sequenced from proximal (hip extensors) to distal (ankle extensors). These three examples show that, despite limitations, forward dynamics can be useful in biomechanical simulations.

Links between biomechanics and the other sports sciences

While biomechanics seeks to determine forces and movements of the human body, it does not say anything about the method of control of these variables. The link with motor control and motor learning is therefore a very important one if the regulation of human movement is an objective. Unfortunately, for many years motor control studies simply examined outcome measures (Schmidt, 1991), and did not seek to examine the methods by which various movements were made. Since the 1980s, however, there has been a stronger interest in the control and regulation of muscle force and segmental movement. Work by authors such as Kelso (1995) has sought to determine the factors that are controlled during human movement, and often uses biomechanical methods and models to examine such questions. The link between these areas will undoubtedly become stronger in the future.

The overlap between biomechanics and exercise physiology is also important. The forces within the human body usually arise from the muscles, and so the timing and magnitude of muscular contraction is important. Monitoring of these factors is usually carried out with electromyography (EMG) and, despite the weak relationship between the EMG signal and muscle force (Burden and Bartlett, 1997), important information regarding muscle recruitment can be obtained via this source. In addition, the use of neuromuscular modelling has helped to develop an understanding of the relative importance of the contractile elements and elastic components within the working muscle. This has also led to an improved comprehension of the importance of the storage of elastic energy during human movement, particularly in walking, running and jumping (Alexander, 1994).

The links between biomechanics and sports psychology are less obvious. One area where the relationship may be seen is that of relaxation. Sports psychologists may use EMG or biofeedback devices to check whether various muscles are relaxed or contracted, either during performance or mental imagery. While relaxation of the antagonist muscles during a dynamic action (except at the end of the movement, where they are used to slow the limbs) may be a sound theoretical concept, there has been little detailed study as to whether this is necessary or achievable in sports performance. It is also unlikely to be of use during slow, guided actions (such as golf putting), as in this type of activity both agonists and antagonists are active.

In summary, it might be argued from a deterministic point of view that biomechanics is the most important of the sports sciences, as the body must conform to Newtonian mechanics during movement. An understanding of biomechanics could therefore be seen as crucial to sports analysis, particularly in technical sports such as gymnastics, track and field athletics and swimming. A more holistic view of the sports sciences would argue that a multidisciplinary approach is required (Nigg, 1993), and the links between each science may be as important as the core fundamentals.

Methods of biomechanical analysis for sports performance

In practice, biomechanical analysis is often divided into two areas; qualitative and quantitative. However, these analyses are not exclusive, and are often performed together as part of a more extensive study.

Regardless of which of the two methods is used, the initial step of biomechanical analysis is the development of a performance model that identifies the relationships between the result and the factors that produce that result (Hay and Reid, 1987). This is often produced as a block diagram, and an example for the high jump is shown in Figure 7.1. This part of a biomechanical analysis is critical, as identification of incorrect factors (or omission of important elements) will invalidate any conclusions drawn about the performance. At this stage it is also possible to treat as constant (and thus rule out) those factors over which the performer has little or no control (for example, the acceleration due to gravity or the effects of air resistance).

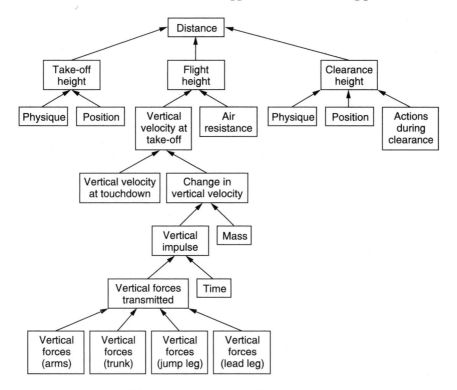

Figure 7.1 Biomechanical factors in the high jump (after Hay and Reid, 1987).

The next step is to observe or measure the performance of the skill. In a qualitative analysis, this will often involve visual observation or video recording. In a quantitative approach, it may involve the use of force transducers and/or digitized video or cine film. Nevertheless, systematic procedures must be applied to both methods in order to allow for the observer's perceptual mechanisms (in the qualitative case) or the equipment design (in the quantitative analysis). The latter case has been clearly understood for many years, with camera parameters, electronics characteristics and system requirements all well determined (e.g. Miller and Nelson, 1973; Winter, 1979; Atwater, 1981). On the other hand, it is only recently that qualitative biomechanical observation systems have come under close scrutiny (Hay and Reid, 1987; McPherson, 1996; Knudson and Morrison, 1997). This research gives useful advice to coaches who wish to examine the technical aspects of performance but do not have access to expensive equipment.

The identification of faults or deviations from the intended actions is usually the next step. Watkins (1987) refers to two methods of qualitative fault analysis; sequential and mechanical. The first method involves the breakdown of the performance into sequential phases containing body positions that are compared to 'ideal' mental images held by the observer (Hay and Reid, 1987). This technique may be seen in gymnastics judging, where correct forms of the movement are awarded points, and incorrect body positions lose points. The limitation of this method of fault analysis is that it does not have any sound theoretical basis, and the ideal image may not be a mechanically sound one. It is also unlikely that revolutionary techniques (for example, the 'Fosbury flop' high jump) would evolve using sequential analysis, as the ideal technique is often simply that used by the current champions. The alternative method of fault diagnosis is mechanically based. Using a model as described above, it is possible to identify which factors are capable of modification for improved performance. This does demand, however, that the performance model be referred to repeatedly during the course of the analysis, and that differences in knowledge, observational skills and experience may mean that coaches may vary in their interpretation of the sports technique to be analysed (Hay and Reid, 1987). The strength of the mechanical analysis (as well as its theoretical soundness) is that it is unlikely that important factors in the performance will be overlooked, as each biomechanical variable in the model will be considered in turn when diagnosing faults.

Once faults are identified, it is necessary to assess their relative level of importance. McPherson (1996) mentions 'primary' and 'secondary' errors, but does not give more information on how these are delineated; however, Hay and Reid (1987) describe faults that are caused by other faults, and it is assumed that these are secondary. Once primary errors have been determined, they must be prioritized. Hay and Reid (1987) state that the prioritization is determined by the variable(s) that would give the greatest improvement in the time available for correction. For example, a 10 per cent increase in the speed of release of a shot putt would typically give an 11 times greater performance increase (in distance thrown) than a 10 per cent increase in release angle. This is due to the distance being directly related to the square of the speed, but only to the sine of the angle.

Once the faults have been prioritized, it is necessary to communicate them to the performer, and to attempt to coach corrections. However, it is not the role of this chapter to review the literature regarding effective coaching communication.

The application of biomechanics to the coaching process

Theoretical knowledge

Fairs' (1987) opinion was that coaching practice has traditionally been based on 'custom, intuition and common sense', rather than on sound training principles, scientific fact or empirical evidence (Cross and Ellice, 1997). This might also be pertinent to the application of biomechanics to coaching. Few authors on the coaching process mention biomechanical principles (for example, Lyle, 1996; Cross and Ellice, 1997), even though they vaguely refer to 'scientific testing'.

Lyle (1996) identifies 12 essential elements in the coaching process. The first (Lyle does not state whether the 12 components are chronological or hierarchical) is that of an information base. While he mentions the athlete's psychological, physical, sociological and educational factors, as well as the sports milieu, nowhere does he identify the source of the theoretical basis for technique. It may be argued that 'for coaches, a knowledge of biomechanics might well be regarded as essential' (Hay, 1994). If a coach does not have a sound understanding of the biomechanical factors underlying successful (and unsuccessful) techniques, then he or she has to resort to three other avenues for teaching technique: aping the techniques of champions (described as 'cookbook science' by Dunbar, 1995); 'educated guesswork' using intuition and experience; or employing a specialist sports biomechanist. None of these methods can be seen as the ideal – whilst the coach may arrive at a successful technique by trial and error, much time and athlete potential may be wasted.

This is not intended to be overly critical of coaches. Biomechanical principles are inherent in the techniques learned by coaches through coach education and experience. It could be true to say, however, that biomechanical analysis has largely been dependent on the coaches' observations, since specialist sports biomechanists are not available to the great majority of coaches. Nevertheless, there is clearly room for considerable improvement in coaching practice.

Over 20 years ago, Norman (1975) sought to make such a contribution. He suggested that there were 10 biomechanical principles that the coach should understand in order to teach sports techniques. These were intended for use with qualitative analysis (often the only methods available to the coach), and were specifically designed for technique error correction. The 10 principles listed by Norman were (Knudson and Morrison, 1997):

1. Summation of joint torques
2. Continuity of joint torques
3. Impulse
4. Direction of force application
5. Equilibrium
6. Summation of body velocities
7. Generation of angular momentum
8. Conservation of angular momentum
9. Manipulation of moment of inertia
10. Manipulation of body-segment angular momentum.

While there is insufficient space to give examples for all of these principles, several will be illustrated with a sporting application. Impulse, the force–time integral (the sum of force × time of force application) and the direction of force application are crucially important in jumping events. The change in momentum (for a body of constant mass, this equals the change in velocity) is equal to the impulse applied. This means that, if a large change in momentum of the body is required, a large impulse must be applied to it. This comes from applying a large impulse to the ground and (by Newton's third law) the ground then applies this impulse back to the body which, being less massive than earth, moves. The large impulse implies a large force, a large time of force application, or both. In high jumping, this is made possible by the heel–toe movement during the take-off stride and by the body position and limb movements maximizing the vertical force and time of application. Unfortunately, in long jumping a large foot–ground contact time acts to brake the body (as the foot is initially ahead of the body), and long jumpers do not maximize the time of force application, but seek to maximize the force applied.

The last four principles listed by Norman are of vital importance during activities involving rotation (such as gymnastic somersaulting). Angular momentum may be understood as the potential for rotation, and this must be maximized at take-off if the gymnast is to complete multiple rotations. The angular momentum is generated by applying a torque at take-off – in other words, the force from the ground is not directed through the body's centre of gravity. The gymnast usually accomplishes this by leaning in the direction of rotation, and by applying a force to the ground in the correct direction. Once in the air, angular momentum is conserved, and the gymnast can only change the rotation by altering one constituent of angular momentum (moment of inertia) by changing body position to change the other component (speed of rotation). Thus, correct amounts of angular momentum are critical for the performance of gymnastic stunts.

The 10 principles identified by Norman (1975) finally became the biomechanical foundation for coach education programmes in Canada (Coaching Association of Canada, 1998).

In Britain, the National Coaching Foundation (NCF) has attempted to improve the biomechanical knowledge of coaches. In its coach education programme there is a home study guide, *An Introduction to Sports Mechanics* (Sprunt, 1993), which seeks to give the coach a basic understanding of the biomechanical fundamentals of various human movements such as starting, stopping, and moving. This is then followed by NCF advanced workshops on Sports Mechanics and Analysing Performance, which endeavour to build on this information. However, the NCF is phasing out the Sports Mechanics workshops and replacing them with Technique Analysis workshops, which will concentrate on the biomechanics of technical sports such as gymnastics, diving and athletics. Whilst this may make the content more comprehensible for coaches, it may also lead to the misunderstanding that biomechanics is not important in other sports.

National governing bodies vary in their teaching of biomechanics within their award schemes. It would be inappropriate to survey all awards for all sports in this chapter, and therefore two schemes are contrasted here. Swimming contains biomechanical factors such as buoyancy, propulsion, resistance, rotation and transfer of momentum in its level II (or NVQ level III) award (Amateur Swimming Association, 1996). In such a technical sport this is not surprising, and a case may be made for introduction of these factors at a lower level. In contrast, volleyball, while examining skilled techniques, does not explicitly mention biomechanical principles. Neither the national association (Scottish Volleyball Association, 1994) nor the international governing body (FIVB) mention biomechanics explicitly in their coach education materials. Vague biomechanical principles ('if players bend their bodies too much or too little, they cannot jump higher at take off', FIVB (Level 1), 1989) are alluded to, but it is surprising that the mechanical fundamentals of balance, force production, linear and angular momentum are not taught to volleyball coaches. Omissions such as these have led to teaching technique errors – many spikers (attackers) are taught hitting actions whilst standing on the ground, when the action must be performed in the air. On the ground, forces and torques can be applied to the earth to maintain body position; in the air, this is simply not possible, and any forces and torques created in one part of the body create an opposite effect on another part. This often leads to unexpected effects in the air (particularly with beginners), and creates problems for the player who wishes to maintain a body position in flight. If coaches were aware of the conservation of angular momentum (once in the air angular momentum stays the same, and any rotation created causes an opposite rotation in another part of the body), they would seek to make all spiking (hitting) technique changes while the player is airborne (or perhaps suspended by a twisting belt). It is recognized, however, that optimum biomechanical learning may have to be balanced against practical organizational demands in participation level coaching.

Biomechanics and performance analysis

Performance analysis was also listed by Lyle (1996) as one of his key concepts of the coaching process. He noted that one of the primary components of sports performance is technique and, as 'biomechanics is the science underlying techniques' (Hay, 1994), it would seem logical that a coach should have a good understanding of not only the biomechanical principles involved in a particular performance, but also of the different methods for biomechanics analysis (as mentioned in a previous section). This is particularly important for the performance coach, for whom small increments of improvement may be very significant.

The main analysis tool available to the coach will usually be visual processes and perception. The addition of video recording and playback facilities (particularly in slow motion) will greatly assist the coach in assessing and improving technique. Qualitative analysis is usually the only technique available to the coach. It is often *more* difficult to identify biomechanical factors by this method than by using quantitative procedures, and the coach must be aware of those biomechanical factors that underpin the technique being studied. This makes it even more critical that a biomechanically accurate model is used as the first stage of the analysis. However, this does not mean that coaches will always have to design a biomechanical model themselves. There are many examples of performance/technique models available in the scientific literature and, as previously mentioned, no biomechanical study (whether qualitative or quantitative) should have been carried out without first identifying the model which is appropriate to the task. As the originator of the biomechanical performance diagram, Hay (1994) is a particularly fertile source for models, and coaches would often benefit from referring to this work.

Naturally, different sports will demand different levels of biomechanical knowledge and analysis. Gymnastics sports, field athletics and swimming are sports in which technique may be seen as the critical factor in a less or more successful performance. Long distance running or cycling, however, may be more dependent on physiological capacities, and other events (such as target sports) may rely on psychological factors. Nonetheless, it could be argued that, as the human being is a mechanical system during motion, biomechanics impinges on all sporting actions and that, in running, cycling or swimming, mechanical efficiency is as important as biochemical and morphological factors when determining success or failure.

Practical use of biomechanics in coaching

A simple example of the use of biomechanics in coaching is that of teaching gymnasts rotational activities (particularly somersaulting). If a gymnast is trying to carry out a somersault but is failing to complete it (either by under- or over-rotation), the coach may look to biomechanical principles to provide an explanation for the errors in technique. Airborne rotational activities require a certain amount of angular momentum to be generated prior to take-off, as once in flight the total amount of angular momentum of the body cannot be changed. Thus, if insufficient angular momentum is created prior to (and at) take-off, certain gymnastic stunts will not be possible. Angular momentum is created prior to take-off by previous rotational moves (such as 'round-offs' or backflips), and at take-off by the conversion of linear momentum (run-up velocity) and by forces directed away from the gymnast's centre of gravity. As previously mentioned, once in the air, although angular momentum cannot be changed, it is possible to manipulate one component of angular momentum (moment of inertia) by changing body position to change the other component (speed of rotation). Thus, gymnasts who 'tuck' in a somersault will increase their rate of rotation. Unfortunately, this sometimes leads inexperienced coaches and teachers to concentrate on the body position in flight, whilst omitting the faults prior to or at take-off that originally caused a lack of sufficient angular momentum. Somersaulting also has the complication that the gymnast must gain enough vertical displacement (flight height) to complete the move and, even if there is sufficient angular momentum, low take-off vertical velocity may lead to inadequate height to execute the move. This is why gymnasts performing double backwards somersaults in floor routines actually take-off leaning slightly forward. Whilst this slightly reduces the angular momentum that has been gained by prior moves and the high speed of approach, it allows the gymnast to time hip, knee and ankle extensions to gain a high vertical velocity, thus maximizing the flight height and giving the gymnast a chance of completing the two rotations. Figure 7.2 illustrates the take-off positions for a backflip, single somersault and double somersault. The biomechanical aims of these three moves are to maximize angular momentum (for the backflip), optimize angular momentum and vertical take-off velocity (for the single somersault), and maximize vertical take-off velocity (while maintaining sufficient angular momentum) for the double somersault.

The following examples illustrate the use of quantitative data in coaching techniques, both in kinetics and kinematics.

Figure 7.3 shows the output from one of a pair of pedals specially designed to measure the forces during cycling. The pedal forces were transformed into effective (those which are at 90° to the crank) and ineffective (those which are directed along the crank) forces. Obviously, it would be of benefit to a cyclist to attempt to maximize the effective forces and minimize the ineffective forces for maximum mechanical efficiency. Unfortunately this is not easy to identify qualitatively, as not only the size of the pedal forces but also the pedal and crank position will affect the effective and ineffective forces. The force pedals therefore provide a way of demonstrating these to the cyclist or coach. An on-line system has been used in our laboratory (Coleman and Hale, 1998) to present real-time displays that allow the cyclist

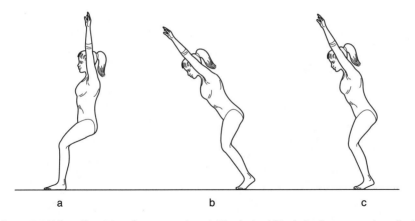

Figure 7.2 Take-off positions for gymnastic activities (a–backflip; b–back somersault; c–double back somersault

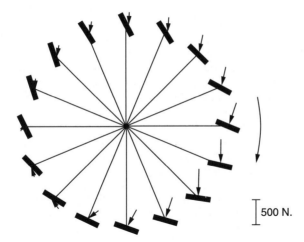

500 N.

Figure 7.3 Output from force pedal

to manipulate the pedal forces and angles and observe the effects on the effective and ineffective forces. It is then possible to employ different techniques and monitor the mechanical changes in pedalling effectiveness.

The next example shows the use of biomechanics in golf. A Scottish golf professional was attempting to modify his technique so that he could eliminate a slight 'draw' (right to left sideways movement of the ball in the air) and play a straight shot or a 'fade' (left to right sideways movement of the ball in the air). A three-dimensional biomechanical video analysis was carried out, and the swing path of the club head was noted. Figure 7.4a shows the swing path viewed from behind the golfer. It can be seen that the club moves on an in-to-out path on the downswing, thus creating a draw. Further biomechanical analysis suggested that this was due to incorrect left shoulder rotation. As the left elbow is kept extended on the downswing, the left arm

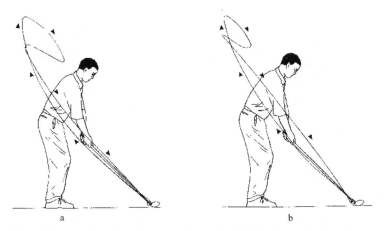

Figure 7.4 a. Swing path before biomechanical analysis b. Swing path after biomechanical analysis.

acts as a single rigid link, and any incorrect movement at the shoulder will be transmitted to the club. Therefore, a suggestion was made to correct this by correcting the left shoulder rotation. The movement of the left shoulder in Figure 7.4b shows the new club-head path being slightly out-to-in after instruction, thus creating a fade. Ten days after this instruction, the professional broke the course record at one of Scotland's top courses, and he attributed a large part of this to the control rendered by the swing modifications. This improvement has so far been retained, and the golfer is considering taking part in the European Tour in the next year.

The final quantitative example illustrates the use that can be made of mathematical data. Shot putting is a fairly simple projectile problem, but it is sometimes difficult for a coach to assess which parameters need to be changed and, if so, by how much. The current Scottish record-holder was analysed prior to the 1996 season to examine biomechanically both his (rotational) technique and important projectile variables (height of release, angle of release and speed of release). These were found to be 1.86 m, 35.41° and 12.86 ms^{-1} respectively. Using the performance model shown in Figure 7.5, and the recommendation of Hay and Reid (1987) that performance improvement should focus upon the variable which gives the greatest result in the time available, it was decided that the athlete needed to increase the speed of release to at least 13 ms^{-1}. Therefore, it was necessary to examine the athlete's technique for possible improvements to this end. The forces applied to the shot (a function of muscle strength and limb movements) and the distance through which the shot travels (and thus the time to accelerate the shot) are seen at the base of Figure 7.5. The muscular strength component was seen as a longer-term change, dependent on strength training in the off-season, and so it was decided to work on increasing the shot acceleration at the beginning of the throw (during the first turn) so that a higher velocity could be reached at release. This entailed altering the position of the limbs (particularly the legs) so that they lay closer to the axis of rotation, thus reducing the moment of inertia and making it easier to turn

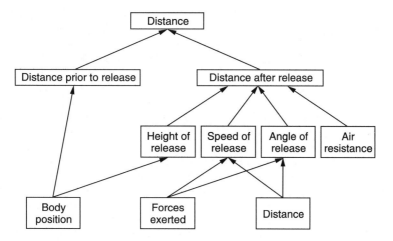

Figure 7.5 Basic factors in shot putting (adapted from Hay, 1994)

faster. The result was that the athlete managed to improve his release velocity, increase his personal best by 0.40 m and set a new Scottish record.

These examples show how biomechanics can assist the coach in improving techniques, thereby making gains in performance.

Issues with biomechanics and applications to coaching

There are two major conceptual problems with attempts to use biomechanics in the coaching process – the understanding of Newton's laws of motion, and the application of mathematics to sport.

Researchers in science education (particularly in physics) have shown that public understanding of Newtonian laws of motion is low (Warren, 1979; Hestenes *et al.*, 1992). There is difficulty in separating real forces from other mechanical variables (mass, momentum, impetus), and there is an intuitive misunderstanding of principles such as Newton's first law of motion (forces *change* motion, not *cause* it). This is not helped by some biomechanics or coaching texts that indicate that forces cause or try to cause motion. When undergraduate sports science students are asked which forces act on a golf ball during its flight, very high numbers (sometimes 100 per cent) indicate that the force of the hit (or impetus) is active throughout the flight. In reality, of course, the force only acts when the club and ball are in contact (Messenger and Sidors, 1994). After the ball leaves the club face, the only forces acting upon it are gravity, air resistance (drag) and lift (due to the Magnus effect). Very few texts seek to correct these intuitive problems, and so beginner coaches often require 'deprogramming' before absorbing correct biomechanical education.

The second problem is that biomechanics is by its nature, mathematical. A correct understanding of Newton's laws of motion, a suitable performance model and qualitative analysis can give important insights into techniques.

However, quantitative analysis requires a sound mathematical underpinning. The relationships between various mechanical variables (such as angular momentum around different axes) are much easier to understand if the practitioner has a working knowledge of calculus and other mathematical techniques. It might be unreasonable to expect the coach to also be a mathematician, and the only option is to work with specialist sports scientists where this kind of analysis is necessary, and for sport biomechanists to improve their dissemination of applications. For example, there has been some interesting work on the mechanical basis of various gymnastics techniques (twisting somersaults, vaulting, bar dismounts), but these research papers require a strong mathematical grounding (Yeadon, 1989). While a coach reading a physiological or psychologically based study might understand a large amount of the content and language, mathematically based biomechanics papers can often appear incomprehensible to the layperson. It is true that these are usually written for specialist readers, but it is not unusual for coaches to sample the sports science literature to improve their knowledge. The intimidation presented by applied mathematics to the average coach should not be underestimated, and a useful suggestion might be for researchers to write less mathematical versions of the same paper for inclusion in technical or professional journals (for example, the papers by Grimshaw *et al.*, 1994 and Salo *et al.*, 1997).

Finally, Bartlett (1998) and Sanders (1998) have used a cautionary account of the propulsive forces in swimming to illustrate that biomechanical analysis does not always lead directly to correct conclusions. Counsilman (1971) and Schleihauf (1974) suggested that elite freestyle swimmers use sculling motions with their hands pitched to use lift forces as the dominant means of propulsion. Despite some arguments about whether Bernoulli's principles (the hand is shaped like an aerofoil and, in moving at high speed through the water, creates low pressure in front of it) or Newton's laws (the hand angle is pitched to gain lift and drag) applied, it was still proposed that lift was used (Sprigings and Koehler, 1990) as the main force for propulsion. This seemed to be supported by the fact that freestyle swimmers create a curved path of the hand through the water. However, papers by Hay *et al.* (1993) and Liu *et al.* (1993) showed that the S-shaped hand path is due to body roll. Instead of an insweep (hand moving towards the body) followed by an outsweep, as originally thought, it was actually observed that the opposite was happening. The swimmers tried to straighten the path of the arm so as to use drag force (from Newton's third law) as the major form of propulsion. In fact, Sanders (1998) reported lift and drag data acquired using a hand model in an underwater testing tank, which showed that the greatest propulsive force was obtained when the hand was pitched at right-angles to the water flow. In other words, all the force came from drag (by Newton's third law, if the hand pushes backwards on the water, the water pushes forward on the hand). When he combined this with three-dimensional kinematic analysis of elite swimmers, Sanders found that the subjects pitched their hands at about 60° to the water, indicating that the dominant force was drag. Bartlett (1998) suggested that the original work by Counsilman and Schleihauf had relied on qualitative analysis that was flawed due to an incorrect analysis of body roll and hand action. Unfortunately, in the absence of contrary evidence from researchers, many swimming coaches had embraced the idea of lift propulsion, and incorrect changes may therefore have been made to a number of swimmers' techniques. It is interesting to note that swimming records still improved over this time, suggesting that successful coaches ignored lift forces, successful swimmers ignored their coaches, that incremental improvements from such changes in technique are relatively small, or that other aspects (such a physiological changes) outweighed the apparently inappropriate technique alterations.

Limitations of biomechanics

Whilst biomechanics can give many important insights into sports techniques, it cannot answer all the questions in this area posed by coaches and athletes. This may be for several reasons.

First, the mathematics may be insolvable or indeterminate, particularly when there are multi-joint motions involved. Each joint has six degrees of freedom and, if full modelling and mathematical solutions are required, complexity can soon become an insurmountable problem. Therefore, there are authors (such as Hatze, 1998) who suggest that, until complete models (including mechanical, neuromuscular, motor control and physiological elements) are available, many questions will remain unanswered. The effort required to find, compute and interpret these models may require a large, multidisciplinary team – an unrealistic expectation for the majority of coaches and athletes in terms of expertise, location and finances, although national institutes of sport may be expected to approach this goal. Other researchers disagree with this mode of approach (Alexander, 1991), and suggest that simple models may give useful insights into sports performance, in addition to being easily solvable.

Secondly, the use of electromyography to examine muscular actions in a sporting performance is a useful tool, but is only an approximation to the actual muscle contractions taking place. As has already been noted, the size of the EMG signal is not directly related to the force exerted by the muscle, and the use of surface electrodes limits accurate recording to those signals emanating from superficial muscles. In-dwelling electrodes are available (Nigg and Herzog, 1994), but are not suitable for analysis of dynamic movements. Consequently, it is difficult to validate muscle models and simulations. The unknown contributions of each muscle means that models have to use reduction (where muscles with similar actions are grouped together), cross-sectional analysis (it is assumed that muscles contribute forces proportional to their cross-sectional area) or optimization (An *et al.*, 1995). These limitations make it very difficult to provide a full muscular analysis of complex sporting actions. This may cause problems when seeking to identify causes of muscular or soft tissue injuries, or when attempting to design weight-training schedules.

Up to the present time, there has been very little biomechanical research carried out on performance variability and its causes. Many biomechanical studies simply analyse a single performance (often best or average), and then use group data to investigate relationships between mechanical variables. This has been called 'correlational research' (Mullineaux and Bartlett, 1997) and, while it may give insights into sports techniques, it may be criticized for three reasons. First, many studies use only a limited sample (for example, elite performers), and so correlational techniques may give reduced r-values due to a limited range in the variables being examined (Howell, 1992). Secondly, correlational studies are sometimes carried out with little consideration for the underlying theoretical relationships. For example, Mero *et al.* (1994) correlated the range thrown during a javelin event with the release speed, when in reality a squared relationship is predicted by Newtonian mechanics (Douglas, 1998). Finally, group research does not say anything about intra-individual variability. One of the most important questions posed by the coach and athlete may be 'why is performance different from day-to-day?' While the superficial answer may be injury, mental state or environment, there is little information concerning the effects these have on the mechanical interactions of the body and imple-ments. Only recently (Morriss, 1997) has this question begun to be answered in a biomechanical way. Morriss' work started from the premise that single variable analysis was insufficient to show changes that affected those actually seen in performance. Therefore, he examined conjugate cross-correlations between pairs of variables for the same athlete over time (from good and poor performances), and identified some important mechanical differences. This links well with some motor control research (Grealy *et al.*, 1999) which looked at 'coupling' between various joints, and found differences between novice and expert gymnasts. This type of research may prove important in future biomechanical analyses, and give useful insights into variability.

Finally, biomechanics has not been greatly used in tactical analyses. It may be useful in sport to be aware of an opponent's technical weaknesses and the tactical opportunities that this offers. However, it is questionable whether a full biomechanical analysis is required for a coach to appreciate tactical advantages, and a qualitative view, backed up by performance statistics, may be sufficient. An example may be useful in illustrating possibilities in this area. During preparation for a European qualifying tie, the England volleyball coach requested a qualitative mechanical analysis of the main opposition attacker. The analysis noted that, due to foot placement and trunk position at take-off, the attacker would have trouble hitting in one particular direction, and this was borne out by previous match statistics. This allowed the coach to set his defence accordingly, and so he was able to neutralize successfully the threat posed by this opponent. Mechanical analysis of sporting objects and implements (balls and rackets/sticks) can also give information about tactical possibilities during matches. The paper by Kao *et al.* (1994) provides a fine example here, showing not only an aerodynamic analysis of a volleyball after impact, but also the coaching implications for hitting over a block or into specific court areas.

Biomechanics and coaching in the future

There have been several papers in the past decade (Yeadon and Challis, 1992; Zatsiorsky and Fortney, 1993; Nigg, 1993) looking toward biomechanics in the future. The only certainty is that some of their predictions will be wrong.

While it is simpler to speculate on advances in equipment and technology in biomechanics, it is much more difficult to hypothesize about the improvements in the knowledge of biomechanics and its use in coaching. As has been previously identified, the way forward may be the combination of support scientists into multidisciplinary teams (including sports science and sports medicine) in order to support one or more athletes. At one time, the team supporting Martina Navratilova had 22 members, ranging from coaching through nutrition to psychology. Whilst sports science support in Great Britain has been provided by the Sports Science Support Programme (and latterly within the World Class Performance Plans), it has often been fragmented and inconsistent. At the time of writing, the introduction of the UK Sports Institute may bring about an improvement in provision at this level, but sports science must be seen as a career if full-time professional support is to be provided to elite athletes and coaches. The alternative is part-time coaches and sports scientists struggling to furnish a variable standard of service to top sportsmen and women. It is unreasonable to expect the coach to be an expert biomechanist, physiologist, psychologist, physiotherapist and nutritionist, but, unless political will exists, this scenario will continue, and many of our sportsmen and women will continue to underachieve in international competition.

Glossary

Acceleration – a change in velocity divided by time. As velocity has size and direction, acceleration can involve a change in speed or direction, or both.

Angular momentum – the moment of inertia of an object multiplied by its angular velocity. Can be thought of as the potential for rotation.

Angular velocity – speed of rotation in a particular direction (e.g. clockwise) about an axis.

Anthropometry – the study of the dimensions of the human body (e.g. mass, height).

Centre of mass – the mathematical (i.e. imaginary) point at which all of the mass of an object or body can be considered to act. Commonly known as the centre of gravity.

Digitization – the conversion of analogue data (e.g. a video picture) into digital form (e.g. a computer picture). Often refers to the collection of image co-ordinates from a computer picture.

Displacement – the size and direction of the change of position of an object or body (not to be confused with the displacement of ships, which describes how much water they move when loaded).

Dynamics – the study of objects or bodies which are accelerating (although more commonly, but incorrectly, used to mean objects or bodies in motion).

Electromyography – the measurement of muscle electrical signals

Equilibrium – when the forces and moments upon an object or body are balanced.

Force – that which when applied to an object or body changes (or tries to change) its motion. Forces can act by touching objects or bodies (contact forces), or at a distance (for example, gravity). Forces in biomechanics are often classified as internal (produced by muscles) or external (produced by other objects or bodies). Force is calculated as mass multiplied by acceleration.

Forward dynamics – the calculation of kinematic data and movement by specifying forces and moments on an object or body.

Gravity – the force of attraction between any two particles (inversely related to the square of the distance between them).

Impulse – the size of a force multiplied by its time of application. Impulse is also the change in linear momentum (*q.v.*).

Inverse dynamics – the calculation of forces and moments (*q.v.*) by using kinematic data combined with masses and moments of inertia.

Kinematics – the study of motions, without necessarily concerning the forces causing the motions.

Kinetics – the study of forces, without necessarily examining the resulting motions.

Linear momentum – the mass of an object or body multiplied by its velocity. Can be thought of as the amount of linear motion a body possesses.

Mass – the property that determines how difficult an object or body is to accelerate. It can be loosely described as the amount of matter in an object or body.

Moment – the turning force on an object or body that is pivoted or moving around an axis. Moments are calculated as force multiplied by the perpendicular distance of the force from the pivot/axis. Moments are also known as torques.

Moment of inertia – the property of an object or body that describes how difficult it is to rotate around an axis.

Statics – the study of objects or bodies at rest or moving with constant velocity – in other words, in equilibrium (*q.v.*).

Torque – see moment (*q.v.*).

Transducer – a device to turn one type of measurement (often force) into another measurable variable (often an electrical signal).

Velocity – a change in displacement divided by time. As displacement has size and direction, velocity is how fast and in which direction.

Weight – the force due to the effect of gravity on the mass of an object or body (i.e. mass × acceleration due to gravity). Should be measured in Newtons (not kg or lb).

References

Alexander, R. McN. (1991). Optimum timing of muscle activation for simple models of throwing. *J. Theor. Biol.*, **150**, 349–72.

Alexander, R. McN. (1994). Human elasticity. *Physics Ed.*, **29**, 358–62.

Amateur Swimming Association. (1998). *ASA Teaching and Coaching Certificates Regulations 1998/99*. Amateur Swimming Association.

An, K.-A., Kaufman, K. R. and Chao, E. S. (1995). Estimation of muscle and joint forces. In *Three-Dimensional Analysis of Human Movement* (P. Allard, I. Stokes and J.-P. Blanchi, eds), pp. 201–14. Human Kinetics.

Ariel, G. and Amherst, C. B. A. (1979). The contribution of biomechanics to equipment design and athletic performance. In *Biomechanics of Sport Games and Sport Activities* (A. Ayalon, ed.), pp. 105–30.Wingate Institute for Physical Education and Sport.

Atwater, A. E. (1981). Kinematic analysis in biomechanics cinematography. In *Proceedings of SPIE; 2nd International Symposium of Biomechanical Cinematography and High speed Photography* (J. Terauds, ed.), pp. 242–60. The International Society of Optical Engineering.

Baltzopoulos, V. and Iossifidou, A. (1998). Muscle length and velocity of contraction during isokinetic knee extension: implications for the estimation of *in vivo* force - velocity relationship. *J. Sports Sci.*, **16**, 4–5.

Bartlett, R. (1998). Does biomechanics improve performance? Communication to British Association of Sport and Exercise Sciences Annual Conference, Worcester.

Bobbert, M. and Van Ingen Schenau, G. (1988). Co-ordination in vertical jumping. *J. Biomech.*, **21**, 249–62.

Burden, A. and Bartlett, R. (1997). Electromyography. In *Biomechanical Analysis of Movement in Sport and Exercise* (R. Bartlett, ed.), pp. 37–52. British Association of Sport and Exercise Sciences.

Challis, J. H. (1997). Estimation and propagation of experimental errors. In *Biomechanical Analysis of Movement in Sport and Exercise* (R. Bartlett, ed.), pp. 105–24. British Association of Sport and Exercise Sciences.

Challis, J. H., Bartlett, R. and Yeadon, M. R. (1997). Image-based motion analysis. In *Biomechanical Analysis of Movement in Sport and Exercise* (R. Bartlett, ed.), pp. 7–30. British Association of Sport and Exercise Sciences.

Coaching Association of Canada (1998). *3M National Coaching Certification Program Levels 4 and 5.* http://www.coach.ca/profdev/level45.html.

Cohen, I. B. and Westfall, R. S. (1995). *Newton.* W.W. Norton and Co.

Coleman, S. G. S. and Hale, T. (1998). The use of force pedals for analysis of cycling sprint performance. In *Biomechanics in Sports XVI: Proceedings of the XVIth International Symposium on Biomechanics in Sports* (H. J. Riehle and M. M. Vieten, eds), pp. 138–41. Univesitätsverlag Konstanz.

Counsilman J. E. (1971). The application of Bernoulli's principle to human propulsion in water. In *First International Symposium on Biomechanics in Swimming* (L. Lewillie and J. Clarys, eds), pp. 59–71. Université Libre de Bruxelles.

Cross, N. and Ellice, C. (1997). Coaching effectiveness and the coaching process: field hockey revisited. *Scot. J. Physical Ed.*, **25(3)**, 19–33.

Douglas, A. (1998). Unpublished BSc dissertation. Moray House Institute of Education, Heriot-Watt University.

Dunbar, R. (1995). *The Trouble with Science.* Faber and Faber.

Fairs, J. (1987). The coaching process: the essence of coaching. *Sports Coach*, **11**, 17–19.

FIVB (1989). *Coaches Manual I.* FIVB.

Grealy, M., Craig, C. and Coleman, S. G. S. (1999). Tau-coupling in novice and experienced gymnasts. *Journal of Motor Behaviour* (submitted).

Grimshaw, P., Marar, L., Salo, A. *et al.* (1994). Biomechanical analysis of sprint hurdles. *Athl. Coach*, **28**, 10–12.

Hatze, H. (1998). Biomechanics of sports: selected examples of successful applications and future perspectives. In *Biomechanics in Sports XV: Proceedings of the XVIth International Symposium on Biomechanics in Sports* (H. J. Riehle and M. M. Vieten, eds), pp. 1–22. Universitätsverlag Konstanz.

Hay, J. G. (1994). *Biomechanics of Sports Techniques.* Prentice Hall.

Hay, J. G. and Reid, J. G. (1987). *Anatomy, Mechanics and Human Motion.* Prentice Hall.

Hay, J. G., Liu, Q. and Andrews, J. G. (1993). The influence of body roll on hand path in freestyle swimming: a computer simulation study. *J. Appl. Biomech.*, **9**, 227–37.

Hestenes, D., Wells, M. and Swackhammer, G. (1992). Force concept inventory. *Physics Teach.*, **30**, 141–53.

Howell, D. C. (1992). *Statistical Methods for Psychology*. Duxbury Press.

Kao, S. S., Sellens, R. W. and Stevenson, J. M. (1994). The mathematical trajectory of a spiked volleyball and its coaching application. *J. Appl. Biomech.*, **10**, 95–109.

Kelso, J. A. S. (1995). *Dynamic Patterns*. MIT Press.

Knudson, D. V. and Morrison, C. S. (1997). *Qualitative Analysis of Human Movement*. Human Kinetics.

Komi, P. V. (1990). Relevance of *in vivo* force measurement to human biomechanics. *J. Biomech.*, **23(S1)**, 23–4.

Komi, P. V., Salonen, M., Jarvinen, N. and Kokko, O. (1987). *In vivo* registration of Achilles tendon forces in man. *Int. J. Sports Med.*, **8**, 3–8.

Liu, Q., Hay, J. G. and Andrews, J. G. (1993). The influence of body roll on hand path in freestyle swimming: an experimental study. *J. Appl. Biomech.*, **9**, 238–53.

Lyle, J. (1996). A conceptual appreciation of the sports coaching process. *Scot. Cent. Res. Papers Sport Leisure Soc.*, **1(1)**, 15–37.

McPherson, M. I. (1996). Qualitative and quantitative analysis in sports. *Am. J. Sports Med.*, **24**, S85–8.

Mero, A., Komi, P. V., Korjus, T. *et al.* (1994). Body segment contributions to javelin throwing during final thrust phases. *J. Appl. Biomech.*, **10**, 166–77.

Messenger, N. and Sidors, D. (1994). Misconception of the Newtonian world. Barriers to communication in biomechanics. In *Proceedings of the BASES Biomechanics Section* (J. Watkins, ed.), pp. 65–8. British Association of Sport and Exercise Sciences.

Miller, D. I. and Nelson, R. C. (1973). *Biomechanics of Sport*. Lea and Febiger.

Morriss, C. J. (1997). Co-ordination patterns in the performances of an elite javelin thrower. *J. Sports Sci.*, **16**, 12–13.

Mullineaux, D. and Bartlett, R. (1997). Research methods and statistics. In *Biomechanical Analysis of Movement in Sport and Exercise* (R. Bartlett, ed.), pp. 81–104. British Association of Sport and Exercise Sciences.

Nigg, B. (1993). Sports science in the twenty-first century. *J. Sports Sci.*, **11**, 265–70.

Nigg, B. and Herzog, W. (1994). *Biomechanics of the Musculoskeletal System*. John Wiley and Sons.

Norman, R. W. (1975). Biomechanics and the community coach. *J. Physical Ed. Rec.*, **46(3)**, 49–52.

Salo, A., Grimshaw, P. N. and Marar, L. (1997). 3D biomechanical analysis of sprint hurdles at different competitive levels. *Med. Sci. Sports Exer.*, **29**, 231–7.

Sanderson, D. (1991). The influence of cadence and power output on the biomechanics of force application during steady-state cycling in competitive and recreational cyclists. *J. Sports Sci.*, **9**, 191–203.

Schleihauf, R. E. (1974). A biomechanical analysis of freestyle. *Swimming Tech.*, **11**, 89–96.

Schmidt, R. A. (1991). *Motor Learning and Performance*. Human Kinetics.

Scottish Volleyball Association (1994). *Club Coach's Award (Course Outline)*. Scottish Volleyball Association.

Sprigings, E. J. and Koehler, J. A. (1990). The choice between Bernoulli's or Newton's model in predicting dynamic lift. *Int. J. Sports Biomech.*, **6**, 235–45.

Sprunt, K. (1993). *An Introduction to Sports Mechanics*. National Coaching Foundation.

Warren, J. (1979). *Understanding Force*. John Murray.

Watkins, J. (1987). Qualitative movement analysis. *Br. J. Physical Ed.*, **18**, 177–9.

Winter, D. A. (1979). *Biomechanics of Human Movement*. John Wiley and Sons.

Yeadon, M. R. (1989). The simulation of aerial movement – I: The determination of orientation angles from film data. *J. Biomech.*, **23**, 59–66.

Yeadon, M. R. (1998). Computer simulation in sports biomechanics. In *Biomechanics in Sports XVI: Proceedings of the XVIth International Symposium on Biomechanics in Sports* (H. J. Riehle and M. M. Vieten, eds), pp. 309–18. Universitätsverlag Konstanz.

Yeadon, M. R. and Challis, J. H. (1992). *Future Directions for Performance-Related Research in Sports Biomechanics.* English Sports Council.

Yeadon, M. R., Atha, J. and Hales, F. D. (1990). The simulation of aerial movement – IV: A computer simulation model. *J. Biomech.,* **23,** 85–9.

Zatsiorsky, V. M. and Fortney, V. L. (1993). Sports biomechanics 2000. *J. Sports Sci.,* **11,** 270–83.

Part 3

Applying the Coaching Process in Specific Contexts

8

Coaching children

Neville Cross and Bob Brewer

- An interdisciplinary account of the coaching process with children
- Government strategies for coaching children
- Policies for physical education and youth sports development
- Standards and moral imperatives in the coaching of children
- Codes of conduct for coaching children
- Competitive and mastery goals in youth sport
- Talent identification and development proposals/issues
- The elite child swimmer as an exemplar
- Growth and development factors, training loads, possible overtraining
- Athlete-centred initiatives for the future

Introduction

The first part of this chapter develops a view on the current priorities that have been established for coaching children in the United Kingdom (UK), and the influence these have had on delineating the special characteristics of the coaching process when implemented in youth sport. The latter part of the chapter considers the nature of the coaching process with elite child athletes. It gives careful consideration to the capabilities of these child athletes, and examines the implications for the coaching process of the physical and physiological demands of competitive swimming. Throughout the chapter, the emphasis is on identifying the relationship between good coaching practice and the special requirements of pre-adult coaching.

Current interest and concerns

Current interest in the United Kingdom about sport and coaching children arises out of two main concerns. The first of these centres on the validity of methods adopted by coaches to nurture young athletes as they move from participatory phases of engaging in physical activity through to the more competitive, more physically and mentally taxing contexts of performance and excellence in sport. The fact that this coincides with a period of rapid and distinct physical growth and development in children is of added significance to the programmes being prepared for them. The second concern is associated with the educational, moral and developmental nature of the coaching process that needs to be adopted with children. This would also be allied to the qualities that are required by coaches in order for these processes to be judged as reasonable and equitable, as well as successful, with such performers. These concerns do not stand alone. They are clearly inter-related, for example, by the moral and ethical complexities implicit in any such interface between adults and children when committing to sports programmes and contexts of more competitive intensity. As a contribution to such a debate, the subject matter of this chapter reflects on the various strands of evidence that can help illuminate the coaching process with children. In doing so, it continues the traditions of interdisciplinary enquiry provided by other writers in this field (for example, Martens, 1990; Lee, 1993a).

Leadership in children's sport: policy and directives for teachers and coaches

The earlier reference to the concerns about coaching children is not without some significance in the UK at the present time. This chapter is being written at a time when the politics of UK sport, and the development of policy and strategies to encourage youth participation, have the considered interest of both academics and practitioners. Policies for children's involvement in sport continue to be informed by a burgeoning research literature which describes aspects of sports participation against a background of evolving social trends and changes to work and leisure patterns (see, for example, Hendry *et al.*, 1993; Mason, 1995; Coalter, 1997; Kremer *et al.*, 1997). In the case of children's participation, research into the level of sports involvement has often been examined with reference to the positive promotion of health, along with concerns over the activity-exercise habits observed in the lifestyles of young people (see, for example, McKenzie *et al.*, 1995; Armstrong and Welsman, 1997; Trew, 1997). Legacies of the anecdotal view that sport is 'good for you', with sports participation providing solutions to perceived social problems of the 'yob culture' (O'Leary, 1994), also form part of this background to policy directives and the influences that are brought to bear on coaches and leaders to deliver a youth sport strategy (see, for example, Scottish Sports Council, 1997a).

In terms of prescribing aims for the coaching process with children, these are important contextual parameters for the types of activities and processes that typically distinguish participation coaching from performance coaching (after Lyle, 1996). As Lyle has explained, there are significant differences between such coaching circumstances. Any serious consideration of regional or national strategies to move children into more performance-specific conditions (as in schools of excellence or sports academies) needs to draw on further sources of information and support (as in sports medicine, for example) to assist in the achievement of competitive standards. TOYA (1992) provides a useful account of such a model of intensive training, which formed the basis of their investigation. Thus, while this is an issue about establishing coaching intentions and subsequent coaching practice, there are other imperatives for the process of providing an environment within which children's coaching can take place successfully. This is evidenced very clearly in the way sport is resourced and prioritized – often a function of political expediency.

Coaching children: the government speaks

A starting point for the concerns we introduced earlier is the backdrop of public opinion and political climate that pleads for something to be done about our competitive merit, particularly in the international sporting world (see Goodbody, 1996). This probably had its most explicit airing in *Sport: Raising the Game* (Department of National Heritage, 1995), in which the then Prime Minister's assertions about the place of sport in society were considered something of a rallying call, not only to the expectant electorate but to the world of school sport in particular. Putting 'sport back into the heart of weekly life in every school', and claiming that 'sport ... is one of the defining characteristics of nationhood and of local pride' (DNH, 1995: 2) formed part of the rationale for a range of policies affecting school provision for sport. More especially, the report charged its government agency, the Office for Standards in Education (OFSTED), with the monitoring of sporting standards achieved in its schools (in England and Wales), and made direct reference to the ways in which teachers in training and in service should be more 'coach qualified' to meet the demands and requirements of the 'blue print for the future of sport in schools' (DNH, 1995: 3).

While changes to the political climate have, to some extent, stalled the policy initiatives framed in the 1995 white paper, it has, nevertheless, put the focus of attention back on the personal and technical qualities associated with good coaching and how 'qualified to coach' can be properly and reliably assured in the contexts of school-age sport leadership. This is sensitive territory, especially in asserting what should be required of coaches, many of whom remain in sport as part of a volunteer-based coaching force. In the case of teachers it has particular relevance, as their contracted obligations to school are primarily described in terms of the tightly defined formal (National) curriculum and the time-tabled hours of employment therein. *Sport: Raising the Game* endorsed the provision of coaching award courses for teachers in training and in service, and furthered the agenda for volunteers and professionals alike to be better equipped and formally qualified to develop sport with children. Such policy statements do raise the very real issue of resourcing relevant courses, as well as freeing up those individuals keen enough to participate in coach education. Given the proper resources, there is recent evidence to suggest that this can be very readily and successfully achieved (NCF, 1998). This drive for qualifications has also, as suggested later, something of a moral prerogative attached to it, especially in terms of establishing some kind of quality assurance where adults are involved in leading children in sport. However, the government's emphasis on 'qualified to coach' suggests a more explicit directive to produce technically competent leadership that will speed the transition of children from participation levels of activity into the standards required at the performance and excellence bands of competition. With this goes the hope that the future medallists and winners will somehow emerge. It will be important to evaluate how teachers and other volunteers associated with school sport respond to any possible compulsion attached to coaching qualifications, for while the circumstances of the extended curriculum have changed since the mid 1980s, these sorts of initiatives should be perceived by adults as incentives rather than anything that could diminish their interest and voluntary commitment to coaching school children.

Schools-sport education and physical education

Events during the 1990s heralded a significant change in the relationship between the key players in coaching programmes for children at a national level. A review of such developments might reinforce the view that resolving a strategy for coaching children is as much a political consideration as it is a delineation of the appropriate processes that might be involved in both teaching and coaching. There have been some noteworthy initiatives that have linked children and schools to sport and coaching schemes. The Champion Coaching scheme, for example, produced a blueprint for inter-agency co-operation in local areas in the UK (apart from Scotland). Under the guidance of a Youth Sport Manager in each locale, nominated athletes were provided with the opportunities to develop skills and attributes that might eventually progress them into more concentrated competitive contexts (NCF, 1993). The success of this strategy was invariably described in terms of the collaboration between physical education teachers and the sports delivery agencies, such as coaches, clubs, sports centres and local authority sports-development units. The extension of the Champion Coaching initiative into the Top Sport programme under the auspices of the Youth Sport Trust is also a significant development in schools-sport education. Similarly, more recent initiatives by the Department for Education and Employment (DfEE) to establish specialist schools-sport colleges based in schools, where appropriate facilities and staff expertise were considered to be in place (eleven were nominated with associated government funding during 1997), might be seen as a natural extension to the Sportsmark award scheme in which schools are encouraged to achieve sports participation criteria overseen by the respective UK Sports Council(s).

Such developments can provoke contention, especially in defusing what are essentially professional sensitivities. Thus, policy directives asserting who should deliver school-age sport tend to get a guarded response. Cairney (1998), for example, commenting on the role of Scottish PE teachers in the wake of new proposals for sports development in Scotland (Scottish Sports Council, 1998a), points up the potential intrusion of a 'sport-driven' curriculum as a 'threat to teachers' in their role of teaching a range of physical activities within the broadly defined expressive arts curriculum (for children of 5–14). This might be particularly relevant when, as he conjectures, coaches increasingly come into schools with a 'sport potential' remit. One might concur with the implicit view here that a different sort of process between adult leader and child athlete is taking place when teachers are teaching, and when coaches are coaching. The relationship between the respective aims and purposes of school-based programmes and youth sport development strategies remains an issue nearly 40 years on from the point of its first reporting (CCPR, 1960). Cooke (1996), in reviewing school sport and the implications of *Sport: Raising the Game*, highlights this distinction and help-fully analyses the processes involved in teaching and coaching. Nevertheless, Cooke reasserts the view that the professionals in physical education and sport should recognize the power of partnership in formulating coaching programmes, and that the processes implied in both teaching and coaching are indeed complementary. Interestingly, the proposed appointment of a school sport co-ordinator to every Scottish secondary school – a New Labour response to earlier Conservative Government-inspired Scottish Office papers on *Scotland's Sporting Future* (Scottish Office, 1995, 1997) – goes some way towards practically realizing the partnership view held by Cooke. Such a model for developing sport in schools, which allows for a teacher's time to be contractually accredited in order to develop work-ing links between the school curriculum and local community sports provi-sion, will be worthy of further analysis in the years ahead (Scottish Sports Council, 1997b).

Competent to coach children: new imperatives for the coaching process

Becoming competent to coach by developing the qualities required to lead young people in purposeful, positive sports activity has been an important feature of recent government policy. The issue of what constitutes safe and responsible conduct with children has always been a central feature of the way National Governing Bodies of Sport (NGB) have continuously revised their coaching awards curricula. Similarly, the generation of industry-led standards in coaching, teaching and instructing (via NVQ/SVQ) has to some degree focused attention onto the professional expectations of coaches and those agencies to which they are ultimately responsible. The Coaching for Teachers programme (1996) in England (see Elder, 1997) and the Sports Coaching Competencies for Teachers initiative being put on trial in Scotland (in 1997–98) are examples of recent coaching development programmes that have their origins in government statements about appropriately qualified leadership for children's sport. Continued support for such schemes will be one way of resolving the difficulties of achieving an adequate provision of coach education, particularly in small communities (as reported in Duncan, 1997). A particular momentum to the reviewing of coaching practice with young children has come about partly as a consequence of Lord Cullen's reporting on recommendations for the vetting and suitability of voluntary leaders (Cullen, 1996), and partly also from a greater public consciousness of how children's rights and welfare should be protected.

The safety of children in the care and charge of coaches has never been under more scrutiny than in the 1990s. It is a state of affairs that fully warrants our previous description of coaching children as a 'special case'. Recent court cases detailing abuse by coaches of young athletes is the most profoundly distressing aspect of this. In linking such cases to the implications arising from Cullen (1996), the notion of being competent to coach children has taken on a new moral imperative that extends the normal frameworks of health and safety generally associated with this area of coaching practice (see, for example, Collins, 1993). The transparency of references to preventative and anticipatory measures adopted by sports agencies in working with young people (for example, Scottish Sports Council, 1997c) is indicative of a period of trying to restore public confidence over standards in coaching practice. In some instances, this has already meant a change to coaching award course formats – witness the development of a Children's Coaching Licence Diploma by the Scottish Football Association (SFA) during 1998 – while, in a similar fashion, the National Coaching Foundation (NCF) has continued to revise the advice made available through its publications on the coach's responsibilities with children (Crouch, 1998). The development of professional practice guidelines for coaches and athletes highlights the responses now required by sporting agencies in a climate of heightened public scrutiny across the world. The pronouncement that a 'national anti-harassment in sport strategy' has had to be declared as part of the guidance in a coaching code of ethics is an indication of the explicit concerns associated with coaching practice with child athletes (Australian Sports Commission, 1998). Perhaps, in the manner described by Gilroy (1993), such developments in the UK might inevitably broaden the scope of protection afforded to children under the legislation of the Children's Act (1989). In many ways these events have compounded the nature of how coaching is delivered to children, a process that continues to be full of dilemmas and difficulties, even for the most experienced of coaches. Attention is now turned to a scrutiny of some of these practical issues.

Dilemmas and difficulties for coaches of children

The standards required of coaches in their working relationship with children in sport have benefited from the current climate of public scrutiny. Many of the changes that have taken place here are entirely consistent with the development of an analytical framework for coaching ethics witnessed in the 1980s (see, for example, Aspin, 1983; Zeigler, 1986). In the UK, the debate about standards and qualifications has given greater authority to those statements of governance by coaching agencies attempting to establish a code of ethics and conduct for its member sports coaches (BISC, 1989). However, such examples of positive declarations of coaching intent (the BISC/NCF has 40 such articles in all, covering a range of qualities including relationships, integrity, safety and competence) might put coaches in something of a moral turmoil as they come to terms with the kind of problems typically confronting them in the world of sport.

'Referee!'

As the element of competition in sport is heightened, so too are the dilemmas facing the coach of child athletes. Consider, for example, the ways in which coaches either encourage or do not encourage the ideas associated with respect for the individual or for the rules. There are well considered examples of 'sports charters' for children, which draw up regulations supporting fair and healthy play (notably through versions of the mini-game – see Lee and Smith, 1993 and Ogle, 1997 for a summary). However, this also has to be seen against a background of regularly expressed warnings about the adoption of adult sports goal orientations in competitive youth sports settings (Roberts, 1980; Martens, 1996). It is difficult to summarize adequately the scope of this argument, but one anecdotal example might be permitted, to assist our understanding. In the film version of *Fever Pitch* (Hornby/Film on 4, 1997), the teacher 'hero', at one point, describes to his schoolboy football team how to play the offside trap in the manner born of his own beloved Arsenal FC. Not only is this carried out with reference to the relevant timing of the defensive player's movement up the field, but it is simultaneously accompanied by the teacher's haranguing of these same players to turn to the officials, wave an arm in the air and shout out, 'hey! offside ref!'. While this may be faintly amusing and even sound familiar, it seems typical of what inappropriate coaching can lead to, with the scale of the wrongdoing increasing in line with the rise in competitive stakes. Indeed, it might even become expected behaviour, with coaches in some contexts under pressure to conform to this type of approach irrespective of their views. The difficulties for coaches of children will be to reconcile these conflicting issues in a way that respects the integrity of the activity and all of the participants (including the coaches themselves). In the instance described, perhaps Arnold's (1997) assertions about sport as a valued practice – 'inherently concerned with the moral' because its participants willingly submit to its rules and obligations (1997: 79) – need to be judged in the changing climate of responses to authority. Invariably this will lead to a review of coaching intention and practice in youth sport contexts. As Lee (1993b) suggests, part of doing this will be to invite everybody to acknowledge more readily the values identified by children for participating in sport and the influence that coaches might have in the formation of these values. His suggested exercise to examine the links between coaching motives, values and behaviour would be a salutary aspect of education for coaches.

'I'm Tiger Woods'

The extent to which sporting values and behaviours are endorsed by coaches and picked up by children has been a regular feature of coach education programmes for working with children (Martens, 1996; NCF, 1997). 'Modelling' is often referred to as a feature of the process by which children gain such attributes, particularly from 'significant others' (Martens, 1996), and in this respect Hemery's (1991) biographical account of 50 world class performers provides a reminder of the place of parental role models in the development of fair play and 'within-the-rules' sports attitudes. Modelling behaviour is a process of learning that finds support across a number of learning dimensions, and particularly in motor learning and skill acquisition (see Magill, 1998 for an overview of this). Many children when they come into sport wish to emulate the prowess of current sporting stars, and this is something that most coaches will recognize and indeed utilize in their instructional strategies to establish the motivational climate to persevere and achieve. 'I'm Tiger Woods' is a modern day slogan for all those wishing for that gift of sporting greatness to be bestowed on them, along with the dream that might inspire them to achieve it.

The influence that coaches will have on the goal orientations of young athletes during the coaching process is a significant issue. Fundamental to the coach's impact is a consideration of the nature of competitive play or performance in youth sport, and the significance of winning to the participants. It is crucial that coaches develop a view on how the attitude to competition evolves in their programmes, and how this will help to prepare children for competition and playing against others in ways that keep them in the sport. This clearly goes beyond physiological or technical accounts of being sufficiently fit to excel in competition (although we refer to it later!). Coaches need to take a broad view of why children enjoy being involved in sport, and be aware that children enjoy sport for different reasons that may change over the duration of their participation (Watkins and Montgomery, 1989; Whitehead, 1993). Differences in goal orientation exist between children and can be very individualized. There is some compelling evidence that also suggests that these differences occur between boys and girls in sport and in other contexts (Mason, 1995; Scully and Clarke, 1997; Moir and Moir, 1998). While Lyle's overview of the coaching process (see Chapter 1) describes the competitive imperative that comes with the concept of performance coaching – 'to improve performance *in competition*' (our italics) – the coaching process adopted with children clearly has to be adjusted as they develop in the sport. Indeed, as Roberts' work over a number of years has shown, in order to prolong children's involvement in sport and to achieve some of the desired health benefits from it, coaches require to be orientated to the ways in which a 'mastery climate' of motivation for children in sports can be sustained in deference to ego or 'did you win?' type targets (Roberts and Treasure, 1992). Similarly, the ongoing and informative work by Duda (1996) on the effects of task versus ego involvement orientations compels coaches to adopt approaches that move beyond the immediacy of results and outcomes if children are to consider themselves successful in sport. The organizational emphasis on amending the scale of playing areas and access to skills, contained in mini games like Pasarelle Basketball and 'Kwik Cricket', provide hints to what coaches and administrators can make possible here. Adjusting the rules and regulations and putting sporting tasks within the reach of children have always been part of the literature of guides to practitioners (e.g. Orlick and Botterill, 1975; Roberts, 1980; NCF, 1997), and perhaps a further contribution to resolving the coaching dilemmas referred to above might be found in the type of coaching process implied in Roberts and Treasure's comment that (1992: 59):

> Persuasive evidence suggests that by making certain cues, rewards and expectations salient, a coach can encourage a particular goal orientation and, in so doing, significantly affect the way a child perceives the sport experience. Practicioners {sic} should therefore work hard to establish a mastery climate by emphasizing short-term goals and learning and skill development. To enhance motivation, children need to be evaluated for their improvement and effort rather than their performance and ability.

Spotting the future – staying on course

Roberts and Treasure's commentary on children's motivation for sport might have particular relevance for coaches considering how their practice with children, who have yet to become committed to performance sport, might be more appropriately sensitized. This is particularly pertinent given the continued interest being shown in the formulation of formalized talent identification and talent development schemes (TID) in the UK. Current UK interest in TID (e.g. a proposed pilot by Scottish Sports Council, 1998b) appears to be based on experiences gleaned from the Australian Sports Search model, in which children's physical potential for sport is judged by a testing protocol linking test achievements, developmental norms and anticipated sports potential to a computer database. However, as Clews and Gross (1995) contend, it is the retention of talented athletes and the ability to persevere with sport that is probably more difficult than the identification of the potential child athlete *per se*. They suggest (1995: 116) that:

> Before large sums of money are spent on identifying this new talent, sporting organizations need to be selective in their talent identification and to be able to target those who are most likely to remain in their sport rather than suffering the large withdrawal rates currently experienced.

As suggested in the next section, there is much to consider in the programmes for developing the child athlete, and never more so than in the management and organization of training over the career span of an athlete. In some activities this has seen the peak performance years actually shift from the early 20s to the late 20s or early 30s (Dick, 1997). The implications of this can be far-reaching, especially in deciding at what point recruitment and selection is actually made. For example, the physical conditioning that has to be assumed for the appropriate development of technique associated with competitive performance will be affected by natural growth spurts. However, in terms of keeping athletes on their respective sports programmes once they have been identified, coaches need to balance very carefully a whole host of variables that could influence the prospects for children staying in sport. Policies extolling 'performance pathways' have to some degree anticipated this requirement (Campbell, 1997), particularly in fitting children to appropriate levels of competition in their sport. Similarly, the continued interest in applying a career perspective to athletes in training is an encouraging point of development in the UK, and follows on from some of the programmes witnessed in Australia (Anderson, 1998).

We suspect that a major requirement for coaches as their athletes ascend the ladder of sporting opportunity will be the way they deal with competition and the winning and losing issues that go with this – a point alluded to earlier. In this respect, Douge (1998) has noted that coaches really do need to work on strategies to ease children from the:

> relatively non competitive exploratory situations defined by the fun games of modified sports to highly competitive situations defined by published scores, ladders, awards and opportunities for performers to progress.

An implicit part of achieving a non-stressful transition into competitive sports will almost certainly be the coach's management of not just their performers' aspirations, but also the expectations of parents. The involvement of parents can work to the advantage of both children and coaches, but, as Lee and MacLean's (1997) study on age group swimmers demonstrated, the precise effect of this involvement requires some careful scrutiny. Their research, based on an analysis of 82 competitive swimmers and their perception of parental pressure, suggested that active parental involvement might be desirable for certain performers, but only if the conditions were such that parents were not perceived to be overly exerting their control (or attempting to), particularly in the actual performing context. The elaboration of such findings is potentially very illuminating for coaching practice with children. For example, it reinforces the view that coaches have to individualize their treatment of athletes – Lee and MacLean (1997) noted the variations between athletes in tolerating pressure, and saw a need for understanding more precisely the causes of this. In those sports where parents might be expected to have a supporting role because of the age of the children (as in transport, finance, kitting out, etc.), coaches will need to be as much involved in nurturing coach–parent relations as they are with the development of athletic performance in their youngsters. Family involvement in the development of sport with children appears to be a critical issue in both initiating and maintaining their interest in sport. The TOYA study, for example, described how families developed and adjusted their approach to supporting family member athletes. Rowley (1989) reported that the nature of this support seemed to evolve in line with the performance status of the athlete and the intensity of training required. Families appeared to 'mature' in their ability to work with and accommodate the athlete in the family! However, what appears to be of continued concern and significance to this aspect of recruitment to sport is the number of athletes from families in the higher socio-economic groups (English Sports Council, 1998). Perhaps one of the tests for assessing the success of the various National Lottery-funded schemes for identifying and funding young athletes will be the extent to which this profile can be adjusted to allow equality of access and development for a greater number of children in sport. Given the basic physical and technical qualities young athletes need to progress into more competitive contexts (Balyi, 1998), the broadening of the sports participation base, allied to structures for identifying and nurturing sporting talent, requires critical and positive prioritizing from policy makers in sport.

The elite child athlete – a case study in competitive swimming

Dick (1989: 133) has noted the multiplicity of factors involved in the pursuit of athletic potential:

> The athlete is the product of nature (the genetic pattern dictated by parents) and nurture (the continuous influence of environment) ... All factors influencing the athlete's internal and external environment may contribute to, detract from, or have no effect upon pursuit of potential.

Dick's reminder of the heredity/environment debate testifies to the diverse nature of the factors to be taken into account when assessing an athlete's circumstances. These circumstances are difficult enough to control and master when related to adult elite athletes, but are infinitely more complicated when related to the child athlete – one who is neither emotionally, physically nor physiologically mature. It makes sense, therefore, for children's psychological, physical and sociological needs, in any specific situation, to be taken into account by parents, coaches and teachers (Tremayne, 1995). Nowhere is this more important than in the elite child athlete coaching situation – one in which 'significant others' exert enormous influence and sway, and where irreparable damage, both psychological and physical, can be inflicted by insensitive and/or uninformed coaches, parents and others with influence.

Wilke and Madsen (1986: Foreword) sum up the paradox thus:

> In our view, the greatest contradictions occur between the considerable time demands which have to be met in accordance with the tenets of training theory and the overall pedagogic/human responsibility towards the young swimmer.

Although the second section of this chapter pays particular attention to the physical and physiological evidence relevant to the coaching process with elite child swimmers, it is essential that the inter-relatedness and interdependence of different features of the research findings are acknowledged. Thus it is anticipated that reference will, on appropriate occasions, also be made to other performance elements, and that their importance to the coaching process is neither denied nor diminished in any way.

Elite child swimmers: an overview

Various texts (Besford, 1976; Davies, 1984) cite examples of extraordinary performances by young swimmers. The majority of these are by females, including: Ilsa Konrads (Australia), world record holder for 800 m freestyle in 1958 aged 13 years; Karen Muir (South Africa), world record holder at 110 yards backcrawl in 1965 aged 12 years; Shane Gould (Australia), who held 11 world records between 1971 and 1973 aged 14–15 years; and Britain's Sharron Davies, who at a mere 11 years of age was picked to swim for her country at senior level. Examples of extraordinary young male performances also exist. Probably the best known of these is John Konrads (Australia), who set six world records in seven days in 1958 aged 15 years and went on to win Olympic gold in 1960.

World records in swimming in the 1990s tend to be set by more mature athletes (i.e. post-puberty) and for a variety of reasons (Costill *et al.*, 1992) – not least that many swimmers are now staying in the sport for longer. However, very young athletes continue to participate at the very highest level. In order to do so, many of these young athletes take part in training regimes that might be considered by many as at least very rigorous, and by some as over-stressful (Cross, 1991). It is these athletes who are the concern of this section, and in order to define for the reader what standard constitutes 'high level' (often described in swimming as 'elite') in this context, qualification for the national age group championships has been chosen as the benchmark. Thus, swimmers falling between the ages of 12 and 17 years who qualify to compete in these championships would constitute the cut-off between elite and non-elite child athletes (note that it is acknowledged that some of these may appear physically to resemble adults). In addition, some of these athletes may also qualify to compete at even higher levels including, in some cases, world championships and the Olympic Games.

Of particular interest here is that it is only in the past decade in the United Kingdom that the problem of 'too much too early' has seriously been considered, and the ages at which children are allowed to compete at national level have been adjusted upwards. In addition to this the European youth championships now acknowledge the differences between boys and girls at various stages in their performance development, with the competition for boys at under 17 years and for girls at under 15 years of age. The Olympic Games and world championships do not segregate athletes by age.

Growth, development and the young athlete

Children and adolescents are not mini-adults (Sharp, 1986; Dick, 1989; Costill *et al.*, 1992; Wilmore and Costill, 1994). Children have some obvious and some less obvious disadvantages (Costill *et al.*, 1992), such as strength differences and lower anaerobic capacity (young children produce less lactate and their muscle fibres are less able to generate large amounts of ATP than adults). However, Wilke and Madsen (1986) have reminded readers that a number of biological advantages in childhood, such as low body weight in relation to body surface and the high trainability of the cardio-circulatory system, still at first sight favour an early start on high-pressure swimming training. In fact, the same factors also favour early specialization in particular swimming strokes and/or competitive disciplines, and they have cited the frequently observed steep rise in performance by age-groupers that often accompanies the early introduction of heavy stress and specialization.

This is not necessarily the best way forward, nor even desirable, but merely highlights the fact that significant increases in performance, using similar methods to training adults, are possible even at the age-group stage of an athlete's development cycle. In addition, Costill *et al.* (1992) compounded the issue when they reminded readers that several recent studies with pre-pubescent boys and girls showed large increases in strength (43 per cent compared to 10 per cent for a non-training group) as a consequence of progressive resistance training (20–30 minutes per day for 3 days per week for 9 weeks), with no evidence of damage to the children's bones, tendons or muscles. They went further by suggesting that the risk of injury and structural damage to children, even from heavy resistance exercise, is extremely low. The recommended use of isokinetic resistance machines for strength training (those where resistance is matched to the force applied) for young athletes, as opposed to the use of free weights or barbells, is principally to eliminate the risk of injury associated with the use of free weights (dropping them on their feet, etc.).

Some of this research seems to contradict the analyses of sport physiologists such as Sharp (1986) and Aldridge (1993) and physical educationalists such as Gilroy (1993), who have described the physical and physiological differences between child and adult athletes and suggested that damage to the bones, epiphyseal plates and joints of children can be caused by both repetition (overuse) and overload stress.

Notwithstanding these contradictions, Costill *et al.* (1992) have also cautioned against the use of stressful training at an early age. The warning was supported by Wilke and Madsen (1986), who quoted the earlier work of Feige (1973) which highlighted that early training and early specialization, sometimes with spectacular short-term results, are often followed soon after with rapid fall-off and premature career ending or burn-out. There is a need therefore to balance the psychological need for observable short-term improvement with a longer-term strategy that considers developmental factors in a sensitive and more holistic way.

Only very recently has such a view been enshrined in an approved code of ethics in which, under the heading of 'relationships', the following requirement appears (ASA/ISTC, 1995: 28):

> The good coach will be concerned primarily with the wellbeing, health and future of the individual performer and only secondarily with the optimization of performance.

Guidance and advice

Published guidelines and advice for age-group swimming training are few and far between. A notable exception is *Splash Out*, a booklet published by the Scottish Sports Council (1995) in conjunction with the Scottish Amateur Swimming Association. Not only does this recognize that:

> Swimming must be adapted to the needs of the developing child and not the child to the dictates of swimming

but it also discusses the important features of the biological development of children, such as growth, puberty and physiology, which have a bearing on both training and potential competitive success in the sport. It also attempts to equate stages of physical development with certain age groupings. Thus, 6–9 years is the age-group associated with basic swimming skills, fun, technique work, low-key competition and training once or twice per week (30–45 minutes per session); the 8–11 years age-group still includes fun, but two to three sessions (45–60 minutes each) of swimming and the introduction of inter-club competition; the 10–13 years age-group is now swimming three to four sessions per week of 60–75 minutes with age-group competition at district and national level; and finally the 12–14 years age-group may undergo training around six times per week with sessions lasting up to 2 hours each, and land conditioning should supplement the swimming programme. Coaches should note that fun and variety should be an integral part of each of these categories.

While to the uninitiated these recommendations (i.e. the amount of training suggested) may at first glance seem somewhat excessive, they should not be considered out of context. For example, each stage must be preceded by the previous one. Moreover, training sessions at all of the stages typically involve a fair amount of socializing, rest periods and periods of instruction and explanation, which together reduce considerably the possible physical loading on the young swimmer.

This is in stark contrast to the chilling example of bad practice quoted by Gilroy (1993: 24):

> one girl took up swimming when she was 5 and quit when she was 14, having done an estimated 10 000 hours of training in the pool. Such a commitment of time and energy would not have been tolerated had the child been at work in a shop, but because sport is seen to be 'play' it escapes our critical eye.

Nevertheless, it must be recognized that competitive success does not come easily. It will only be achieved at the highest level by a dedicated and comprehensive application to appropriate training theory and practice (Wilke and Madsen, 1986; Bompa, 1994). The 10 000 hours of training in 9 years quoted in Gilroy's example is not itself necessarily excessive, equating to approximately 21 hours per week. Many elite athletes often exceed this total. However, the age at which it is done and the stage in the athlete's development at which it is undertaken is extremely critical. The example quoted is a classic case of too much too early!

Development-related swimming training

According to Wilke and Madsen (1986), a training programme that is planned in the interests of the age-group swimmer, with optimum success in mind, must be designed to make full use of the individual's surges in natural growth. Thus, young swimmers should be encouraged to practise technique continuously from an early age in order to maximize time for the co-ordination skills to develop in line with maturational developments. In addition, it would be advantageous to introduce training practices for the development of the biomotor abilities (flexibility, endurance, strength etc.) some time prior to the final growth spurt which occurs at approximately 14–16 years. A further consideration is necessary. Although children are relatively lacking in anaerobic capacity and power (Sharp, 1986), it is important to incorporate sprinting practices into their training programmes from an early age. Not only are these enjoyable for the young swimmer, but children are well equipped to handle activities which require short but intensive exertion, utilizing the phosphagen energy system (Armstrong and Welsman, 1993).

Finally, flexibility is a component that is crucial at this time. Although girls have more elasticity and flexibility up to the age of 10 years, the elasticity of the capsular and ligament tissue of the joints declines for both sexes from about the tenth year (Weiss, 1980, cited in Wilke and Madsen, 1986), and flexibility exercises should therefore be included in every age-grouper's programme from the outset. However, Armstrong and Welsman (1993) have highlighted the lack of scientific research into how training of flexibility affects children, and have advised caution in this area. Despite their misgivings, they have suggested that training for increased joint mobility should start before puberty. In addition, Wilmore and Costill (1994) have noted that flexibility can be lost very quickly during inactivity, and that reduced flexibility can increase athletes' susceptibility to injury.

Loading factors

The requirement to relate training to maturational development will necessitate both the volume and intensity of training being systematically increased and distributed differently. For example, an age-grouper would spend more time on developing strength with correspondingly less time on recovery and maintenance work compared to a more mature athlete, who would spend more time on maintaining strength and on recovery. Similarly, an increase in intensity can be achieved simply by swimming at a higher average speed in training from year to year as a result of progressive coaching stimuli, attention to the principle of progressive overload, and the beneficial effect of correct training loads being applied at previous stages.

Swimming at faster speed even for the same periods of time will, of course, also result in greater volume, and progressively increasing volume (e.g. moving from one training session per day to two sessions) is an accepted strategy over an extended planning cycle. However, Wilke and Madsen have been at great pains to remind readers that (1986: 12):

> ... quality comes before quantity, i.e. the greater volume must not be achieved with poor execution of the movements.

Overtraining

No analysis of coaching children would be complete without some reference to the possibility of overtraining. While it is unlikely that most age-group programmes would be of sufficient stress to lead to the pathological state of training known as 'overtraining syndrome' (an imbalance between stress and adaptability over a prolonged period), many age-group programmes, especially those in which talented age-groupers are training alongside elite adult athletes, may result in short-term imbalance. This is sometimes referred to as 'over-reaching' (Fry *et al.*, 1991). If this is allowed to continue for an extended period, it can result in 'burnout', in which young athletes become disillusioned by lack of improvement and constant tiredness and can be tempted to leave the sport prematurely.

It is important for coaches to recognize that there are two different roads to overtraining. These are, according to Bompa (1994), addisonoid overtraining caused by excessively high volumes of training, and basedowoid overtraining, which is the result of overstressing the emotional processes, usually through overemphasizing high intensity stimuli in training. Both may apply in the case of age-groupers, even though young athletes are essentially aerobic performers. The best predictors of the onset of overtraining syndrome, in addition to drop-off in performances, appear to be heart rate, oxygen uptake and blood lactate responses to a standardized bout of work (Wilmore and Costill, 1994). Taking blood from very young swimmers is not always recommended, and concerned parents will often refuse permission for coaches to do so. In addition, young children, essentially 'aerobic performers', produce very little lactate in comparison with adults. This fact, when considered in tandem with the other limitations of using lactate levels to signpost overtraining, such as diet (low carbohydrate intake equates to low glycogen levels and hence low lactates) and prior stressful exercise (also resulting in depleted glycogen stores and lower lactate levels), together render the use of lactate levels to indicate overtraining as problematic (Mackinnon and Hooper, 1991; Gregg, 1995). It would appear therefore that heart rate, both post-exercise and at rest (normally taken first thing in the morning), is one of the few physiological ways (monitoring mood state is a psychological method) of predicting approaching problems of overtraining with young athletes. However, heart rates can be erratic, change for the same workload from the morning to the afternoon, are affected by illness, excitement, anxiety and fear, and, particularly in the case of young athletes, may be difficult to count and sometimes even to find. In addition, as Wilmore and Costill (1994) noted, maximum heart rates are higher in children than in adults, and comparing the heart rates of children and adults after similar workloads may be misleading. Nevertheless it is worth persisting with heart rates, as practice can result in reasonably accurate records of training intensity levels and responses to training, and thus contribute to an early warning system.

In perspective

Although it is unlikely that an unqualified coach (swimming is well-supported by a comprehensive coach education structure) would be employed as a chief coach in any of the hundreds of clubs in the United Kingdom, incidences of bad practice can and do still occur. These are not exclusive to age-group swimming nor to coach behaviour, but are compounded in the case of age-group swimming by the child's relative lack of maturity, which may contribute to an inability to cope with the resultant stress (Gilroy, 1993).

The young athlete is physiologically different to the adult, and must be considered differently (Wilmore and Costill, 1994). Although children adapt well to the same type of training regime and stimulus as used by adult elite athletes, coaches should ensure that programmes for children and adolescents are designed specifically for each age group, and take account of the developmental factors (growth spurts, etc.) associated with a particular age range.

The principal focus of this latter section of the chapter has been on the physical and physiological aspects of elite age-group swimming, but coaches should be aware of all the stress factors involved. As we have noted, high on this list is competitiveness and the accent on winning (Lee, 1993b; Shields and Bredemeier, 1995). Not only should age-group athletes be encouraged to set performance or process goals for themselves which are not exclusively centred on winning, but coaches should also reflect carefully on their own coaching philosophies and objectives. In this respect, the often quoted, 'athletes first, winning second' (Martens, 1988) is still worthy of our attention, and there is sufficient evidence to suggest that coaching practice should adhere constantly to this maxim, particularly when coaching children.

Summary

This chapter has reported on a number of current and critical accounts of the coaching process with children. It has reaffirmed the fundamental principle that children are not mini-adults. In addition, it has examined some of the important issues that require resolution as policies for the development of coaching practice with youth sport performers are being formulated. The richness of debate found in the research literature investigating children's participation and development in sport will continue to engage both researchers and practitioners alike. Recent directives towards developing children *in* sport (as opposed to 'sport for all') might be an indication of how the reporting of research has come to impact on sports development policy in the UK (Ogle, 1997). Removing the barriers to participation, as well as extolling the virtues of being personally involved in a sport of a child's choosing (and at a level the child can sustain), appears to be indicative of a 'child first' priority for coaching sport, in the same way as an 'athlete-centred' approach to the coaching process is currently being promoted by the most enlightened administrators in contemporary sport. What are the implications for the future? For example, how might children's sport evolve or change in the era of TID (Talent Identification and Development) currently about to be launched? How will the coaches of children have to respond as they advise young athletes on the prospects of a 'career in sport', as well as develop programmes to help them achieve this? These are some of the compelling issues of the moment for coaches of children, and it is suggested that they are also the factors that place coaches in the sorts of moral dilemmas alluded to earlier in the chapter. We suggest that the greatest challenge for the UK will be in how education and training strategies can assist the large proportion of volunteer coaches to maintain their credibility in, and interest for, coaching. Such a view is predicated on the basis that it is not only children that have to be kept in sport, but their coaches also.

References

Aldridge, J. (1993). Skeletal growth and development. In *Coaching Children in Sport* (M. Lee, ed.), pp. 51–78. EFN Spon.

Anderson, D. (1998). Athlete career and education programme. Scottish Sports Council Workshop with National Governing Bodies. Murrayfield Stadium, Edinburgh 1st July 1998.

Armstrong, N. and Welsman, J. (1993). Children's physiological responses to exercise. In *Coaching Children in Sport: Principles and Practice* (M. Lee, ed.), pp. 64–77. EFN Spon.

Armstrong, N. and Welsman, J. (1997). *Young People and Physical Activity*. Oxford University Press.

Arnold, P. (1997) *Sport, Ethics and Education*. Cassell Education.

ASA/ISTC. (1995). Code of ethics for swimming coaches and teachers. *The Swimming Times*, **LXXII(10)**, 28.

Aspin, D. (1983) Towards a curriculum for the education of coaches: some principles and problems. *Physical Ed. Rev.*, **6(2)**, 92–100.

Australian Sports Commission (1998). Harassment-free sport – questions and answers. *Sports Coach*, **21(2)**, 12–15.

Balyi, I. (1998). Long-term planning of athlete development. *Faster Higher Stronger*, **1**, 8–11.

Besford, P. (1976). *Encyclopaedia of Swimming*. Robert Hale.

BISC (1989). *Code of Ethics and Conduct for Sports Coaches*. National Coaching Foundation.

Bompa, T. O. (1994). *Theory and Methodology of Training* (3rd edn). Kendall Hunt.

Cairney, J. (1998). Sport 21 a threat to teachers. *The Herald*, 23rd May 1998, p. 11.

Campbell, S. (1997). The role of the coach in the development of the young athlete. *Coach '97: Into the New Millennium*. Conference Proceedings, pp. 4–11. Scottish Sports Council/Glasgow City Council.

CCPR (1960) *Sport and the Community – The Report of the Wolfenden Committee on Sport*. The Central Council of Physical Recreation.

Clews, G. and Gross, J. B. (1995). Individual and social motivation in Australian sport. In *Sport Psychology Theory, Applications and Issues* (T. Morris and J. Summers, eds), pp. 90–121. John Wiley and Sons.

Coalter, F. (1997). Sport and recreation in the United Kingdom: flow with the flow or buck the trends ? Paper presented at the ANZALS Conference *Leisure: People, Places, Spaces, Newcastle, New South Wales*, July 1997.

Collins, V. (1993). Coaching and the law. In *Coaching Children in Sport: Principles and Practice* (M. Lee, ed.), pp. 289–95. EFN Spon.

Cooke, G. (1996). The power of partnership – sport, coaching and physical education. *Supercoach*, Summer, 10–11.

Costill, D. L., Maglischo, E. W. and Richardson, A. B. (1992). *Swimming*. Blackwell Scientific.

Cross, N. (1991). Arguments in favour of a humanistic coaching process. *The Swimming Times*, **LXVIII(11)**, 17–18.

Crouch, M. (1998). *Protecting Children: A Guide for Sportspeople*. National Coaching Foundation.

Cullen, Hon. Lord (1996). *The Public Inquiry into the Shootings at Dunblane Primary School on 13 March 1996*. The Scottish Office.

Davies, S. (1984). *Against the Tide*. Willow Books.

Department of National Heritage (1995). *Sport: Raising the Game*. Department of National Heritage.

Dick, F. W. (1989). *Sports Training Principles*. A. C. Black.

Dick, F. W. (1997). Strength training in the young athlete. *Coach '97: Into the New Millennium*. Conference Proceedings, pp. 64–77. Scottish Sports Council/Glasgow City Council.

Douge, B. (1998). Progressing from non-competitive to competitive activities. *Sports Coach*, **21(2)**, 16–17.

Duda, J. L. (1996). Maximizing motivation in sport and physical education among children and adolescents: the case for greater task involvement. *Quest*, **48**, 290–302.

Duncan, J. (1997). Focus group interviews with elite young athletes, coaches and parents. In *Young People's Involvement in Sport* (J. Kremer, K. Trew and S. Ogle, eds), pp. 152–77. Routledge.

Elder, C. (1997). Coaching call. *On Track*, Autumn, 14–17.

English Sports Council (1998). *The Development of Sporting Talent 1997. An Examination of the Current Practices for Talent Development in English Sport*. English Sports Council.

Feige, K. (1973) (ed.) *Report on the 3rd European Congress on Sports Psychology*. Schorndorf.

Fry, R., Morton, A. and Keast, D. (1991). Overtraining in athletes: an update. *Sports Med.*, **11**, 21.

Gilroy, S. (1993). Whose sport is it anyway? Adults and children's sport. In *Coaching Children in Sport: Principles and Practice* (M. Lee, ed.), pp. 17–26. EFN Spon.

Goodbody, J. (1996) Olympic shame over Britain's medal tally. *The Times*, 5th August 1996, p. 7.

Gregg, J. (1995). Optimizing performance in swimming. Coaching Seminar, September 1, 1995, Aberdeen.

Hemery, D. (1991). *Sporting Excellence: What Makes a Champion*. Collins Willow.

Hendry, L. B., Shucksmith, J., Love, J. G. and Glendinning, A. (1993). *Young People's Leisure and Lifestyles*. Routledge.

Hornby, N. (1997). *Fever Pitch*. Film Four Distributors.

Kremer, J., Trew, K. and Ogle, S. (eds) (1997). *Young People's Involvement in Sport*. Routledge.

Lee, M. (ed.) (1993a). *Coaching Children in Sport: Principles and Practice*. EFN Spon.

Lee, M. (1993b). Why are you coaching children? In *Coaching Children in Sport: Principles and Practice* (M. Lee, ed.), pp. 27–38. EFN Spon.

Lee, M. and MacLean, S. (1997). Sources of parental pressure among age group swimmers. *Eur. J. Physical Ed.*, **2**, 167–77.

Lee, M. and Smith, R. (1993). Making sport fit the children. *Coaching Children in Sport: Principles and Practice* (M. Lee, ed.), pp. 259–72. EFN Spon.

Lyle, J. (1996). A conceptual appreciation of the sports coaching process. *Scot. Cent. Res. Papers Sport Leisure Soc.*, **1(1)**, 15–37.

Mackinnon, L. T. and Hooper, S. (1991). Overtraining. *State of the Art Review*, **26**. National Sports Research Centre.

Magill, R. A. (1998). *Motor Learning: Concepts and Applications*. WCB/McGraw Hill.

Martens, R. (1988). Helping children become independent, responsible adults through sports. In *Competitive Sports for Children and Youth: An Overview of Research and Issues* (E. W. Brown, E. Wand and C. F. Branta, eds), pp. 297–307. Human Kinetics.

Martens, R. (1990). *Successful Coaching*. Leisure Press.

Martens, R. (1996). Turning kids on to physical activity for a lifetime. *Quest*, **48**, 303–10.

Mason, V. (1995). *Young People and Sport in England, 1994.* Sports Council.

McKenzie, T., Feldman, H., Woods, S. *et al.* (1995). Children's activity levels and lesson context during third-grade physical education. *Res. Q. Exer. Sport,* **66(3),** 184–93.

Moir, A. and Moir, B. (1998). *Why Men Don't Iron.* Harper Collins.

NCF (1993). *Champion Coaching 1993 : More Recipes for Action.* National Coaching Foundation.

NCF (1997). *Making Sport Fun – Helping Children to Get the Most from Sport.* National Coaching Foundation.

NCF (1998). What is coaching for teachers? *Br. J. Physical Ed.,* Autumn, 33–4.

Ogle, S. (1997). International perspectives on public policy and the development of sport for young people. In *Young People's Involvement in Sport* (J. Kremer, K. Trew and S. Ogle, eds), pp. 211–31. Routledge.

O'Leary, J. (1994) Bannister hails sport as answer to yob culture. *The Times,* 23 September 1994.

Orlick, T. and Botterill, C. (1975). *Every Kid Can Win.* Nelson Hall.

Roberts, G. C. (1980). Children in competition: a theoretical perspective and recommendations for practice. *Motor Skills Theory Pract.,* **4(1),** 37–50.

Roberts, G. C. and Treasure, D. C. (1992). Children in sport. *Sport Sci. Rev.,* **1(2),** 46–64.

Rowley, S. (1989). Intensive training and its effect on family life. *The Growing Child in Competitive Sport.* BISC International Congress Proceedings 1989, pp. 50–56.

Scully, D. and Clarke, J. (1997). Gender issues in sport participation. In *Young People's Involvement in Sport* (J. Kremer, K. Trew and S. Ogle, eds), pp. 25–56. Routledge.

Scottish Office (1995). *Scotland's Sporting Future – A New Start.* HMSO.

Scottish Office (1997). *Scotland's Sporting Future – Towards the Goal.* HMSO.

Scottish Sports Council/Scottish Swimming Association (1995). *Splash Out.* Scottish Sports Council.

Scottish Sports Council (1997a). *Youth Sport Strategy.* Scottish Sports Council.

Scottish Sports Council (1997b). *School Sport: A Co-ordinated Programme for School Sport Co-ordinators.* Briefing notes – Paper 1. Scottish Sports Council.

Scottish Sports Council (1997c). *Safe and Secure: Young People in Sport.* Scottish Sports Council.

Scottish Sports Council (1998a). *Sport 21 Nothing Left to Chance.* Scottish Sports Council.

Scottish Sports Council (1998b). *Talent Identification and Development: Consultation Paper.* Scottish Sports Council.

Sharp, N. C. C. (1986). Some aspects of the exercise physiology of children. In *The Growing Child in Competitive Sport* (G. Gleeson, ed.), pp. 100–12. Hodder and Stoughton.

Shields, D. L. L. and Bredemeier, B. J. L. (1995). *Character Development and Physical Activity.* Human Kinetics.

TOYA (1992). *Training of Young Athletes Study: Project Description.* Sports Council.

Tremayne, P. (1995). Children and sport psychology. In *Sport Psychology Theory Applications and Issues* (T. Morris and J. Summers, eds), pp. 516–33. John Wiley and Sons.

Trew, K. (1997). Time for Sport ? Activity diaries of young people. In *Young People's Involvement in Sport* (J. Kremer, K. Trew and S. Ogle, eds), pp. 126–51. Routledge.

Watkins, B. and Montgomery, A. B. (1989). Conceptions of athletic excellence among children and adolescents. *Child Development,* **60,** 1362–72.

Weiss, U. (1980). Belastbarkeit und Trainerbarkeit des Bewegungsapparates bei Kindern und Jugendlichen. *Jugend und Sport,* **37(8),** 254–8.

Whitehead, J. (1993). Why children choose to do sport – or stop. In *Coaching Children in Sport: Principles and Practice* (M. Lee, ed.), pp. 109–21. EFN Spon.

Wilke, K. and Madsen, O. (1986). *Coaching the Young Swimmer.* Pelham Books.

Wilmore, J. H. and Costill, D. L. (1994). *Physiology of Sport and Exercise.* Human Kinetics.

Zeigler, E. F. (1986). Dimensions of an ethical code for sport coaches. *Proceedings VIII Commonwealth Conference on Sport, Physical Education, Dance, Recreation and Health – Coach Education Preparation for a Profession,* pp. 79–90. EFN Spon.

9

Individualization of training programmes

Neville Cross

- The uniqueness of each individual athlete
- Coaching principles relevant to individualizing the coaching process
- Constraints on individualizing the process optimally
- Psychological support, coaching philosophy and individualization
- Swimming as an exemplar
- Some individualization research findings
- Nutrition and individualization practices

Introduction

Individualization is an essential element of the coaching process, and has been identified as a key concept (Lyle, 1996). In addition, Lyle (1996: 23) noted that:

> Each coaching process is unique for a number of reasons. Athlete aspirations, capabilities and personal circumstances will differ as will the organizational, resource and occupational circumstances within which the coach operates.

An effective coaching process aims to develop an athlete physically, technically, tactically, psychologically and in terms of theoretical knowledge of the sport – areas which are all-important in an athlete's readiness for competition (Bompa, 1994). With this range of objectives, and because each athlete is unique, the coach has both an opportunity and a responsibility to individualize training. After all, the essential elements and features that make up the framework of the sports coaching process, along with the idiosyncrasies of the individual athlete and/or coach, suggest that no two coaching situations will be the same, and hence demand some form of individualization (see also Mathers, 1997). Harre (1982) has identified these idiosyncrasies or individual performance factors of each athlete as:

- The personality of the athlete
- Physical condition
- Technique and co-ordination
- Tactical ability and mental preparation.

In addition, Trebels (1992: 12), in analysing movement pedagogy, suggested that:

> In the context of the general concept of sport, sport performance cannot be detached from the individual practising it: it cannot be viewed as a product independent from the person who produces the performance ...

The fact that each athlete is unique in terms of physiology is also important in this context. For example, Costill *et al.* (1992: 133) have noted that:

> There is a limit to the physiological and anatomical development that can be achieved with training – a factor that is probably determined by genetics. Swimmers [athletes] are not created with the same ability to tolerate training.

Consequently, coaches planning the training programme of an individual athlete must be aware that all of the performance factors may need individual attention, both separately and in concert. As far as the athlete is concerned, the tangible impacts of the coaching process will include a set of goals, training targets incorporated in personally tailored training schedules, monitoring reports and feedback, psychological support and technical advice and instruction. In both individual and team sports, coaches should seek to individualize each of these aspects in ways that are truly meaningful for each athlete.

This chapter discusses the various factors that contribute to the individualization debate. Although the sport of swimming is the principal focus of the discussion, most of the factors identified apply across all sports. However, it is acknowledged at the outset that some differences between sports (e.g. between team sports and individual sports) may have a considerable impact on both the type of individualization possible and how often this occurs. Despite these differences, there are performance and training parameters in which a substantial amount of individualization should take place. Some of these are directly controlled by the coach (training session practices, etc.), while others are much more under the athlete's control, with the coach having to rely on a degree of trust in the athlete to adopt the correct approach. Examples illustrating this point include the coach having to trust the athlete to work at the correct and individually appropriate training intensity (in this instance, the coach is in partial control), or having to trust the athlete to adopt the most appropriate nutritional strategy for the individually chosen and preferred event. In this latter example, the coach has little control, particularly in part-time sport. However, the coach may be able to monitor and regulate such factors more rigorously with professional athletes. Nutritional aspects of individualization are pursued at some length later in this chapter.

Individualizing the coaching process

The effectiveness of the coaching interventions made in relation to performance factors will be, to a large extent, dependent on the level of process specificity and individualization that the coach employs. Rushall (1985a, 1985b) has identified seven principles of coaching, including two principles most apposite for the concept of individualization; the principle of specificity, and the principle of individuality. He suggests that these factors will have a significant impact on the athlete's performance. Consequently, tailoring the coaching process to the needs of individual athletes, taking into consideration age, degree of previous training and current level of skill, should assist in the achievement of challenging but realistic individual performance goals. In addition, adjusting the coaching intervention strategies to allow some of the training sessions to replicate the demands of the individually chosen event in competition (described in training theory as specificity and/or modelling) should also help to optimize athlete performance development. In an individual sport like swimming this would lend increasing significance to an event-specific training approach, where the actual event to be swum in competition and its particular energy requirements would take precedence. In the team sport situation this would be compounded by the need to consider also a player position-specific approach, which would recognize the differences between and training requirements of forwards and backs, attack and defence etc. It is important to realize that any training model adopted should be specific to the individual or to the team. Thus, coaches should resist the temptation merely to copy the training model of an already successful athlete (Bompa, 1994). Instead, they should use their knowledge of each athlete's psychological and physiological potential to construct a model that is individually tailored to the needs of each athlete.

Thus coaches will have to individualize training programmes for different events (100 m freestyle, 200 m backstroke, 400 m individual medley, etc.) because of their different physiological, skill and strategic requirements, and/or for different positions in team sports (forward, back, goalkeeper etc.) that might also require completely different skills and tactics. While athletes will have personal preferences regarding the particular event or events on which they wish to concentrate, in many cases this will be tied to physiological make-up. For example, those athletes well-blessed with a high proportion of type II (fast twitch) muscle fibres may very well have had success in explosive events such as sprints, and are therefore predisposed to these. Those with a preponderance of type I fibres (slow twitch) may have developed a predisposition for middle-distance and/or distance events. These differences have important implications for individualization. Not only will the coach have to consider the best strategies for preparing for the different events, but training loads will also have to be carefully planned in line with the relevant energy systems appropriate for both types of muscle fibre. Thus, appropriate ratios of the components of training – volume (how much? i.e. duration, distance covered, number of repetitions etc.), intensity (how hard? i.e. the qualitative component of work performed in a given period of time) and density (how often? i.e. frequency of exposure per unit of time) – should be calculated for each and every athlete (Bompa, 1994). These in turn should be based on the type of overload (either aerobic or anaerobic) appropriate to the particular event, and the physiological and psychological make-up of the individual. Training loads will also have to be considered in tandem with the personal goals of the individual athlete and the particular sport's competition pattern. For example, a world class athlete who has an Olympic final as a goal may need a plan that includes a progressive increase in training load over a 4-year period (despite some important competitions during the 4-year period) to ensure that peaking does not occur too early. For the team athlete who may be required to perform maximally every weekend, progression is a far more complicated issue, but must be considered just the same.

While it is inconceivable that a performance coach in any competitive sport would deny the need for individualizing training in one way or another, only where the coach/athlete relationship is on a one-to-one basis is it always guaranteed. Thus, individualization in all team sports is problematical and, even where the sport is an individual one, being responsible for a large number of athletes may make it difficult here too. Personal experience as a swimming coach at the elite level for more than 20 years has taught me that swimming training programmes are seldom as individualized as much of the swimming and applied literature suggests should be the case (see, for example, Costill *et al.*, 1992; Bompa, 1994; Wilmore and Costill, 1994; Colwin, 1995). This might seem strange, given that the general coach education literature identifies training principles (one of which is the principle of individualization) to guide coaching practice. However, despite the fact that many elite coaches are aware of the necessity for individualizing training, various factors (e.g. having to deal with large numbers of athletes, insufficient training time and inadequate facilities etc.) in actual practice often militate against it. Failure to individualize training adequately may inadvertently contribute to less than optimum coaching effectiveness (Cross, 1995a, 1995b).

One further distinction needs to be made at this point. Although some individual sports employ specialist event coaches (for example, in the areas of sprints, hurdles, throwing events, jumps etc.), which in itself contributes to a more individualized coaching approach, many other sports generally do not. Swimming is one sport in which a single coach is often in control of all aspects of performance and is responsible for the preparation of all competitive strokes and race distances. Exceptions include when athletes are on duty with national teams, and when they are based at national institutes of sport. In such circumstances, particular coaches will be responsible for certain strokes (backstroke, breaststroke etc.) or particular race distances (1500 m freestyle, 400 m individual medley, etc.). Obviously, most coaches will have particular areas of expertise, and it is doubtful if one coach can attend adequately to all swimmers in a squad in order to individualize training optimally, given the range of individual strokes and preferred racing distances. One would expect that the same problems might arise in the team sport situation. Although professional team sports will often have not only a head coach in overall charge but also additional coaches for particular aspects of performance (e.g. a professional rugby team may have a forwards coach, a backs coach and a 'kicks' coach), many amateur sports teams do not. Field hockey is a team sport where a single coach is often required to cater to all aspects of performance. This may be detrimental to the potential performance of some or even all of the players, and to the ultimate effectiveness of the coaching process itself.

Although there is a varied and diverse literature in the area of the coaching process (see for example, Franks *et al.*, 1986; Fairs, 1987; Sherman and Sands, 1996; Lyle, 1996; Cross and Lyle, 1996), there is a paucity of information on actual elite coaching behaviours. Hardy (1995), for example, has noted the lack of information regarding the behaviour of swimming coaches. There is even less information available about their extended coaching management role, which should include strategies aimed at individualizing training. (For some swimming coaching examples see Cross, 1995a.) An example of the coach's extended management role is given by Scobie (1991: 8), who has noted that there are various ways of securing the same training effect in athletics, and that the coach's extended management role might include 'a selection from his repertoire not only to achieve the physiological or psychological benefits, but also to meet the needs of particular athletes'. As Scobie's article reminds readers, good coaching goes beyond physiological, psychological and technical considerations, and includes advice and direction in a large number of different areas. These areas might include advice on injury problems, career and finances, counselling, advice on how to deal with the opposition, and praise and consolation, most of which are personal to the individual athlete.

Some examples of individualization practices in team sports also exist. For example, Cooke (1990) has noted that the England rugby union team's physical fitness training has, since 1987, included fitness training programmes based on individual player strengths and weaknesses. However, it is not clear whether this is generally replicated at club level. McGowan *et al.* (1990) have reported that some individualization took place in the training of the 1984 United States Olympic volleyball team. This team, which took the gold medal, had trained together from 1981 and had spent approximately 3500 training hours (4 hours per day) in its preparation for the Olympic competition. Approximately 30 minutes each day was spent on purely individualized training practices, with a further 90 minutes spent on small group practices. As this team won the gold medal, it could be argued that these individualization practices provide an example of best practice.

In addition to a variety of constraints encountered in the coach's working environment (large groups of athletes, poor facilities etc.), coaching effectiveness and the degree of individualization possible in any specific coaching circumstance have also been affected, in some cases, by the behaviour of the athletes themselves (Cross, 1997a, 1997b). For example, some athletes actually train at an intensity higher than that requested by the coach. Cross (1997a) has suggested that many of the recorded instances of British swimmers suffering from overtraining syndrome are due to too high an intensity in training for too long a period, rather than too high a volume in training. Other athletes do not pay enough attention to advice on factors such as nutritional requirements, rest and lifestyle etc. (Cross and Lyle, 1996). As mentioned earlier, coaches would wish to be in a position to trust athletes to act in their own best interest. Unfortunately, coaching elite athletes for many years has shown me that this trust is often not well founded. Not only do some train at the wrong intensity but, when left to their own devices, many also spend large amounts of time practising those aspects of their sport that they are good at rather than their weaknesses. Thus in swimming, athletes who are good kickers will spend, if given a choice, long periods of time on kicking practice rather than working on their arms (referred to as 'pulling' practices), and flexible athletes will engage in a lot of stretching practices when it might be better to concentrate on strength exercises, etc. Consequently, it is possible for even the best-intentioned coaching strategies for individualization to be undermined, in many cases by the very athletes for whom they are designed.

Psychological support is an important aspect of the coaching process, and is especially relevant to the individualization of the programme. Not only does a humanistic psychological approach to the coaching process (Whitson, 1980; Lombardo, 1987; Cross, 1990, 1991) testify to the uniqueness of each athlete, and to the desirability of coaches catering for the individual needs of each athlete, but it also suggests that any training programme should also offer a collaborative approach between athlete and coach. Collaboration here would be to ascertain and agree upon a strategy aimed at optimal effectiveness for the particular athlete. The strategy agreed upon might not guarantee success, but it affords the athlete some personal control over the process. Note, however, that while the humanistic approach has been described here, other psychological approaches may also involve collaboration. Collaboration in this way is not always sought by elite athletes, who have come over time to trust the judgement of the coach and wish to concentrate solely on the physical and technical work to be done (Cross, 1995a). However, it does suggest the need for at least a collaborative goal-setting strategy that is individually tailored to the needs, aspirations etc. of each athlete (Hogg, 1995). Although not addressing humanistic coaching directly, Troup and Reese (1983) have suggested that what they call a co-operative style of coaching will ensure that the coaching process is individualized far more than when an authoritarian style is in operation. This is an important point. One would expect an authoritarian or autocratic style to assume less consultation and collaboration, but not necessarily less individualization. However, in situations of little consultation, there must be a danger that the coach may not realize the importance for an individual athlete of certain aspects of the coaching process. This is not exclusive to individual sports, and athletes in the team situation are also likely to have different motivations and needs. Irrespective of the psychological approach adopted by the coach, treating everyone in the team in exactly the same way is unlikely to result in optimum performance.

Within any coaching situation, whether in an individual or a team sport, it is extremely difficult to satisfy the needs of all athletes at all times, and it is inconceivable that some will not be concerned that their precise coaching needs are not always being met. Failure to satisfy the needs of athletes can lead them to suffer from lack of confidence, reduced motivation, decreased levels of performance and even to dissatisfaction with their sport. If allowed to continue for any length of time, it can even result in premature 'drop-out' or early retirement from the sport. Obviously in the team sport situation, the loss of a experienced and/or particularly skilful team member can have dire consequences for team morale and potential success.

Athletes may need individualized attention in several different areas. Obviously, the athlete's particular weaknesses will dictate areas for individualized treatment. Some athletes will require particular work on technique development, which may even involve help from a specialist sports scientist such as a biomechanist, etc. Others may need the specialist help of a sports psychologist, counsellor, exercise physiologist, physiotherapist, nutritionist or medical practitioner. In many cases, especially in amateur sport, the coach will personally have to adopt some of these roles. Only in professional or international sport is it common practice to elicit the help of individual specialists to complement the role of the coach. Individualized attention is compounded by some athletes needing frequent monitoring in one or more areas of the coaching process, and some of these for extended periods of time.

Swimming as an exemplar

Many swimming coaches operate under conditions that necessitate them having to work with fairly large groups of athletes (20 or more is not uncommon) in the pool at the same time. Therefore, it is difficult to cater for the individual needs of each and every athlete all of the time. Consequently, the majority of coaches have to compromise on their desire to individualize training programmes for the full range of athletes in order to accommodate adequately the needs of those athletes whom they consider to have priority in one way or another. Rushall (1985a: 4) has noted that priorities will arise because '... attention to individual requirements becomes more important as the level of performance of the athlete improves'. The necessity of having to compromise on individualization strategies raises several important questions to which there are few answers at present. For example, what measures do coaches take, if any, to accommodate the needs of priority athletes? If elite coaches are conscious of the need to individualize training, how do they go about it, given a large group size? Do they concentrate on the needs of the most elite athlete(s) by adopting a demanding schedule, and hope that this does not damage the chances of the others too much, or do they cater to the needs of the weakest in the group, whose need for the coach's attention is after all undeniable? Do some coaches rely on the very best athletes to look after themselves, or do they compromise on both the strongest and the weakest? Swimming coaches have a large variety of individualization practices to choose from. For example, training sessions may be individualized on the basis of stroke lanes (lanes for freestyle, backstroke, etc.), according to the energy requirements of particular events (lanes for sprinters, middle distance and distance athletes), or on areas of strength and/or weakness.

Very little research (some are discussed in the next section) has been carried out in this area. For example, even where coaches do try to individualize training, it is not known whether the measures that they use to individualize training are always put into practice. Periodization is a process of breaking up the training year into manageable sections with specific training or competition objectives etc., and is an almost universal practice for swimming coaches. Different periods in the coaching process may therefore demand more or less attention to individualization within the training year. Are some periods more important than others? For example, the mesocycle immediately preceding a major competition in swimming, in which the training load is reduced gradually (commonly referred to as the 'taper' or as 'peaking'), is normally a period in which swimming programmes receive much more attention to individualization. This is perfectly understandable when one considers the competition requirements of the different swimming events. Obviously a distance athlete (e.g. 1500 m freestyle), while reducing the volume of training drastically in the taper period, will still need to maintain aerobic conditioning, as this is the major player in this event. Sprinters (e.g. 50 m freestyle) will also reduce volume, but will have to 'sharpen up', as their event is explosive and heavily dependent on strength and anaerobic conditioning.

Some athletes may be treated differently depending on status. Most swimming programmes in the United Kingdom consist of disparate groups of athletes working together – that is, athletes not only grouped according to stroke or distance, but also including some who are more successful (elite) than others. It seems likely that these 'higher status' individuals will receive more specialized and individualized programmes than their less successful compatriots. Age too is likely to be a consideration. Certainly, Cross (1991) and Hogg (1995) have suggested that older athletes merit a more collaborative coaching approach than do immature age-groupers. While this may not result in more individualization, it will provide an opportunity for these athletes to express their needs in this regard.

Several constraints acting upon the coaching process will negatively affect the individualization process. Numbers of athletes, size of pool, availability of pool time, pool equipment, conflict with school requirements etc. are all constraints that previous research has identified as having a negative effect on coaching effectiveness in swimming (see, for example, Cross, 1995a, 1995b). These constraints will also limit the amount of individualization possible in this sport. Tensions will arise because of these and other constraints. For example, single or combinations of different constraints have the capacity negatively to affect the individualization strategy. These constraints can be manifested both at the level of practice (for example, a pool without starting blocks will mean no meaningful practice on starts is possible) and at the psychological level (for example, too many athletes or not enough water time may curtail or even prevent individualization taking place, resulting in frustration for both coach and athletes).

Some recent swimming research findings

Recent research (Wright, 1998) carried out with a number of Great Britain's full-time professional swimming coaches (60 completed questionnaires and 18 in-depth interviews) has helped to answer some of the questions posed earlier in this chapter. The questionnaires sought to establish what type of individualization practices coaches employed, and the in-depth interviews discussed not only what kinds of individualization took place, but also the reasons behind the decisions taken. All of the coaches were coaching swimmers at least at national age-group level (i.e. with swimmers who had qualified for the Amateur Swimming Association's National Age-Group Championships), with many also coaching at the elite senior level. As the individualization of training is particularly important for established performance athletes, it was important to ensure that all of the coaches involved in the research were working at an appropriate level. Of course, it is likely that some of them were also coaching some athletes at the participation level. Although 56 of the 60 questionnaire respondents and all of the interviewees were male, this appears to provide a not inaccurate reflection of the present gender composition in full-time professional swimming coaching in Britain at this time. For example, in an earlier swimming research exercise, only 11 females were found in a sample of 76 full-time professional swimming coaches (Cross, 1997b).

The difficulty of always individualizing training in swimming has already been acknowledged, with the frequently large numbers of athletes in each training group cited as a constraint. This was confirmed by the research, which identified that the coaches trained a mean average of 21.6 swimmers in their training group, of which an average of 13.65 were at the elite level. These are very large numbers to handle at the same time, and individualization would be difficult. Additional constraints identified by the coaches centred on differences in ability across the squad, inadequate facilities, insufficient time for adequate training, and lack of finance for sports science support and hiring adequate pool time.

As one might have expected, coaches tended to individualize training more as athletes became older, gained more experience, improved their performance levels and became more mentally and physically mature. While most coaches might attempt to set the correct training loads for each athlete, both Maglischo (1993) and Colwin (1995) have noted that it takes several years before a coach can fully comprehend how each individual athlete reacts and responds to different training loads. In addition, Wright's (1998) interviews with 18 head coaches indicated that most individualized training more if the athlete was committed, older or of high status, and some individualized training more if the swimmer demanded more attention. This last aspect is extremely worrying. If those who demand more attention get it, are some of those who do not make a fuss receiving even less of the individualized attention they deserve?

The research also confirmed that different periods in the training year demanded higher levels of individualization, and the taper period (that period immediately before a major competition when athletes reduce training load substantially) was identified as the most significant period when a large amount of individualization took place.

Considering the importance that each of the coaches gave to the physiological aspects of training, including focusing their planning on the physiological requirements of the particular event chosen by the athlete (e.g. 200 m butterfly, 800 m freestyle, 50 m backstroke, etc.) and the relevant energy system(s), it was surprising to find that diet was one of the most poorly monitored aspects of training. Twenty years' personal experience in swimming coaching supports this finding. Although many coaches understand the importance of a well-balanced diet for athletes, and despite advice provided for elite swimmers at centres of excellence, on national training camps and by team nutritionists, most coaches generally rely on the athletes' parents to provide what is required in the home environment. For this reason, the second part of this chapter focuses on nutrition and its importance to an appropriately individualized training programme.

Individualization and nutrition

Because the individualization of training programmes for elite athletes requires detailed and comprehensive planning, it is surprising that so many coaches appear to take the nutrition of their athletes somewhat for granted. Although an appropriate nutritional strategy is relevant for most sports, swimming coaches in particular often rely principally on parents and the athletes themselves, and occasionally on nutritionists associated with the national team, to look after this aspect of training (Cross, 1997b). However, this is not to deny that many coaches do, in fact, recognize its importance. Indeed, much of the current coach education literature highlights the benefits to be gained from paying proper attention to the recommended proportions of carbohydrate, fat and protein in the athlete's diet. Wellington (1996) has recommended a diet of approximately 60 per cent carbohydrate, 15 per cent protein and 25 per cent fat for swimmers. In addition, Maglischo (1993) has suggested that adult male swimmers (18–25 years) training for 4 hours per day will require between 4000 and 5400 calories per day. Females in the same age range, he contends, will require between 3400 and 4000 calories per day. Unfortunately, very few athletes actually calculate either percentage contributions of the different fuels or overall calories, and this may be compounded by diets often being culture-specific. In the British culture, this often equates with a diet too high in fat and too low in carbohydrate. Carbohydrate is generally accepted as being the 4-star fuel for athletic performance, with ingestion of low glycaemic index (GI) complex carbohydrates recommended 30–60 minutes before exercise or competition. These carbohydrates minimize the hypoglycaemia that can occur at the start of exercise, increase the concentration of fatty acids in the blood and, by increasing fat oxidation, reduce reliance on carbohydrate fuel (Bledsoe, 1997; Rankin, 1997). McArdle *et al.* (1996: 118) have reinforced the important role of carbohydrates, noting that 'lipids [fatty acids] burn in a carbohydrate flame'. Examples of low glycaemic index foods include pasta, soya, apples, peanuts, etc. The glycaemic index of food actually consumed during exercise is, as Rankin (1997: 5) noted, 'probably not critical because the insulin response is muted during exercise'. In addition, the consumption of high glycaemic index foods shortly after exercise (rice cakes, biscuits, etc.) may assist in faster muscle glycogen restoration. However, Bledsoe (1997) notes that this may not be too important if the next exercise bout is more than 24 hours away.

Another advantage of complex carbohydrates over simple carbohydrates is that they also contain an abundance of vitamins and minerals, which the simple sugars do not. One of these minerals is chromium (from beans and peas), a trace mineral which, along with the hormone insulin, unlocks cells and allows sugar to enter, thus contributing to the use of carbohydrate for energy (Applegate, 1998). Finally, they generally contain less fat than the simple variety, and they break down over a longer period. Note, however, that even carbohydrate, if eaten in excess, will be deposited as fat. While few elite athletes could be considered overweight, balancing the requirements of sufficient carbohydrate ingestion to supply the energy needs of training and competition with the obvious advantages to be gained by not carrying too much weight is an aspect of individualization that should be considered carefully by all coaches.

Despite being armed with this kind of knowledge, the multifaceted nature of the coaching process (Lyle, 1992; Cross and Lyle, 1996) and the large amount of time required to cover all aspects of the process often militate against coaches actually finding the time to construct a detailed and individualized nutrition programme for each of their elite athletes. This failure is in turn compounded by the general nutrition literature, where reference is often made to the need for a balanced or varied diet (see for example, Paish, 1979: 60; Wootton, 1989: 154; Williams, 1995: 14) which, it is suggested, will provide not only enough calories but also all of the nutrients needed for athletic performance. While this well-intentioned advice may very well be true for the general population, and even for some elite athletes, it is not always necessarily appropriate in the case of the elite athlete for whom one or more additional factors may contribute to a need for nutritional supplementation of some kind. Indeed, the concept of a varied or balanced diet does nothing to highlight and accentuate the importance of consuming enough liquid during exercise. Waiting until they feel thirsty before taking on fluid is a common mistake exhibited by inexperienced athletes, and is often synonymous with early dehydration.

Some examples of the circumstances in which an elite athlete might need dietary supplements include: when the athlete is on a diet that is low in calories or lacking in certain areas; when the athlete is a vegetarian; when the athlete does not naturally produce high creatine levels; when an overstressed athlete has a particularly low glutamine level; when there is an iron or vitamin deficiency; or when low glycogen levels are found. All of these may, either separately or collectively, require special attention to contribute to optimal performance. Indeed most people, including elite athletes, will have personal likes and dislikes which may detract from a diet that is optimal for the athletic performance required. Not only will personal likes and dislikes affect intake, but so too will individual financial circumstances. For example, many athletes, even in our British culture, cannot always afford the very best or the most desirable of foods. This is particularly true of some of the more popular ergogenic supplements currently on offer, such as creatine, which are expensive. However, the increasing level of lifestyle subsidy being made to elite and potentially elite athletes since the introduction of National Lottery funded support programmes should redress this problem to some extent. Professional sports clubs are also increasingly making attempts to control more directly the dietary intakes of their performers.

Anderson (1997) has testified to the cornucopia of supplements available on the open market, identifying a bewildering array of more than 25 different ergogenic aids currently on offer. Such a large range enables the coach to individualize supplementation. Some of the products, such as creatine and glutamine, were supplements taken by individuals on the 1996 British Olympic swimming team (Cross, 1997b), while the majority of the others were not. With one supplement in particular, Endurox, reported to lower heart rate, lift lactate threshold and help the athlete to burn 43 per cent more fat when training, it is surprising that many more supplements were not found to be in use at this elite level. It has been suggested that this particular supplement should not be incorporated into the athlete's diet until further research has been carried out. Incidentally, Anderson's list did not include reference to specific vitamin supplementation, for which there is evidence (vitamins E and C) of benefits to the immune system (Pyne and Gray, 1994), nor to additional iron supplementation, also important in immune function (Brock, 1992).

Although not important for immune function, Anderson's (1997) list also ignores one of the very latest advertised ergogenic aids; medium chain triglycerides (MCTs), an alternative energy fuel to carbohydrates, which are purported to boost endurance performance (Jeukendrup, 1996). An MCT, produced from coconut oil, is a fatty acid with a small molecular size, is liquid at room temperature, is much more miscible in water than long chain triglycerides (LCTs) and is apparently rapidly digested and absorbed in the intestine. After absorption, these fatty acids are transported directly to the liver and later, at cell level, are apparently easily absorbed and oxidized, providing twice as much energy per gram as glucose. As such, they may serve an important function in reducing muscle glycogen breakdown and so delay the onset of exhaustion. However, Jeukendrup (1996) suggests that the possible benefits are as yet not supported by enough scientific evidence to recommend general use.

Even caffeine has been suggested to be a possible ergogenic aid (Graham, 1998). Graham's article cites research that has apparently shown that caffeine supplementation may have resulted in trained swimmers being 1 s faster over 100 m. In these circumstances, it is almost certain that some coaches will be interested in using it in this way. Graham has suggested that caffeine may be the most commonly used or abused drug in sport, and that this may be because it is socially accepted (coffee and chocolate), readily available, inexpensive and easily orally ingested. Despite there being stipulated levels permissible under current doping control regulations, these are significantly in excess of the levels necessary for gaining substantial ergogenic assistance.

One further consideration should be taken into account. Peak performance is thought to be dependent on an environment where external pressures and anxiety are minimized. Therefore, taking supplements such as multivitamins or creatine or other substances (whether actually needed or not) may be just one way of reducing such anxiety. Where excess levels are harmlessly passed in the normal way (e.g. via the urine) and where expense is not an issue, the psychological benefits may very well be justified for some athletes. This is another example of the potential individualization of aspects of the coaching process.

What does the research show us about supplements?

Creatine
Cross (1997b) found that six females (two of whom described themselves as vegetarians despite both eating fish) and eight males from the total sample of 28 (13F, 15M) swimmers on the British swimming team reported taking creatine in supplement form in preparation for the 1996 Olympic Games in Atlanta.

Creatine, an amino acid, is a naturally occurring substance found in considerable quantities in meat and fish (Thomson, 1995; Greenhaff *et al.*, 1996). However, Greenhaff (Edinburgh University presentation, May 11, 1998) has noted that white meat (both fish and chicken) has higher levels of creatine than does red meat. Incidentally, at the same presentation Greenhaff suggested that it might be more beneficial to take creatine in conjunction with carbohydrates. Although vegetarians may receive no creatine from the diet, it can be manufactured by the body, primarily by the liver. According to Greenhaff *et al.* (1996), the total creatine pool in a 70-kg male amounts to approximately 120 g, of which 95 per cent is found in muscle. Note, however, that some individuals will have much lower levels than others. The major proportion of the muscle creatine is found in fast twitch skeletal muscle rather than in slow twitch or heart muscle, a fact that would appear to support its relationship with power rather than endurance. In fact, Greenhaff *et al.* (1996: 224) found that the availability of creatine phosphate in type II (fast twitch) muscle fibres is of critical importance to the maintenance of performance during maximal, short-lasting exercise. In terms of individualization, there may be important implications here for sprinters in general and for vegetarian sprinters in particular.

Despite the various natural sources of creatine, many athletes at the elite level are concerned that they might need more than that available from primary sources. This is to provide additional creatine/creatine phosphate stores in order to improve ATP production during the first 10 s or so of exercise, and in the hope that, by increasing these stores, the anaerobic glycolysis optimum 'production run' will be prolonged beyond its normal 20 s or so. If these benefits have been accurately assessed, creatine supplementation may be of advantage during single high-intensity bouts of exercise of short duration (all of the 50 m sprint events in swimming; 100 m and 200 m sprints in athletics) and, by acting as a buffer for lactic acid, may also help to delay the onset of fatigue in all anaerobic events and training.

How much should athletes take? In terms of individualization, this is a difficult question to answer, and it is not something that should be tried for the first time just before a major competition. As Greenhaff *et al.* (1996) have noted, different individuals have different natural levels of muscle creatine concentration, although there appears to be an upper limit that cannot be exceeded by supplementation. Consequently, it is possible that creatine supplementation will not have a positive effect with individuals who have naturally high levels, but may be of significant value where individuals have lower levels (e.g. vegetarians). Their suggested dose for the latter is 20 g per day for 5 days, followed by 2 g per day thereafter, over a 4-week period. However, the results of a very recent survey into creatine use in sport, reported in the *The Independent* newspaper (December 8, 1998), suggest that the supplement's long-term use has yet to be tested and that, with some doctors suggesting that it can cause kidney damage, cramping and dehydration, athletes should approach its use with caution.

Glutamine
Only one athlete in Cross' (1997b) research, a female, was found to be taking glutamine as a supplement at the time. Glutamine is a neutral amino acid with an important function in maintaining immunity to infection during repeated high intensity exercise (Pyne and Gray, 1994; Rowbottom *et al.*, 1996). In fact, Pyne and Gray (1994) reported research by Parry-Billings *et al.* in 1992 which demonstrated that glutamine supplementation prevented the plasma concentration of glutamine from markedly decreasing for 48 British athletes (runners, swimmers and rowers) when they were exercised to exhaustion. Decreased levels of plasma glutamine (below 80 per cent of normal) inhibit lymphocyte function, leading to a reduction in the efficiency of the immune system. This adds to the risk of infection, especially during periods of 'overload' training (Rowbottom *et al.*, 1996).

Natural sources of glutamine include meat and fish, with wheat providing a source for vegetarians. Note that glutamine is the most abundant amino

acid in human muscle and plasma. Some manufacturers are currently producing supplements containing both glutamine and creatine packaged together.

Vitamins
Cross' (1997b) research with the 1996 British Olympic swimming team discovered that a total of 21 swimmers (11F, 10M) were taking vitamin supplements of one kind or another. Although the majority of these were either
taking multivitamins (6F, 6M) or vitamin C tablets (7F, 7M), other named
vitamins included vitamin E (1F, 2M), cod liver oil with vitamins A and D
(1F), and cod liver oil with zinc and vitamins B12 and B6 (1M).

Vitamins are a group of unrelated organic compounds that perform specific functions to promote growth and maintain health (Wilmore and Costill,
1994). Although most vitamins have some function important to the athlete,
only the B-complex vitamins and vitamins C and E have been extensively
investigated for their potential to facilitate athletic performance. For example,
according to Wilmore and Costill, the importance of the vitamin B complex
should not be underestimated for its role in cellular metabolism and for the
vitamins in this complex to act as co-factors in various enzyme systems
involved in the oxidation of food and the production of energy. Where
there is a deficiency of the vitamins in this complex, supplementation of
one or more of the B complex vitamins can facilitate performance.

Vitamin C is essential for healthy bones, ligaments and blood vessels, and
is also of importance to the athlete because of its functions in metabolizing
amino acids, synthesizing some hormones and promoting iron absorption
from the intestines. Pyne and Gray (1994) have also highlighted the importance of iron in immune function. Although many people believe that vitamin
C assists healing, combats fever and infection and prevents or cures the
common cold, Wilmore and Costill (1994) have reminded readers that the
evidence to date is inconclusive.

Vitamin E's most important role is as an antioxidant (Wilmore and Costill,
1994). For example, Dowden (1996) highlights the importance of this vitamin
in the body's antioxidant defences. Despite this, various swimming coaches
(e.g. Maglischo, 1982) had previously suggested that it should be used with
caution as megadoses of this vitamin have been reported to have a detrimental effect on the athlete, with headaches, blurred vision, gastrointestinal
disturbances and low blood sugar the possible results of its use.

The natural sources for most vitamins, including the main antioxidants
such as vitamins C and E and betacarotene, are fruits and vegetables, especially the brightly coloured ones such as carrots, peppers, broccoli and apri-
cots (Dowden, 1996).

Carbohydrate loading

Although only four female swimmers on the 1996 British Olympic swimming
team (Cross, 1997b) admitted using pre-competition carbohydrate loading –
that is, increasing the amount of carbohydrate as a percentage of the overall
diet just before competition – 8 of the 13 regularly used carbohydrate drinks
during training and/or competition. This trend was reversed for the males,
with 6 using pre-competition carbohydrate loading but only 5 admitting to
using carbohydrate drinks. There was no particular drink common to either

group, with a wide variety of the current brands being named. Although the somewhat dated practice of starving the athlete of carbohydrate for the first 3 days of the final week before a major competition and then overcompensating for the last 4 days is no longer popular (Wilmore and Costill, 1994), it is still beneficial to maintain or increase carbohydrate intake (in tandem with more rest and less intense training) during the final week before a competition to ensure glycogen levels are high. In addition, replacing glycogen stores occurs faster if carbohydrate intake is sooner rather than later following exercise. It is not always practical to take solids immediately after exercise, and this is where carbohydrate drinks can make a significant difference. Even here, coaches should be aware that not all athletes can digest the same carbohydrates equally. For example, although bananas have a reputation for being an ideal complex carbohydrate for athletes (complex carbohydrates break down slowly and do not contain as much fat as simple sugars), experience has shown that several swimmers have experienced difficulties in digesting them quickly. Consequently, different types of food should be tried and tested by individual athletes in training before being used in the competitive environment.

It would appear from Cross' research that, despite well-intentioned nutritional advice from various quarters which advise a varied or balanced diet as being all that is needed for athletic performance, many elite athletes are taking supplements of one kind or another. The reasons for this are not always clear-cut, with some supplements used for their performance enhancing properties, others because of a perceived dietary deficiency and some for their placebo effect. Whatever the reason, the fact that several are taking supplements at present, and that others are considering taking them (in some cases, should the substances be shown to have a beneficial effect), testifies to the need for coaches to treat this aspect of training seriously. While the suggestion that a varied and/or balanced diet is all that is needed for sporting performance might be a safe option for general health, it may not be the best option for all of our very elite athletes. Many elite athletes, because of personal likes and dislikes, and some because of the expense involved, might benefit from a variety of supplements. Certainly, many will be competing against athletes from those parts of the world where scientific backup is ensuring the very best in terms of legal ergogenic aids for their athletes. When individualizing training programmes, our coaches too, have a responsibility in this regard.

Summary

This chapter has highlighted the importance of individualization as a principle of both coaching and training theory (Rushall, 1985a; Bompa, 1994). The analysis has sought to reinforce the importance of coaches routinely individualizing training and other aspects of the coaching process. The importance of individualizing training in terms of physiology, age and maturation, experience and current skill levels, and training state and stage in the coaching process, has been identified. Additional factors such as athlete status, commitment and responsibility have also been highlighted. Considerable attention was given to the problems that coaches encounter when attempting to match the process to individual athletes. Constraints that limit or compromise the amount of individualization possible with elite athletes were discussed and some recommendations made.

One particular aspect of the coaching process was used as an exemplar. The coaches' attention (often inattention) to the individual nutritional requirements of their athletes was shown to be very important, but also to be a rather neglected element of the individual athlete's overall preparation for training and competition. Sufficient variety in athletes' basic and supplementary dietary intake was illustrated to suggest that the individual athlete's specific needs can and should be catered for. An example of current practice was provided by referring to some fairly recent research carried out with several of Great Britain's top swimmers and coaches.

The analysis, particularly that to do with the nutritional and ergogenic aspects of training, is not intended to be a blueprint for coaches' action. However, it does demonstrate that, even at the highest levels, there is considerable scope for improved practice. It is a plea for coaches to move beyond inaction, and to be aware that this is an important aspect of an all-embracing coaching process. The early part of the chapter demonstrated clearly that individual specialization, technique development, competition requirements, and physical, psychological and emotional makeup must be taken into account if the coaching process is to be optimally effective for each athlete. Nevertheless, this has to be balanced against the practicalities of completely individualizing training, particularly in the team sport situation. Further research is required into coaching behaviour, particularly in team sports, to establish good practice. For the performance coach and for the performance athlete, a number of individualization strategies are possible. These will range from individual goal-setting, individually focused drills, monitoring to provide individual feedback and analysis, personally tailored schedules, and a clear distinction between group and individual psychological intervention. Individualization is problematical, but this must not be used as an excuse for lack of detailed planning or a failure to consider the particular needs of individual athletes.

References

Anderson, O. (1997). Ergogenic aids: Don't be taken in too soon by the claims of this latest 'magic potion'. *Peak Perf.*, **86**, 2–6.

Applegate, L. (1998). Nutrition: Looking for a boost. *Runner's World*, **33(9)**, 24–6.

Bledsoe, J. (1997). Things mother forgot to tell you about the glycaemic index of your food – and how it influences your training. *Peak Perf.*, **93**, 4–8.

Bompa, T. O. (1994). *Theory and Methodology of Training* (3rd edn). Kendall Hunt.

Brock, J. H. (1992). Iron and the immune system. In *Iron and Human Desease* (R. B. Lauffer, ed.), pp. 161–78. CRC Press.

Colwin, C. (1995). Gold that doesn't glitter. *Swimming Tech.*, **32(2)**, 7–8.

Cooke, G. (1990). A scientific approach to rugby excellence. *Coaching Focus*, **15**, 10.

Costill, D. L., Maglischo, E. W. and Richardson, A. B. (1992). *Swimming*. Blackwell Scientific.

Cross, N. (1990). Terry Denison: An insight into a coaching philosophy. *Swimming Times*, **LXVII(4)**, 17–19.

Cross, N. (1991). Arguments in favour of a humanistic coaching process. *Swimming Times*, **LXVIII(11)**, 17–18.

Cross, N. (1995a). Coaching effectiveness and the coaching process. Part 1. *Swimming Times*, **LXXII(2)**, 23–5.

Cross, N. (1995b). Coaching effectiveness in hockey: A Scottish perspective. *Scot. J. Physical Ed.*, **23(1)**, 27–39.

Cross, N. (1997a). Overtraining: A swimming coach perspective. *Scot. Centre Res. Papers Sport Leisure Soc.*, **2**, 114–25.

Cross, N. (1997b). Nutrition and the elite athlete: Implications for the management of coaching practice. *Swimming Times*, **LXXIV(6)**, 25–6.

Cross, N. and Lyle, J. (1996). Overtraining and the coaching process: Implications for the management of coaching practice. *Scot. J. Physical Ed.*, **24(3)**, 28–43.

Dowden, A. (1996). Upping the anti oxidant. *Ultrafit*, **6(5)**, 51–3.

Fairs, J. (1987). The coaching process: The essence of coaching. *Sports Coach*, **11(1)**, 17–20.

Franks, I., Sinclair, G. D., Thompson, W. and Goodman, D. (1986). Analysis of the coaching process. *Science Periodical on Research on Technology in Sport*. CAC, Paper A.

Graham, T. (1998). Caffeine and coffee: a useful supplement? *Insider*, **6(2)**, 1–7.

Greenhaff, P., Bodin, K., Casey, A. *et al.*, (1996). Dietary creatine supplementation and fatigue during high-intensity exercise in humans. In *Biochemistry of Exercise* (R. J. Maughan and S. M. Shirreffs, eds), pp. 219–42. Human Kinetics.

Hardy, C. A. (1995). The realities of coaching swimming: A systematic observation study. *Swimming Times*, **LXXII(11)**, 25–8.

Harre, D. (Ed.) (1982). *Trainingslehre*. Sportverlag.

Hogg, J. M. (1995). *Mental Skills for Swim Coaches*. Sport Excel Publishing.

Jeukendrup, A. E. (1996). MCT and the athlete's diet. *Insider*, **4(3)**, 1–6.

Lombardo, B. J. (1987). *The Humanistic Coach: From Theory to Practice*. Charles C Thomas.

Lyle, J. (1992). Systematic coaching behaviour: An investigation into the coaching process and the implications of the findings for coach education. In *Sport and Physical Activity* (T. Williams, L. Almond and A. Sparkes, eds), pp. 463–9. EFN Spon.

Lyle, J. (1996). A conceptual appreciation of the sports coaching process. *Scot. Centre Res. Papers Sport Leisure Soc.*, **1**, 15–37.

Maglischo, E. W. (1982). *Swimming Faster*. Mayfield Pubs.

Maglischo, E. W. (1993). *Swimming Even Faster*. Mayfield Pubs.

Mathers, J. F. (1997). Professional coaching in golf: Is there an appreciation of the coaching process? *Scot. J. Physical Ed.*, **25(1)**, 23–35.

McArdle, W. D., Katch, F. I. and Katch, V. L. (1996). *Exercise Physiology: Energy, Nutrition and Human Performance* (4th edn). Williams and Wilkins.

McGowan, M., Sucec, A. A., Frey, M. A. B. *et al.* (1990). Gold medal volleyball: The training program and physiological profile of the 1984 Olympic champions. *Res. Q. Exer. Sport*, **61(2)**, 196–200.

Paish, W. (1979). *Diet in Sport*. EP Publishing.

Parry-Billings, M., Budgett, R., Koutedakis, Y. *et al.* (1992). Plasma amino acid concentrations in the overtraining syndrome: Possible effects on the immune system. *Med. Sci. Sports Exer.*, **24**, 1353–8.

Pyne, D. B. and Gray, A. B. (1994). Exercise and the immune system. *State of the Art Review*. Australian Sports Commission: National Sports Research Centre.

Rankin, J. W. (1997). Glycemic index and exercise metabolism. *Sports Sci. Exch.*, **10(1)**, 64.

Rowbottom, D. G., Keast, D. and Morton, A. R. (1996). The emerging role of glutamine as an indicator of exercise stress and overtraining. *Sports Med.*, **21(2)**, 20–2.

Rushall, B. S. (1985a). Several principles of modern coaching. *Sports Coach*, **8(3)**, 40–4.

Rushall, B. S. (1985b). Seven principles for modern coaching: Part II. *Sports Coach*, **8(4)**, 21–3.

Scobie, B. (1991). Coaching the elite athlete. *Coaching Focus*, **16**, 7–9.

Sherman, C. and Sands, R. (1996). Thinking ahead – a new perspective. *Sports Coach*, **19(1)**, 31–4.

Thomson, K. (1995). Creatine supplementation in swimming: Does it give you an edge? *Swimming Times*, **LXXII(5)**, 25–6.

Trebels, A. (1992). Individualizing of movement actions – a fundamental problem of movement pedagogy. *Int. J. Physical Ed.*, **XXIX(4)**, 9–14.

Troup, J. and Reese, R. (1983). *A Scientific Approach to the Sport of Swimming*. Scientific Sports Inc.

Wellington, P. (1996). Nutrition preparation of the GB swimming team for the 1996 Olympic Games. *Swimming Times*, **LXXIII(9)**, 27–8.

Whitson, D. (1980). Coaching as a human relationship. *Momentum*, **5(2)**, 36–42.

Williams, C. (1995). Nutrition and sports performance. In *Nutrition and Sport* (J. J. Strain, ed.), pp. 3–20. SCI.

Wilmore, J. H. and Costill, D. L. (1994). *Physiology of Sport and Exercise*. Human Kinetics.

Wootton, S. (1989). *Nutrition for Sport*. Simon and Schuster.

Wright, I. (1998). Individualization of training programmes in competitive swimming. Unpublished MSc thesis, Faculty of Education, University of Edinburgh.

10

Overtraining and the coaching process[1]

Neville Cross and John Lyle

- The concept of overtraining
- Defining and explaining overtraining, its causes and symptoms
- Stress hormone activity and overtraining
- Incidence of overtraining in the sport of swimming
- Monitoring for signs of overtraining
- The need to treat coaching as a process
- Approaches to prevent overtraining: periodization, cyclic training etc.
- Nutritional considerations
- Summing up of overtraining issues

Introduction

Overtraining is a process which, when combined with ineffective management of the stresses acting on the athlete, ultimately results in what is commonly referred to as 'overtraining syndrome'. In this state, physical, psychological and emotional factors contribute to a chronically depressed athletic performance. In this chapter, a number of elements of the coaching process that have the capacity to prevent overtraining are discussed. Strategies are suggested for monitoring training status and, thus, for avoiding some of the dangers of overstressing the athlete. For example, coaches have a responsibility to implement a coaching process, especially with elite and high-level performance athletes, which is comprehensively planned, adequately and frequently monitored and in which, through careful regulation of the training loading factors, the athlete's progress and wellbeing are constantly emphasized. Although the great majority of the principles discussed in this chapter are appropriate to all sports, and to all levels of athletic performance, the sport of swimming and elite competitive swimmers are used throughout the chapter as a focus for the discussion. The sport of swimming has been chosen as an exemplar because one of the authors has considerable experience of coaching this sport at the very highest level, and has carried out considerable research in the past in this area (see Cross, 1997, in particular). Examples will be given in the chapter of particular circum-

---

[1] This chapter is an extension of our thoughts on overtraining and the coaching process first reported in *The Scottish Journal of Physical Education*, **24(3)**, 28–43.

stances in the sport of swimming in which athletes have been reported to have suffered from 'overtraining syndrome'.

Elite athletes are most at risk from overtraining. This is not really surprising when one considers the motivational reward environment fostered by our performance and excellence sport sub-system. With substantial National Lottery grants being made to successful athletes, and with a variety of other financial incentives including sponsorship, appearance money and win bonuses etc. on offer, commitment to training and competition is, as a result, often extremely intense. In addition, coaches and athletes operating at the elite level are well aware that the small increments in performance standards that are possible at the highest level will require training programmes that are both extensive in scale and may also need to be conducted at a high level of intensity.

The difficulty of balancing the perceived need for high-intensity, high-volume loadings with adequate periods of rest and recovery creates the potential for a less than optimal 'adapted performance state', with concomitant effects on the health and wellbeing of the athletes involved. At the final chronically depressed performance stage, the athlete is usually said to be suffering from 'overtraining syndrome'. This chapter will suggest that overtraining can best be conceptualized and understood as the outcome of a process (albeit a mismanaged one), and that the prevention of overtraining is influenced most significantly by the quality of coaching direction and practice (i.e. coaching effectiveness), which itself also constitutes a process.

Overtraining and coaching: a coincidence of interests

The interdependency between the concepts of overtraining and the management of the coaching process are at the heart of the discussion in this chapter. It is necessary therefore to identify the assumptions upon which the argument is based and to demonstrate the similarity of the contexts within which both the overtraining syndrome and a developed coaching process are most likely to occur. The common denominator in each case is the performer who, in order to secure improvements in performance, undertakes a series of intensive training loads. Where there is insufficient time between these training loads (which may include competition) for rest and recovery, their cumulative effect can lead to a diminution in the adaptive training state of the performer and, ultimately, 'overtraining syndrome'. The frequency, duration and intensity of training and commitment implied in this scenario are also characteristic of the essential elements of the performance coaching process. Coaching here refers to the serial, goal-directed, interdependent, multivariable accumulation of training, competition and other units or episodes that together constitute a process. How the coach manages this process through planning, monitoring and regulation will have a direct bearing upon the training state of the athlete.

The overtraining syndrome, whatever the causal mechanism, is the final stage in a process that passes through either (or both) overstraining (sometimes referred to as 'local overtraining') and overreaching (short-term imbalance between stress and adaptation). The term 'syndrome' itself connotes a characteristic grouping of factors within which a continuous, cumulative and perhaps predictable succession of events leads to the characteristic outcome. It will be argued that:

1. Overtraining often results from an inappropriate implementation of the coaching process
2. Overtraining can be prevented by the effective implementation of appropriate planning, monitoring and regulation procedures
3. Detailed attention to performance goals, training theory principles and individualized training programmes is essential in order to avoid overtraining at the elite level
4. Unmanaged, episodic coaching will not produce the continuity of data awareness necessary to provide an adequate early warning system
5. Attention to the breadth of variables encompassed in the coaching process provides a richer source of potential influences on the performer's adapted training state than does a narrower focus based solely upon the physical conditioning programme.

The defining element of the coaching process is the attempt to control the variables that influence athletic performance. If it can be shown that overtraining results from the mismanagement of some of these variables, it seems likely that attention to good coaching practice, which should include appropriate attention being paid to all of the constituent parts of the coaching process, will be a strong preventative measure in reducing the incidence of overtraining.

Overtraining defined

Overtraining is a pathological state of training (Bompa, 1983; Fry *et al.*, 1992a; Wilmore and Costill, 1994). Exhaustion, which is also the consequence of an imbalance between accumulated training stress and the adaptability of the body, is the organism's response to *short-term* imbalance, sometimes referred to during a training programme as overreaching (Fry *et al.*, 1991). Overtraining (better referred to as overtraining syndrome) is generally the system result of an imbalance accumulated *over a prolonged period*.

The cumulative or processual element of overtraining is important. For example, Chogovadze and Butchenko (1992) have noted that the 'insidious road to overtraining' is often signposted at the end of training sessions by residual fatigue and soreness, persistent minor injuries, loss of self-motivation and/or lack of progress. Unfortunately, as Wilmore and Costill (1994) have noted, most of the apparent symptoms that arise from and during overtraining, such as those identified by Chogovadze and Butchenko and other symptoms such as sleeping difficulties, loss of appetite and unexplained weight loss, are often subjective in perception and interpretation. They can also be highly individualized and are therefore not always susceptible to an all-embracing diagnosis. In fact, the picture is further complicated by Wilmore and Costill, who have also reminded us that the underlying causes of overtraining syndrome are, as yet, not fully understood. However, they have suggested that it is likely that *physical* or *emotional* overload, or a *combination of these two stresses*, is most likely to trigger the overtraining condition. The symptoms identified above would seem to support the notion of a combination of different types of stress.

The distinction between physical and emotional or psychological stress is an important one (Counsilman, 1968; Maglischo, 1982), and highlights the importance of coaches considering both psychology and physiology in any analysis of overtraining. In fact, Maglischo draws attention to the confusion regarding the origin of overtraining by informing us that 'it is difficult, if not impossible, to determine whether overtraining is psychological or physiological in origin' (1982: 368). Many of the analyses that address the psychological aspects of overtraining further complicate the picture by usually referring to *resultant* rather than *causal* symptoms (although some of these may be appropriate in either case).

Resultant symptoms such as depression, anxiety, insomnia, boredom and lack of motivation have been identified (Madrigal, 1985; Feigley, 1985; Fry *et al.*, 1991), and overtraining in this context is often referred to as 'burnout' or 'staleness'. Fry *et al.* (1991) also identified some of the emotional factors which may contribute (i.e. are causal symptoms) to the overtraining state, and cited the work of Costill (1986) and Selye (1957) in this regard. Thus, the demands of competition, such as the desire to win, fear of failure, setting unrealistically high goals and the high expectations of coach and/or family, may also contribute to the overtraining state inasmuch as they also contribute to the overall psychological stress placed on the athlete.

Morgan *et al.* (1987, 1988) lend support to our argument that the concept of overtraining is best understood as the outcome of a *process* with their important work on 'mood states', both before and after the critical onset of overtraining. They have suggested that the distinction should be approached in terms of product and process. Thus, they suggested that the onset of overtraining might be better referred to as staleness (a common term in North America), and that the term overtraining, as it really reflects a process, should indicate the stimulus or antecedent variables leading to the ultimate state of staleness. Note that this ultimate state is normally referred to as overtraining syndrome in the United Kingdom (see for example, Budgett, 1995 and Newsholme, 1995).

Despite Wilmore and Costill's (1994) assertion that the actual mechanisms to explain overtraining are not yet clear, Chogovadze and Butchenko (1992) went some way to explaining what is happening during the process with their reference to the control systems involved with human movement. Like Kuipers and Kiezer (1988), they noted that overtraining syndrome is a dysfunction of the neuro-endocrine system, localized at the hypothalamic level (the hypothalamus is that area of the brain concerned with regulating homeostasis). Further, they identified two types of overtraining; local and general. Local overtraining affects a specific part of the body, whereas general overtraining affects the whole body and results in overall stagnation and/or a decrease in performance. As far as Chogovadze and Butchenko (1992) were concerned, the presence of local overtraining (referred to as 'overstrain' by Fry *et al.*, 1991) is relatively simple to recognize, since it is often accompanied by stiffness or soreness in a particular muscle group in which the symptoms do not dissipate with alternate days of work and rest. However, the presence of general overtraining is not always so easy to detect and requires some knowledge of those parts of the body involved in adaptation to stress. For example, adaptation to physical, psychological and environmental stress depends on the links between the central nervous system (CNS – termed the 'fast control system of the body') and the endocrine system (termed the 'slow control system').

The endocrine system is a major player in the management of stress. This system controls a complex group of glands whose hormones are vital to all aspects of life, including preparation of muscle for physical activity in the face of stress (adrenal glands), anti-stress responses at cell level including demands for extra energy (thyroid gland), and a variety of other glands involved in producing human growth hormone, insulin and testosterone. Thus, two categories of general overtraining have been identified (Chogovadze and Butchenko, 1992; Bompa, 1994):

1. A-overtraining (addisonic overtraining) which is associated with diminished activity of the adrenal glands and is difficult to detect early (performance may merely remain static)
2. B-overtraining (basedowic overtraining) which is associated mainly with thyroid hyperactivity, leading to the classic symptoms of overtraining such as tendency to tire easily, susceptibility to colds, depression etc.

One of the few ways of detecting A-overtraining early is by an increase in diastolic blood pressure during and after physical stress (Chogovadze and Butchenko, 1992) – not something that is normally part of an average coach's monitoring behaviour!

According to Bompa (1994: 113), addisonic overtraining (or addisonoid as he labels it – sometimes referred to as parasympathetic overtraining), which results in an increase in inhibition processes, is normally caused by an excessively high volume of training. Basedowic (or basedowoid) overtraining (sometimes referred to as sympathetic overtraining), on the other hand, is normally associated with hyperexcitability and restlessness (Flynn, 1998) and is the result of over-stressing emotional processes, usually through over-emphasizing high intensity stimuli in training.

'Stress hormone' activity in relation to overtraining has been noted by various researchers (Burke *et al.*, 1982; Troup, 1986; Kuipers and Keizer, 1988; O'Connor *et al.*, 1989; Hooper *et al.*, 1993; Wilmore and Costill, 1994). For example, O'Connor *et al.* (1989) found that salivary cortisol, global mood disturbance and depression were significantly raised in American female college swimmers during overtraining. In addition, although many of the results were inconclusive, Hooper and co-workers' (1993) research carried out with 14 elite Australian swimmers did appear to suggest that monitoring the level of plasma norepinephrine in athletes might be a useful way of assessing an athlete's risk of overtraining. In their study, three of the elite swimmers identified as suffering from the overtraining syndrome (based on performance decrements and high, prolonged levels of fatigue) exhibited higher norepinephrine levels than the other swimmers from mid-season onward, and significantly higher levels during the taper period. Acknowledging that further work was required to confirm their data, the results were positive enough for them to suggest that, because norepinephrine levels of 'stale' athletes were elevated at the same time points in the season, monitoring norepinephrine levels might provide an objective means of monitoring the overtraining syndrome. However, Wilmore and Costill have pointed out that the measurement of hormone concentrations such as norepinephrine is expensive, complex and time-consuming, and therefore unlikely to be widely used (1994: 305). Similarly, they suggested that measuring blood enzyme levels (for example, creatine phosphokinase levels suggest muscle cell membrane damage) is also both difficult and expensive, and may even confuse the issue. While blood enzyme levels may increase and muscle damage occur during overtraining, both occur frequently during intensive eccentric exercise, regardless of the state of training (1994: 306).

At this point, it is worth commenting on what is sometimes anecdotally referred to as post-viral syndrome (*The Independent*, Tuesday 7 November 1989). This 'mystery illness', which can attack athletes in hard training, involves extreme exhaustion and a susceptibility to common ailments, and is not unlike the appearance of glandular fever. In this case it is the concentration of glutamine in the lymphocytes (a subset of leucocytes, the white blood cells) that appears to be the indicator of potential trouble. A concentration of 80 per cent of normal levels inhibits lymphocyte function, leading to a reduction in efficiency of the immune system and, hence, to post-viral syndrome. Glutamine is an amino acid essential for making proteins, and is needed in large quantities. Unfortunately, it is processed in the large muscles and is often depleted after severe exertion (Rowbottom *et al.*, 1996). Therefore it is rest, not work, which is the key; not enough rest means that the concentration remains low, near the 80 per cent mark, and the syndrome persists. Koutedakis *et al.* (1990) have highlighted the importance of rest in underperforming competitors.

Pyne and Gray (1994) have also highlighted the role of iron in immune function, citing the work of Brock (1992). Not only do lymphocytes require iron in order to increase in number, but the effectiveness of both leucocytes and neutrophils (which ingest and destroy foreign particles) is also directly related to the availability of iron. As intensive exercise is generally associated with immune suppression and increased risk of upper respiratory tract infection (Mackinnon, 1998), oral supplementation of glutamine and/or iron may prove beneficial in the prevention of infection during periods of intensive exercise. The role of nutrition in the prevention of overtraining is covered in more depth later in this chapter.

Incidences of overtraining in swimming

Overtraining syndrome can be the result of either physiological or psychological overstress, or a combination of both, and the locker room slogan 'No pain, no gain' has just enough truth in it to be dangerously misinterpreted by both coaches and athletes (Feigley, 1985). Because many high-level swimmers have a particularly high work ethic, they often apply this slogan in an effort to realize maximum potential. For some of them, the price is too high and overtraining syndrome is the result. For example, Mackinnon and Hooper (1991) and Budgett (1995) have suggested that 10 per cent of elite competitive college swimmers in the United States can be described as 'burning out' each year, and Hooper *et al.* (1993) described three out of 14 elite

Australian swimmers in their research group preparing for the national trials as being 'stale'. In Great Britain, Wilson (1995), himself an Olympic swimming finalist and European silver medallist, has documented his own debilitating experience of the syndrome, and Cross (1997) discovered that the 76 swimming coaches he surveyed estimated that, between them, they had coached a minimum of 80 swimmers suffering from overtraining syndrome. In addition, Pyne (1989) has suggested that overtraining may occur far more frequently than has been recognized to date.

Despite the large research literature on overtraining, high-level athletes continue to be put under, and to place themselves under, considerable stress in order to improve competitive performance. As Denison (1995: 10), one of Britain's most successful swimming coaches, has noted, 'there is a fine line between achieving peak fitness and becoming overtrained'. It is clear that the coach's responsibility is to guide each athlete along this fine line so that there are maximum benefits in physiological adaptation without pushing the athlete into the overtraining zone. However, some of the very qualities of elite athletes – such as determination, preparedness to endure pain and discomfort, a great work ethic etc. – can and sometimes do actually encourage it. In addition, Hooper *et al.* (1993) have noted that some elite athletes, already 'stale' and hence performing poorly in training and competition, sometimes actually intensify training instead of reducing it in the mistaken belief that more, rather than less, work is called for to rectify the situation.

Consequently, in order to address the problem of overtraining (either athlete or coach initiated), coaches should individualize coaching practice and provide a planning strategy for each athlete aimed at achieving the most effective balance between stress and overstress. Such a structured training programme (Kuipers and Keizer, 1988) should avoid excessive increases in training load, vary training loads in terms of volume and intensity, and include regular monitoring of the programme so as to avoid the onset of overtraining.

Overtraining and coaching practice

Waiting until the performer reaches the overtraining state (staleness or overtraining syndrome) before taking remedial action is often too late for success to be achieved in that particular season. Coaches should therefore implement procedures that help to signpost the approach of staleness and allow remedial action to take place before it reaches chronic proportions (see National Coaching Foundation, 1995 for an overview). Blood testing for abnormally high levels of stress hormones such as norepinephrine may be one way although, as Wilmore and Costill (1994) have recognized, it is expensive, complex and time-consuming. Although testing for high levels of salivary cortisol (O'Connor *et al.*, 1989) does offer a non-invasive method of monitoring stress levels, it too is expensive and time-consuming. What is needed is a relatively simple and reliable test (or battery of tests) that can be conducted weekly or fortnightly during the hard training phase of the season in order to monitor training adaptability and training state. Wilmore and Costill (1994: 307), in weighing up the options, suggested that:

The best predictors of overtraining syndrome appear to be heart rate, oxygen uptake, and blood lactate responses to a standardized bout of work. Performance decrements are also good indicators.

In addition to these recommendations, Dressendorfer *et al.* (1985) and Kuipers and Keizer (1988) have suggested that a clinical feature of staleness (especially that related to large volumes of work) is an increased resting heart rate. Monitoring performers' resting heart rates may therefore provide a very simple and effective method of anticipating overtraining syndrome and act as an early warning device. However, Noakes (1986: 230) noted the work of Czajkowski (1982) with cross-country skiers, which suggested that the morning resting heart rate (lying in bed) and another taken exactly 20 seconds after getting up might provide a better indicator of approaching staleness. Not only was staleness exhibited by a higher resting heart rate, but also by a bigger difference between lying and standing rates. Despite this, coaches should proceed with caution when using resting heart rate as an indicator of overtraining. Budgett (1995: 11) has noted that it is perfectly normal for resting heart rate to rise during a period of hard training.

Of Wilmore and Costill's predictors, those most appropriate for swimmers appear to be heart rate and blood lactate response to a standardized bout of work. The protocol for this type of testing is described in Costill *et al.* (1992: 70), and is detailed as a standardized swim of 200 m or 400 m performed at approximately 95 per cent of the swimmer's best time for the distance. This is repeated each week at the same pace, with blood lactate post-swim and/or heart rate during and/or post-swim recorded. A reduction in lactate level (similarly a drop in heart rate) over subsequent weeks for the same effort will normally indicate that the swimmer has become more efficient, has improved aerobic capacity, produces less lactate (higher anaerobic threshold) and is able to remove lactate faster (i.e. has gained in conditioning). In contrast, an increase would suggest a loss of conditioning. Should this occur when it is known that the athlete has maintained or increased training volume and/or the general intensity of training has been increased, it may indicate the onset of overtraining syndrome or staleness.

Some of the limitations of using lactate levels to signpost overtraining have been highlighted by Mackinnon and Hooper (1991) and Snyder *et al.* (1993), and by Gregg (1995), who has advised caution in interpreting training lactate concentrations too freely. The first two have noted that *lower* blood lactate levels during submaximal (Costill advised 95 per cent of best time for the standardized bout of work) and maximal exercise have been observed during overtraining, which would appear contrary to what is suggested in the previous paragraph. The latter joined them in drawing attention to the fact that blood lactate levels can be affected by several factors, such as diet (low carbohydrate intake equates with low glycogen levels and hence low lactates) and prior exercise (glycogen levels depleted), which renders lactate level use in indicating overtraining as somewhat problematic.

Costill *et al.* (1992) noted the limitations associated with measurement of heart rate post-exercise, and swimming coaches should also take these into consideration. Not only are some swimmers' pulses difficult to find manually and to count accurately without sophisticated equipment but, because heart rate initially declines very quickly post-exercise, the figure arrived at may underestimate the actual heart rate achieved during the exercise. Thus, heart rates recorded actually during the exercise provide the best indicator of stress, and some of the latest heart rate monitors (taped to the chest) are presently being used successfully for this purpose, despite the discomfort. One additional consideration for swimming coaches in particular is necessary. Measurements of heart rate during water exercise will be 8–10 beats per minute lower than similar levels of effort on land. Thus, a swimmer working with a heart rate of 170 beats per minute in the pool would actually be working harder than on land with the same heart rate. Many coaches attempt to relate heart rate to anaerobic threshold (training at or slightly above anaerobic threshold can result in large gains in aerobic capacity), and it is important therefore to establish what this rate is for each individual athlete and in the environment of the actual sport. In addition, Maglischo (1993) has noted that swimmers' heart rates equivalent to a lactate concentration of 4 mmol/l rise as the season progresses. Thus, as the swimmer gets fitter, a higher heart rate will be required to reach anaerobic threshold and provide an overload stimulus. Of course, 4 mmol/l is not exactly equivalent to the anaerobic threshold for all athletes. For example, Maglischo (1993: 145) reported that his research has shown that 4 mmol/l approximated the individual anaerobic threshold for 50–60 per cent of his swimmers, with significantly lower values for another 20–30 per cent and somewhat higher values for the remaining 10–20 per cent. None the less, the basic principle remains the same.

While the above tests may offer a useful physiological method for anticipating overtraining, sympathetic and/or empathetic coaches, using nothing other than their eyes and ears, may also use psychological indicators (mood swings etc.) as an early warning device. As Morgan *et al.* (1988) have noted, swimmers asked to endure increased volumes of work over a 10-day period (from 4000 m to 9000 m per day at a constant intensity equal to 94 per cent of VO_2 max.) showed significant psychological changes. The alterations in mood states recorded (for the Profile of Mood States {POMS}, see McNair *et al.*, 1971) equated significantly with physiological changes recorded during the same period. Thus, swimmers' ratings of exercise intensity and muscle soreness during the 10-day period equated with mood state changes such as increased depression, anger, fatigue and global mood disturbance. Watching for mood swings such as these when volume and/or intensity of training is increased may therefore also contribute to an early warning system. Other instruments for measuring mood swing have been suggested by Collins (1995), who has suggested the use of a shorter psycho-behavioural overtraining scale (POTS), and by Dr. Richard Cox who suggests a different instrument in Chapter 4, 'Psychological Considerations of Effective Coaching', earlier in this book.

Coaching as a process

Thus far in this chapter, a case has clearly been made that overtraining is associated with a number of process-related factors such as:

1. The quality of performance monitoring
2. The use of precise and individualized training loadings

3. The need for observation of athlete behaviour
4. The influence of psychological and emotional responses
5. Goal-related behaviour.

Furthermore, the end state (staleness or, in some cases, clinical depletion of faculties) is an outcome of a process of overtraining. It is appropriate at this point to examine coaching practice more closely and to demonstrate that good practice does not consist merely of episodic attention to variables, but forms part of a systematic regulated process. Addressing the dangers of overtraining requires that a processual approach to coaching practice be adopted.

In an exploratory paper, Lyle (1984) proposed that coaching could best be understood as a process. This conceptualization now characterizes the literature (Woodman, 1993; Salmela, 1995; Lyle, 1996), and the relatively few papers which have attempted to model the process stress the interdependency of the variables, albeit the models themselves are generally episodic (Franks, 1986; Fairs, 1987; Cote *et al.*, 1995). Sports coaching is concerned with improving sports performance in a way that is not reflective of chance factors. Thus, the coach's role is to 'direct a process that results in the unpredictability of performance being minimized' (Lyle, 1996: 18). This role describes that of the performance coach, whose context is notable for its stability and continuity over an extended period of time, commitment to a goal-orientated relationship, regular and frequent performer participation, planned progression in work-loads and attempts to control the many variables influencing performance. As indicated in the early part of this chapter, such circumstances are redolent of the high-level (elite) performance athlete, whose intensity of commitment and training demands give the potential for overtraining to develop.

Any attempt to describe a process, such as coaching in action, often fails to convey the complexity of interaction, the finely balanced interdependency of contributory factors and the dynamic immediacy of practice. The clear message is that coaching practice that, through oversight or ignorance, ignores the complexity and interdependence of the elements of the process is unlikely to cope adequately with monitoring the accumulation and aggregation of causal factors which result in the overtraining state.

A fuller conceptual description of the coaching process has been offered by Lyle (1996). He identified the key concepts of the process as:

- An information base
- The knowledge and skills of the coach
- The performer's capabilities
- Performance analysis
- Mechanisms for regulating the process
- Systematic progression
- Operationalization
- Goal-setting
- Planning
- The preparation programme
- The competition programme
- Individualization.

Some of these key concepts are obviously pertinent to coaching *per se*, but there are generic sub-processes without which the coaching process and coaching practice would become less systematic and less controlled. A contextual interpretation of these key concepts might indicate that overtraining, as a failure of the management of performance variables, depends for its prevention on the coach's capacity to ensure that systematic progression is achieved through the operationalization of mechanisms for regulating the process. The mechanisms depend on information availability, planning and monitoring.

This may seem distant from much actual coaching practice, and there can be little doubt that coaches do not always operate in a systematic fashion (Lyle, 1992). Some may even appear to ignore planning and regulation, and seem more to work to short-term horizons with short cuts that would seem to imply a more intuitive decision-taking form (Schon, 1983, 1987; Cross, 1995). This is particularly true of many team sports which, for example, appear to offer a model in which the complexity of team preparation and the need for individual athlete considerations together constrain the systematic approach (Lyle, 1996). Unlike individual sports, where planning and regulation are often extremely detailed and where poor performance often elicits an immediate response in terms of adjustments to the programme, team sports need to be understood in a wider context, where improvement in performance is non-linear and variability is to be expected. As Lyle (1996: 25) noted, in team sports, 'schedules and training session plans are not constructed or amended on the basis of the fluctuations in [individual] athlete status or performance'.

The implication from this is that, even in sports in which top level performers train on a full-time or near full-time basis, merely collecting data from a well-regulated coaching process is not sufficient on its own to spot all of the dangers. A degree of interpretation or evaluation of data is required, and this has implications for coach education. Nevertheless, systematic coaching practice is more likely to provide meaningful data for the coach to evaluate. A process that is insufficiently regulated may not provide the monitoring output with which to detect the onset of overtraining. Adequately planning the training and competition programme, particularly the physical conditioning element, is vital. Although the principles of training theory are readily available (e.g. Bompa, 1994), coaches often tend to operate much more in a 'recipe' fashion, rather than devising schedules from first principles on each occasion. Using recipes for action in this way can be risky, as some aspects of the coaching process are not only difficult to devise accurately on any particular occasion, but also do not lend themselves to repetition other than in only the most general terms. For example, the business of peaking (which refers to the optimal state of readiness for competition) through a tapering process (reducing training load immediately prior to competition) is far from an exact science (Francis, 1990: 100–8). In addition, the need to individualize training schedules within group settings, the demands of representative teams and the contingency/crisis planning required to cope with injury, illness, individual athlete response etc. adds to the difficulty of effectively managing any training programme. In relation to overtraining, the coach needs:

1. To know what to look for
2. To make an early diagnosis
3. To have sufficient data for comparison purposes
4. To have sufficient control of loading variables to take preventative and/ or remedial action
5. To have a sufficiently comprehensive knowledge and understanding of the performer to be able to respond to non-performance as well as performance cues, and thus allow for a more intuitive sense that something may be wrong.

Systematic coaching conceptualizes performance enhancement as the result of a process in which the coach has sufficient data and monitors progress on a regular basis. However, the coaching process is concerned with all of the variables that influence performance, and these include the performer's lifestyle and aspirations. Coaching is also an interpersonal relationship or set of relationships, and the quality of interaction is important insofar as it allows the coach to detect, amongst other things, psychological or emotional factors that either cause or result from overtraining. Thus it is obvious that the performer's contribution and reaction to the process is important, and the coach should pay particular attention to responses to training and to training diaries. For example, Mackinnon and Hooper (1994) have suggested that one of the best ways for monitoring for overtraining in swimming would be through monitoring swimmers' log books. Despite this, Cross' research with 76 predominantly full-time professional British swimming coaches did not identify this as general practice. Instead, several coaches spoke of 'knowing the swimmer' and 'regular discussions with swimmer and parents' (Cross, 1997: 119) rather than monitoring swimmers' log books.

For the high-level performer there will be times of the year when high volume or high intensity work is required, often in circumstances of perceived pressures arising from elevated competition expectations. If coaching is approached as a process, the potential difficulties arising from such an intensely focused part of the programme will be monitored more frequently by the coach and the 'crisis thresholds' lowered accordingly.

Training approaches to prevent overtraining

Moving now to more specific coaching practices, we begin with the basic premise that it is more important to prevent overtraining than to treat it (Crampton and Fox, 1987; Fry *et al.*, 1991). Since overtraining can be caused by both overdistance work and too high an intensity for too long a period, coaches need to balance the components of training (volume, intensity and density) in order to promote optimal training adaptation and prevent overtraining. Careful planning is therefore essential. Appropriate loads have to be calculated for each and every athlete (notwithstanding the difficulties of individualizing training in the team sport situation), and adequate regeneration periods planned to avoid excessive fatigue.

Various techniques have been adopted by swimming coaches to bring the appropriate balance to training. Probably the best known and most widely used of these are periodization (Bompa, 1987; Fry *et al.*, 1991, 1992a, 1992b,

1992c) and cyclic training. Fry *et al.* (1991: 55), citing the influence of Bompa (1983, 1987) and Harre (1982), defined periodization in the following terms:

> Different types of training are emphasized at appropriate phases of the training year and an athlete's career, in recognition that the development of some abilities are prerequisite to the development of others and that neuromuscular, cardiorespiratory, anatomical, biochemical, physiological, psychological and other developmental functions are achieved progressively over a long period of time.

Periodization therefore leads to modification of training within well-established guidelines, and based on a continuous evaluation of training progress. As Fry *et al.* (1991: 57) noted:

> It provides a framework for incorporating intensive training and regeneration periods in the appropriate ratio and volume in a training programme.

Normally, periodization involves dividing the 52 weeks of the training year into phases of training called macrocycles. Note that training may vary considerably within the different macrocycles, and is dependent on the position of the macrocycle in relation to the major competition(s). Usually, each week of a macrocycle is termed a microcyle, and four microcycles are normally grouped together as a mesocycle so that the training load can be varied between weeks of high training load and weeks of reduced load (Scholich, 1994).

Cyclic training, although somewhat similar to periodization, usually refers to a variety of different cyclic patterns at the microcycle level. Thus, patterns such as hard day–easy day, two hard workouts–one easy workout, etc. can be used to avoid the pitfalls of excessive stress and its concomitant failing adaptation (Madrigal, 1985).

Madrigal has also noted that not all swimmers react to the same training stress equally and that, rather than basing training loads on distance to be swum in a set time, it might be better to base training loads on the three energy systems used in swimming and the degree to which these might contribute towards the specific event(s) chosen for preparation. Thus, a 1500 m swimmer (essentially an aerobic event) would train for long periods at or near anaerobic threshold (equates with large gains in aerobic capacity), whereas a 200 m swimmer (whose energy requirements are almost equally anaerobic and aerobic) would train both near anaerobic threshold and above threshold, but for much shorter periods of time (swimming at speeds above anaerobic threshold is extremely stressful).

In fact, Madsen (1983) has suggested that much swimming training at the elite level is undertaken at an intensity that is too high to achieve its desired effect. He is not suggesting that high intensity training is unnecessary, but that it does not contribute optimally to taxing the aerobic system (the major player in most distances over 200 m in swimming), and that too much intensity causes acidic overtraining (lactic acid). To this end, he suggested that, for a 400 m swimmer, a 7-day cyclic programme with the main training sets based on lactate levels and anaerobic threshold (anaerobic threshold is the point during exercise at which the production of lactate exceeds the body's ability to dispose of it) might be most beneficial. For example, Monday might be at threshold, Tuesday below threshold, Wednesday progressive with some training below and some above threshold, Thursday below threshold,

Friday at and slightly above threshold, Saturday progressive with some below and some above threshold, and Sunday a rest day. Adopting a cyclical programme such as this would allow the body time to recover adequately and encourage optimal adaptation.

Both Madsen and Madrigal have stressed that cycles of this type are contingent upon the establishment of a sound aerobic adaptation during an early macrocycle. In addition, Madrigal (1985: 29) quoted Frederick (1978), who suggested that cardiovascular training adaptations occur in 3-week cycles and that increases in volume and intensity should reflect this pattern. He also suggested that increases in training resistance of no more that 5 per cent per week might be a good way to avoid overtraining. Dramatic increases in either volume or intensity are therefore far more likely to lead to the onset of overtraining.

Before leaving this section, it is important to note that training volume and intensity are not the only types of stress that contribute to the possibility of overtraining. As Rowbottom *et al.* (1998: 57) have reminded us, a combination of extraneous stresses – including environmental, occupational, educational or social stresses – has the propensity to add to the physical stress from training and cause failing adaptation. Should this be allowed to continue, there is a potential risk of overtraining.

Nutritional considerations

All the adenosine triphosphate (ATP) required for muscular activity is derived, with the exception of a very small amount provided by a breakdown of phosphocreatine, from glycogen (muscle sugar), either anaerobically (glycolysis) or aerobically (aerobic metabolism). Glycogen (or glucose) is derived from food consumed (carbohydrates, fats and proteins), with carbohydrates, particularly complex carbohydrates with a low glycaemic index (Salo, 1992), being the best providers and fastest muscle glycogen restorers. Increased training loads (both increased volume and increased intensity) will serve to reduce and ultimately deplete muscle glycogen reserves (Costill *et al.*, 1992). Failure to replenish these stocks adequately before the next training stimulus can inadvertently contribute to overtraining syndrome. Consequently, no training programme should ignore the need for athletes to consume adequate quantities of carbohydrate, preferably of the complex variety.

In addition, coaches should note that it is plausible that creatine supplementation (contributing to an increase in creatine/creatine phosphate stores) may actually improve ATP production during the first 10 seconds of exercise, either by increasing ATP stores or by maintaining ATP turnover for longer (Thompson, 1995). Increases in muscle creatine may also act as a buffer for lactic acid, and so help to delay the onset of fatigue. According to Greenhaff *et al.* (1996: 230), creatine ingestion can significantly increase exercise performance by sustaining force or work output during exercise. However, not everyone responds to it equally and not everyone needs it, and creatine supplements currently available are expensive. Creatine is only naturally available in the diet from meat and fish (white meat has a high percentage of creatine), and vegetarians, who generally have low creatine levels, may wish to consider creatine supplements at the elite athlete level. There is some speculation that ingesting creatine together with carbohydrate may be of added benefit.

Finally, bearing in mind what has been said about the importance of iron (mandatory for lymphocyte increases) and the role of the amino acid glutamine in immune function, attention should also be paid to green vegetables and to meat and/or wheat in the athlete's diet. Note that nutrition is considered in greater detail in Chapter 9, *Individualization of Training Programmes*.

Summary

Despite the underlying causes of overtraining not being as yet fully understood, it is likely that both emotional and physiological factors contribute to the overtraining state. Some of the emotional factors – for example, boredom or frustration – may both contribute to overtraining syndrome and be the result of it. The physical and physiological factors involved in training loads devised in line with the principle of progressive overload may be either local or general in nature, and these, where the training results in failing adaptation, may be differentiated by the terms overstrain, overreaching and overtraining syndrome. Increased training loads in the form of increased volume and/or increased intensity may contribute to overtraining syndrome if not matched by adequate periods of rest and recovery.

'More and harder' is not always better. This chapter has sought to demonstrate that the prevention of overtraining lies with the attention to the performer's response to training loads that can only come from a processual approach to coaching. The availability of information, sound planning and continuous monitoring, particularly at periods of high training load demand or at times of intense lifestyle demands, are essential parts of an effective coaching practice. More specifically, Fry *et al.* (1991: 53) identified three important factors in the prevention of overtraining:

> (a) the structure of the training programme must allow adequate regeneration and prevent injury and excessive fatigue due to extreme levels of training stress; (b) a scientific testing programme ... for the detection of overtraining must be developed ...; and (c) the testing procedures must be incorporated in such a way that the normal fatigue associated with training is not confused with the fatigue associated with overtraining.

The implementation of a systematic coaching process will ensure an appropriately planned and periodized training calendar. Attention to training theory principles should ensure that adequate regeneration accompanies the progressive, but periodized and cyclical, periods of high demand. The monitoring element of the coaching process should create data with which to detect the onset of overtraining. Two useful systematic methods for detecting the approach of overtraining syndrome involve blood lactate and heart rate response to a standardized bout of work (notwithstanding the critical comments noted earlier). In addition, the monitoring of resting heart rate and mood state may also provide useful clues, as may sleeping difficulties, loss of appetite and, in some cases, unexplained weight loss.

Finally, despite Costill's (1992: 140) assertion that it is tempting to suggest that elite swimmers should confine their training to one training session of 3000–5000 m per day, it is not unlikely that some coaches will plan to exceed these figures by some considerable margin. This in itself is not problematic, provided that strict attention in planning is paid to appropriate blends of volume, intensity and density (Bompa, 1994), and adequate periods of rest are written into the programme. Of course, these principles apply equally to other sports, and all coaches should plan in the best interests of each particular athlete.

Overreaching and overstrain are short-term imbalances that can be fairly easily remedied. Overtraining, on the other hand, may both lead to and/or reflect a set of circumstances in which the physical, psychological or emotional state of the performer is a matter of serious concern. This is not simply the likely failure to achieve the goals for that year but, more importantly, has implications for the performer's overall health and welfare. All elite athletes have the right to expect that the coach in whom they place considerable trust and control is approaching the coaching process in such a way as to ensure that deviations from the planned and anticipated performance and behaviour will be detected early, interpreted correctly and remedied appropriately.

References

Bompa, T. O. (1983). *Theory and Methodology of Training*. Kendal/Hunt.

Bompa, T. O. (1987). Periodization as a key element of training. *Sports Coach*, **11(1)**, 20–33.

Bompa, T. O. (1994). *Theory and Methodology of Training* (3rd edn). Kendall/Hunt.

Brock, J. H. (1992). Iron and the immune system. In *Iron and Human Disease* (R. B. Lauffer, ed.), pp. 161–78. CRC Press.

Budgett, R (1995). The doctor's viewpoint: Case Study Ian Wilson. *Coaching Focus*, **28**, 11.

Burke, E. R., Falsetti, H. L., Feld, D. F. *et al.* (1982). Blood testing to determine overtraining in swimmers. *Swimming Tech.*, **18(3)**, 29–33.

Chogovadze, A. V. and Butchenko, L. A. (eds) (1992). *Sports Medicine*. Meditsina (1984). Reviewed in *Fitness Sports Rev. Int.*, **27**, 19–21, 31–2.

Collins, D. (1995). Early detection of overtraining problems in athletes. *Coaching Focus*, **28**, 17–20.

Costill, D. L. (1986). *Inside Running – Basics of Sports Physiology*. Benchmark Press.

Costill, D. L., Maglischo, E. W. and Richardson, A. B. (1992). *Swimming*. Blackwell Scientific.

Cote, J., Salmela, J. H., Trudel, P. *et al.* (1995). The coaching model: A grounded assessment of expert gymnastic coaches' knowledge. *J. Sport Exer. Psychol.*, **17(1)**, 1–17.

Counsilman, J. E. (1968). *The Science of Swimming*. Pelham Books.

Crampton, J. and Fox, J. (1987). Regeneration vs burnout: Prevention is better than cure! *Sports Coach*, **11(2)**, 7–10.

Cross, N. R. (1995). Coaching effectiveness in hockey: a Scottish perspective. *Scot. J. Physical Ed.*, **23(1)**, 27–39.

Cross, N. (1997). Overtraining: a swimming coach perspective. *Scot. Cent. Res. Papers Sport Leisure Soc.*, **2**, 114–25.

Czajkowski, W. (1982). A simple method to control fatigue in endurance training. In *Exercise and Sport Biology* (P. V. Komi, ed.), pp. 207–12. International Series on Sport Sciences, 10. Human Kinetics.

Denison, T. (1995). Case history – Ian Wilson: the coach's viewpoint. *Coaching Focus*, **28**, 10.

Dressendorfer, R. H., Wade, C. E. and Scaff, J. H. (1985). Increased morning heart rate in runners: A valid sign of overtraining? *Phys. Sports Med.*, **13(8)**, 77–81, 86.

Fairs, J. (1987). The coaching process: The essence of coaching. *Sports Coach*, **11(1)**, 17–20.

Feigley, D. A. (1985). Psychological burnout in high-level athletes. *Swimming Tech.*, **21(3)**, 19–24.

Flynn, M. G. (1998). Future research needs and directions. In *Overtraining in Sport* (R. B. Kreider, A. C. Fry and M. L. O'Toole, eds), pp. 373–83. Human Kinetics.

Francis, C. with Coplan, J. (1990). *Speed Trap*. Grafton Books.

Franks, I., Sinclair, G. D., Thompson, W. and Goodman, D. (1986). Analysis of the coaching process. *Science Periodical on Research on Technology in Sport*. CAC, Paper A.

Frederick, E. C. and Welch, J. (1978). Work and rest. In *The Complete Marathoner* (J. Henderson, ed.), pp. 153–60. World Publications.

Fry, R., Morton, A. and Keast, D. (1991). Overtraining in athletes: An update. *Sports Med.*, **12(1)**, 32–65.

Fry, R., Morton, A. and Keast, D. (1992a). Overtraining: Considerations for the coach. *Sports Coach*, **25(1)**, 3–9.

Fry, R., Morton, A. and Keast, D. (1992b). Periodization of training stress – a review. *Can. J. Sports Sci.*, **17(3)**, 234–40.

Fry, R., Morton, A. and Keast, D. (1992c). Periodization and the prevention of overtraining. *Can. J. Sports Sci.*, **17(3)**, 241–8.

Gregg, S. (1995). The physiologist's view. A presentation given at the *Optimizing Performance in Swimmers* seminar, Aberdeen, Scotland, 1 September.

Greenhaff, P. L., Bodin, K., Casey, A. *et al.* (1996). Dietary creatine supplementation and fatigue during high-intensity exercise in humans. In *Biochemistry of Exercise* (R. Maughan and S. Shirrefs, eds), pp. 219–42. Human Kinetics.

Harre, D. (1982). *Principles of Sports Training*. Sportverlag.

Hooper, S. L., Mackinnon, L. T., Gordon, R. D. and Bachmann, A. W. (1993). Hormonal responses of elite swimmers to overtraining. *Med. Sci. Sports Exer.*, **25(6)**, 741–7.

Koutedakis, Y., Budgett, R. and Faulman, L. (1990). Rest in underperforming elite competitors. *Br. J. Sports Med.*, **24(4)**, 248–52.

Kuipers, H. and Keizer, H. A. (1988). Overtraining in elite athletes. *Sports Med.*, **6**, 79–92.

Lyle, J. (1984). Towards a concept of coaching. *Scot. J. Physical Ed.*, **12(1)**, 27–31.

Lyle, J. (1992). Systematic coaching behaviour: An investigation into the coaching process and the implications of the findings for coach education. In *Sport and Physical Activity* (T. Williams, L. Almond and A. Sparkes, eds), pp. 463–9. EFN Spon.

Lyle, J. (1996). A conceptual appreciation of the sports coaching process. *Scot. Cent. Res. Papers Sport Leisure Soc.*, **1(1)**, 15–37.

Mackinnon, L. T. and Hooper, S. (1991). Overtraining. *State of the Art Review*. No. 26. National Sports Research Centre.

Mackinnon, L. and Hooper, S. (1994). Training logs: An effective method of monitoring over-training and tapering. *Sports Coach*, **17(3)**, 13–18.

Mackinnon, L. T. (1998). Effects of over-reaching and overtraining on immune function. In *Overtraining in Sport* (R. B. Kreider, A. C. Fry and M. L. O'Toole, eds), pp. 219–41. Human Kinetics.

Madrigal, R. (1985). Problems with overtraining. *Swimming Tech.*, **21(3)**, 25–30.

Madsen, O. (1983). Aerobic training: Not so fast, there. *Swimming Tech.*, **19(3)**, 13–18.

Maglischo, E. W. (1982). *Swimming Faster*. Mayfield Pubs.

Maglischo, E. W. (1993). *Swimming Even Faster*. Mayfield Pubs.

McNair, D. M., Lorr, M. and Droppleman, L. F. (1971). *Profile of Mood States Manual*. Educational and Industrial Testing Service.

Morgan, W. P., Brown, D. R., Raglin, J. S. *et al.* (1987). Psychological monitoring of overtraining and staleness. *Br. J. Sports Med.*, **21(3)**, 107–14.

Morgan, W. P., Costill, D. L., Flynn, M. G. *et al.* (1988). Mood disturbance following increased training in swimmers. *Med. Sci. Sports Exer.*, **20(4)**, 408–14.

National Coaching Foundation (1995) Focus on: Overtraining and fatigue. *Coaching Focus*, **28**, National Coaching Foundation.

Newsholme, E. A. (1995). Possible biochemical causes of failure of the immune system and of fatigue in the overtraining syndrome. *Coaching Focus*, **28**, 14–16.

Noakes, T. (1986). *Lore of Running: Discover the Science and Spirit of Running* (2nd edn). Leisure Press.

O'Connor, P. J., Morgan, W. P., Raglin, J. S. *et al.* (1989). Mood state and salivary cortisol levels following overtraining in female swimmers. *Psychoneuroendocrinology*, **14(4),** 303–10.

Pyne, D. (1989). Monitoring overtraining in elite thletes. *Sports Coach*, **13(1),** 18–21.

Pyne, D. B. and Gray, A. B. (1994). Exercise and the immune system. *State of the Art Review*. National Sports Research Centre.

Rowbottom, D. G., Keast, D. and Morton, A. R. (1996). The emerging role of glutamine as an indicator of exercise stress and overtraining. *Sports Med.*, **21(2),** 80–97.

Rowbottom, D. G., Keast, D. and Morton, A. R. (1998). Monitoring and preventing of over-reaching and overtraining in endurance athletes. In *Overtraining in Sport* (R. B. Kreider, A. C. Fry and M. L. O'Toole, eds), pp. 47–66. Human Kinetics.

Salmela, J. H. (1995). Learning from the development of expert coaches. *Coach. Sports Sci. J.*, **2(2),** 3–13.

Salo, D. (1992). The importance of a proper diet. *Swimming Tech.*, **29(1),** 7.

Scholich, M. (1994). *Circuit Training for All Sports: Methodology of Effective Fitness Training*. Sport Books Publisher.

Schon, D. A. (1983). *The Reflective Practitioner: How Professionals Think in Action*. Basic Books.

Schon, D. A. (1987). *Educating the Reflective Practitioner*. Jossey Bass.

Selye, H. (1957). *The Stress of Life*. Longmans Green.

Snyder, A. C., Jeukendrup, A. E., Hesselink, M. K. C. *et al.* (1993). A physiological/psychological indicator of over-reaching during intensive training. *Int. J. Sports Med.*, **14,** 29–32.

Thompson, K. (1995). Creatine supplementation in swimming: Does it give you an edge? *Swimming Times*, **LXXII(5),** 25–6.

Troup, J. (1986). Setting up a season using scientific training. *Swimming Tech.*, **23(1),** 8–16.

Wilmore, J. H. and Costill, D. L. (1994). *Physiology of Sport and Exercise*. Human Kinetics.

Wilson, I. (1995). Case history – Ian Wilson: The athlete's viewpoint. *Coaching Focus*, **28,** 75–6.

Woodman, L. (1993). Coaching: A science, an art, an emerging profession. *Sports Sci. Rev.*, **2(2),** 1–13.

11

Coaches' decision making

John Lyle

- The coach's role and decision making
- Characteristics of decision making
- Naturalistic decision making
- Decision making and coaching research
- Intuition, awareness and anticipation
- Models of decision making applied to coaching
- Key features of coaches' decision practice
- An integrated Natural Decision Making model
- Decision making and coach education

Introduction

One of the characteristics of expert coaches is that they make decisions in an apparently effortless, intuitive manner. Students of coaching who identify communication skills as the most important coaching quality fail to realize that this transmission stage is dependent upon the correct decisions having been made. It may be a sterile exercise to debate what is the most important coaching quality, but in performance coaching there can be no doubt that decision making is essential. Consider the decisions to be taken: selecting performers, devising training programmes, organizing training drills, evaluating progress, selecting game strategies, managing tactical variations and substitutions. Indeed, if the model of the coaching process identified in the opening chapter is adopted, it is clear that planning, monitoring and evaluating the process involves almost continual decision making. Beckett (1996: 135) says that one of the 'central distinguishing features of the professional's work is that of discretionary judgements'. In other words, decision making is a mark of the professional, and the way the decisions are taken may be the benchmark of the expert (Dreyfus and Dreyfus, 1986; Chi *et al.*, 1988; Eraut, 1994).

It would be inappropriate to suggest that all decision making is similar in nature. The coach who has to deal with a squad member who is disrupting the harmony of the squad will engage in a different process to that used when planning a competition preparation microcycle. A distinction can be drawn between coaches' decisions for which there is relatively little time pressure (Jones *et al.*, 1995) and those characterized by the need for an immediate or almost immediate response (i.e. non-deliberative). Sports coaching practice reflects this distinction. The coach's functions can usefully be categorized into three levels:

1. Direct intervention (the coach and performer working together in training or competition)
2. Indirect responsibilities (planning, monitoring, negotiating)
3. Managing the external environment (equipment, finance, facilities, recruitment etc.).

It is immediately obvious that the coach's 'direct intervention' behaviour is most likely to be characterized by non-deliberative behaviour. Some decision making (for example, planning the programme) will be sufficiently non-time-constrained to be deliberative. Much of this decision making will be characterized by routine activity. Where there are substantive issues to be resolved, such as with the disruptive squad member, it is likely to be termed problem solving. There are many instances, however, when coaches must make instant decisions – the need for time-outs during competition, dealing with injury, player substitution, control of practice drill loadings, contingency reactions to tactical crises, etc.

The need for non-deliberative decisions is to be found more extensively in some sports than others. This is dictated by the role of the coach during competition and the interactive nature of training, and is more prevalent in team sports. In these circumstances there is a continuous and contested 'momentum flow' between two players or teams, and a high degree of uncertainty about outcomes and performance. One of the coach's roles is to manage this competition context. It is also this context about which there has been little research. How can the coach cope with such complexity? This chapter will demonstrate that coaches, like other experts, devise professional shortcuts to minimize the number of substantive contingency decisions to be taken, and operate within routines. There is no doubt about the uniqueness in each coaching environment. Workers who have studied 'hot action', the term given to behaviour under conditions of time pressure (Schon, 1983; Beckett, 1996), emphasize the fluid and dynamic nature of such a context. Lyle (1996) demonstrated that coaching is characterized by its multivariable nature, uncertainty of outcome, non-linearity of stimulus–response, the influence of human consciousness, the effect of the instrumental competitive action by others and the interdependence of performance variables. The difficulty of control and prediction in such circumstances of complexity and potential novelty precludes a simplistic, analytical approach. The complexity of the process is, therefore, a fertile ground for professional shortcuts and apparently intuitive behaviour. An awareness of this complexity is at least a partial explanation for the dearth of coach education practice related to non-deliberative decision making. This is one of the failings of coach education for experienced coaches, and demonstrates why attention has been focused on technical content and declarative knowledge rather than decision-making skills and procedural knowledge.

The way coaches make decisions is important because the methods they use should form the basis of a significant element of coach education. This chapter, therefore, examines the decision making of coaches in non-deliberative contexts, such as match coaching, and considers the implications for

coach education. It will become evident that situational awareness, anticipation, modelling, rules of thumb and the contested nature of the task environment are all important features. The explanations for the coach's decision
making are best considered within a Naturalistic Decision Making (NDM)
framework (Zsambok and Klein, 1997).

What do we mean by decision making?

The issue of what constitutes decision making appears to be deceptively
simple. However, this is not the case. Svenson (1996) identifies four types
of decision problems, each requiring appropriate psychological processes:

1. Automatic and unconscious decisions involving no reference to alternative choices (expanded on later in reference to Klein's (1998) recognition-primed decision making).
2. Decisions about which there is no conflict between attributes and attrac-
   tiveness, and the solution is obvious. These include meta-strategic decisions and repetitive decisions.
3. Decision making where there is a choice between alternatives with goal
   conflicts. ('Most of the existing decision research literature treats problems at this level' (1996: 254).)
4. Decisions in which neither the alternatives nor the attributes are fixed.
   Svenson characterizes the latter as 'real-life' decisions, and comments
   that, in these situations, there may be 'just one alternative that is considered and the decision therefore concerns a choice between the *status
   quo* alternative and one other alternative' (1996: 256).

Goldstein and Weber (1995) proposed four categories of decision making
based on the way knowledge is employed to evaluate alternatives: non-
deliberative, associative, rule-based and schema-based. Each of these implies
a different cognitive organization. The non-deliberative category deals with
routinized decisions and the use of stereotypes and episodic memory to
generate the actions taken and their consequences. Goldstein and Weber
compare this to the expert's intuitive decision making. Associative deliberation is also close to intuitive behaviour. An associative semantic network
provides a 'stream-of-consciousness' flow, which may be the mechanism
for providing feedback on a course of action in interactive coaching. Rule-
based deliberation includes explicit and implicit use of plans or procedures
to guide decision making. This category can include both analytical and more
intuitive strategies. In the final category, schema-based deliberation owes
much to 'explanation-based decision making' (Pennington and Hastie,
1993) and involves the construction and testing of models or structures of
declarative knowledge. Scripts, mental models and categories are special
cases in this model, and these more technical terms will be considered
later. First, it is necessary to introduce Naturalistic Decision Making (NDM).

The distinction between decision making as a 'choice' activity, with structured alternatives and clear goals and less well structured 'problem decisions',
is at the heart of alternative research paradigms in this field. Teigen (1996)
distinguishes between the traditional experimental, laboratory-based judge-
ment/decision making research (J/DM) with structured, contrived problems,

and naturalistic decision making (NDM) which is ill-structured, 'messy' and untidy, and with less 'givens'. He contrasts the 'choice tasks' of the experimental tradition with the daily life decision characteristics identified by Karlsson (1988): one alternative, a creative act, and imbued with self-investment. A similar distinction was identified by Devine and Kozlowski (1995). The traditional problem-solving literature is characterized by them as having 'typically studied expertise in the context of tasks with formal, quantifiable rules, established procedures and demonstrably "correct" answers' (1995:295). In the more traditional J/DM experimental paradigm (with 'static' tasks), time pressure brings with it the need for increased speed of information processing and more non-compensatory judgements, and increased risks are taken if negative outcomes are anticipated.

However, there is no doubt that much of sports coaching has the 'untidiness' of the naturalistic paradigm. Orasanu and Connolly (1993) identify a list of factors that are central to NDM: uncertain dynamic tasks, multiple event feedback loops, meaningful consequences, multiple goals, time constraints, decision complexity, multiple players, the level of congruence of organizational and personal goals, quantity of information, and level of expertise. NDM researchers are said to be more concerned to describe patterns in decision behaviour rather than to identify normative behavioural rules within prescribed choices. Cannon-Bowers and colleagues (1996) cite the work of Brehmer and Allard (1990), who draw a link between the real-life timing inherent in dynamic tasks and the concept of an 'action decision' rather than a choice of options.

The term 'naturalistic' has come to be used for decision making that deals with evidence of 'how decisions actually are made, rather than on how they "should" be made' (Beach, 1997: 9). This naturalistic approach is less suited to the controlled experimentation of the normative rules associated with problem solving. The rational, logical and detached nature of such problem solving research contrasts with realistic decision making, which is highly involved, and influenced by passions, desires and motives (Strack and Neumann, 1996). Although Fischhoff (1996) points to the limitations of 'standard' decision making research for producing applied and applicable findings, the options which characterize such research may be rather more clear-cut than the action context of decision making, such as coaching. This is more creative, value-laden, and apparently has few realistic, viable alternatives. Teigen (1996:250) agrees that real-world research is necessary to capture the richness of this decision making: 'real world situations are not easily and certainly never completely captured by the vocabulary of the lab (these situations) form a gold mine for extracting new questions' (1996: 251).

NDM is in the process of being established as a force within psychological research (see Flin *et al.*, 1997; Zsambok and Klein, 1997; Klein, 1998). Although the boundaries of the research field are still being established, the general approach is already evident. The often unrealistic, static, experimental approach of the traditional behavioural decision theorists is eschewed for explaining how experienced or expert decision makers make decisions in conditions of stress: 'NDM is directed at understanding the demands the task domain places upon the decision maker' (Klein, 1997: 17). At this stage in its development, NDM is more concerned with descriptive models of decision making (Rasmussen, 1997). Klein (1998: 24–8) has provided a model of decision making which has been influential in NDM, and to which we will return later. The version of decision making normally given in all secondary sources is of pattern recognition of a situation that leads to a known course of action. However, Klein has integrated into his model how it might deal with complex situations of the sort that arise in coaching. These require greater diagnosis (including misdiagnosis not spotted until the expectancies are violated) and those in which the course of action needs to be given further consideration.

In a very useful conceptualization of decision making for coaching, Brehmer (1992) describes it as that of 'an attempt to gain control i.e. as an attempt to achieve some desired state of affairs' (1992: 212). He stresses the point that 'dynamic decision making' is an on-going process, and that decision-makers are constrained by the environment. Decisions are made 'when the environment demands decisions from them' (1992: 213). The dynamic nature of the environment was also studied by Kersholt (1994) in an experimental task involving judgements about an athlete's fitness level. In dynamic task environments (which he characterized as demonstrating continuous change, currency of information flow and uncertainty), he comments that time pressure is caused by the developing situation and not by artificial deadlines, and that action rather than judgement strategies are required. His findings suggested a speeding up of information processing, the use of thresholds ('waiting until a specific value was reached' (1994: 101)), and attempting to increase 'waiting time' by beginning to monitor the situation earlier. He concluded that individuals achieve an 'illusion of control'. Before attempting an explanation of decision making in coaching, it will be valuable to examine the existing literature on sports coaching.

Sports coaching literature and decision making

Almost 30 years ago, Cratty (1970), an eminent sports psychologist, identified the problem: 'coaching decisions must be made rapidly', the value of research 'depends first upon deciding what types of decisions coaches must make. A second step is to explore the degree to which research has or has not provided information leading towards more productive decision-making behaviour' (1970: 46). It is clear from the literature, however, that there has been little theoretical development of coaching behaviour (Lyle, 1996). Abraham and Collins (1998) suggest that little progress has been made in clarifying the relationship between the cognitive skills of the coach and the most prevalent approaches to coaching research. It will become clear from this brief review of the literature that there is some recognition of the issue, but that the central question of non-deliberative decision making remains unexplored.

In its current stage of development, some basic questions about coaching practice have yet to be asked or answered. However, a number of writers have interpreted coaching as a dynamic, largely cognitive process which, *prima facie*, requires constant regulation and, therefore, implies the pre-eminence of decision making (Cote *et al.*, 1995; Salmela, 1995; Lyle, 1996; Abraham and Collins, 1998). There is an increasing recognition that coaching is a cognitive activity. Franks *et al.* (1986) constructed a quasi-quantifiable coaching model to assist direct-intervention decision making by the coach. Having reviewed the research literature on coaching behaviour, Abraham and Collins (1998) conclude that coaching expertise is 'a knowledge of making correct decisions within the constraints of the session. Thus coaching is not a behaviour to be copied but a cognitive skill to be taught' (1998: 68). Cote and co-workers (1995) used knowledge-elicitation procedures to structure the knowledge of expert coaches into a conceptual model. They found that coaches constructed a mental model, which was used as a working model to guide the coaches' day-to-day decisions in a deliberative context. Although the authors discuss some of the properties of knowledge schemata, this is not based on any findings. In a similar type of study, Salmela (1995) interviewed 21 expert coaches, each of whom had coached for over 10 years. While Salmela did not present any specific insights into non-deliberative decision making, he summarized in a way that makes it clear that coaches operate as experts, using tacit knowledge which can be accessed and non-conscious procedures that are difficult to investigate. They have 'a metacognitive form of knowledge which experts possess and are able to verbalize. A number of contingencies are brought into play which allow their decision making and operational styles to be precisely formulated into effective ways of coaching' (1995: 13). To some extent this helps to explain the reaction of Gould *et al.* (1990), who were disconcerted that 'less than half of the coaches sampled felt that there exists a well-defined set of concepts and principles for coaches' (1990: 337), in their study of elite American coaches. However, the coaches also cited experience and interactions with other coaches as their primary means of developing knowledge. It seems highly likely therefore that the coaches operate to such concepts and principles, but that their use is more implicit than explicit.

The nature of the competition and the coach's role is very sport-specific (Cote *et al.*, 1995), and it was this that forced Bloom *et al.* (1997) to focus on pre- and post-competition behaviours. Perhaps the key is that there have been few studies of coaches' operating practices that have focused on decision making, and even fewer naturalistic studies of coaches. Lyle (1992) investigated the coaching practice behaviour of 30 experienced coaches of national and international performers. He concluded that 'there seems to be little doubt that the detailed implementation of the coach's intentions and the crisis management of the process is not approached in an overtly systematic fashion. Coaches take decisions based on feelings or intuitions' (1992: 467). This balance of rational intention and apparently intuitive implementation has been replicated in several follow up studies (Cross, 1995a, 1995b).

In an interesting study, Duke and Corlett (1992) investigated the factors influencing basketball coaches' time-out decisions. They cite Leet *et al.* (1984) as reinforcing the potentially important nature of coaching decisions on performance. Commenting on the lack of previous research, they say: 'despite acceptance of timeouts and substitutions as important parts of many sport contests, the circumstances surrounding how coaching intervention decisions are made have been studied very little and we have limited insight into how coaches themselves understand their own decision making' (1992: 334). The study investigated why, rather than how, coaches made decisions, and identified the physical state of the players as most often leading to a timeout. The authors acknowledge that coaches will employ heuristic approaches to make sense of the 'chaotic stimulus array' in the game, and are likely to reduce their game interpretation to relatively few factors in order to engage in more logical decision making.

Jones and co-workers (1997) investigated the interactive decision making and behaviour of experienced and inexperienced coaches. In an earlier paper (Jones *et al.*, 1995), they had demonstrated that experienced coaches used contextual information (enabling conditions) more so than inexperienced coaches. This work replicated and supported other studies on physical education teachers (Housner and Griffey, 1985; Griffey and Housner, 1991; Byra and Sherman, 1993) that suggested that 'experienced physical education teachers appear to make use of routines or mental scripts that include specific task structures, management strategies and instructional statements' (1997: 456). In the 1997 study, Jones and his colleagues found that experienced coaches made fewer changes to plans and had more alternatives available. However, the studies were no more than behavioural analyses and very limiting: future research should 'move beyond assessments of the type and frequencies of behaviours and cognition and begin to address how experts integrate and apply knowledge' (1997: 467).

These studies are reflective of a more general approach to teaching expertise, although it is worth noting again the confused conceptualizations of teaching and coaching. The work in this field is similar in nature to the contrived conditions noted in experimental decision theory research. For example, in the Housner and Griffey (1985) study, which is very widely cited, the teachers taught only four children and there were only six subjects (three experienced and three inexperienced). More naturalistic studies would be welcome in order to reduce this artificiality.

There is no doubt that coaches are required to engage in complex cognitive activity and that such cognitive behaviour is under-researched. There is a limited literature or research tradition in this area, although more recent writing is identifying the problem. There is an appreciation that a 'form of cognitive organization' (or more than one) is engaged, but at present no synoptic conceptualization of how this (or these) are operationalized. The importance of interactive decision making is often identified but rarely, if ever, explained.

Intuition, awareness and anticipation

Before moving to a potential explanation for the way in which coaches make decisions, it would be valuable to clarify a number of concepts that will be involved. One of the assumptions on which this chapter is based is that coaches make what appear to be intuitive decisions. What is intuition? The characteristics of intuition in relatively routine decisions made by professionals are discussed by Easen and Wilcockson (1996) in a review paper. They conceive of intuition as a 'spontaneous, effortless, non-conscious, unexplained (to the intuiter) phenomenon' (1996: 670). This is explained by Claxton (1998) as a product of non-conscious neural associations. He suggests that this has been an uncomfortable subject for psychology, but that cognitive science is 'resuscitating the idea of the intelligent unconscious' (1998: 220). When problems are well defined and susceptible to decomposition in verbal–symbolic terms, the more deliberative cognitive strategies will be appropriate and efficient. In less well-defined problems, key parts of the problem act as a catalyst to a level of neural activity within which associations are formed to existing memory and knowledge stores. Much of this activity may be below a 'notional level of consciousness', but the result is that the coach comes to a view of the appropriate action, or even initiates it, without being aware of having generated the solution. Claxton distinguishes 'speedy association' from the slower 'creative' intuition.

There is little doubt that many coaching contexts will be susceptible to intuitive decision making. Compare Hammond and co-workers' (1993) list of contributory factors to the coach's interactive practice context. If the task presents many redundant cues, the cue values are continuous, the cues are displayed simultaneously and are measured perceptually, and the subject has available no explicit principle, scientific theory, or method for organizing cues into a judgement, then the subject will be much more likely to employ intuitive cognition. Klein attempts to disabuse us of intuition's mysterious qualities: 'intuition depends on the use of experience to recognize key patterns that indicate the dynamics of the situation' (1998: 31). It will be seen later that recognizing the situation brings with it a very speedy awareness of the appropriate solutions.

It would appear then that developing an awareness of any situation is likely to be an important part of decision making. What is important is that this is a learned capacity. When reviewing the nature of expertise, Chi *et al.* (1988) found that 'experts perceive large meaningful patterns in their domains' (1988: xvii). This has also been demonstrated in a naturalistic setting with the cognitions of fire-fighters (Klein, 1990). Chi and colleagues also note that 'experts see and represent a problem in their domain at a deeper (more principled) level than novices; novices tend to represent a problem at a superficial level' (1988: xix). The place of early recognition of patterns is often emphasized. Adelson (1984) suggests that experts perceive patterns in 'abstract conceptually based representations' (1984: 483), whereas novices organize their perceptions at a much more superficial level. She suggests that the expert represents information as a procedure and can, therefore, recognize and match more quickly because the process is not confused by the details (1984: 495). This will make sense to inter-active games coaches, who seem able to analyse matches with a level of interpretation which differs markedly from the more superficial description of the novice coach.

Similarly, the expert coach, when making decisions, will focus on the initial analysis in order to identify the problem accurately. The novice will focus unduly on the choice of solutions. Randel *et al.* (1996) describe an experiment into expert behaviour in the Naturalistic Decision Making tradition. They employed an electronic warfare task to study the decision making process of more and less expert technicians. Their findings were that 'experts put their emphasis on deciding on the nature of the situation, while novices are more concerned with deciding the course of action' (1996: 593). The previous experience and stored solutions of the experts allowed them to concentrate on appraising the situation. The authors also identified a capacity to focus on the most meaningful elements of the display and to have more developed memory structures: 'expertise appears to take the form of a complex model of potential situations' (1996: 595). These mental simulations allow experts to interpret their perceptions and to predict outcomes with minimal effort. This capacity of the expert to focus on and make use of situation assessment to shortcut the decision making process clearly has implications for coach education.

Sports coaching also involves situations in which decisions have to be taken very quickly. In the paper described above, Randel *et al.* (1996) point to the criticality of the time factor in complex, dynamic settings and emphasize the situational assessment element of recognition-primed decisions in such circumstances. The correct assessment of the situation reduces the need for multiple options to be considered. In complex dynamic situations, however, there is a need for the coach to continue the monitoring of the unfolding situation for two reasons: first, because the action decision 'point' may be the crucial issue, and secondly, because amendments to the solution may be required. Therefore, some form of forward modelling seems likely in the explanation of decision making. It is worth reiterating the point that the coach's most immediate problem may be whether to act or when to act, rather than what the action should be. This reinforces the need for an accurate assessment of the initial situation.

Of course, individuals may selectively attend to the environment on the basis of experience, and may operate a 'crisis threshold' approach to cope with the scale and complexity of the information. It has been suggested that coaches operate on a system of performance triggers or thresholds (Lyle, 1996: 25). In a coaching context, for example, the coach may not react to lack of improvement in performance whilst it remains within a broad band of acceptability, but following continued monitoring it may eventually lead to action.

Some consideration needs to be given to the coach's anticipation of events. Decision making in uncertain environments involves making estimations about the future, and in these situations is not helped greatly by probability judgements. Some insight can be achieved from considering the use of the term 'reflection'. Donald Schon (1983, 1987) used the term 'reflection-in-action' to describe how professionals deal with conditions in which artistry and intuition play a part. He suggests that they use reflection to reframe the problem and move to a speedy resolution. Eraut (1994) is critical of Schon, but his comments are very apt for an insight into this study. He suggests that reflection is more appropriately thought of as a 'metacognitive process in which the practitioner is alerted to a problem, rapidly reads the situation, decides what to do and proceeds in a state of continuing alertness' (1994: 145). This is a form of rapid hypothesis testing, employing a tacit personal interpretation of the relevant action. Beckett (1996) is also critical of Schon's assumptions. In a very closely argued paper, his view is that there is 'no such thing' as reflection-in-action. He suggests that the professional is making a judgement to continue (or not), and that this is linked reflexively to an aggregation of events as they happen, but not reflectively. This is similar to the coach's intuitive association described earlier. Beckett makes a case for anticipative action. He suggests that a concept of 'feedforwardness' might be a useful one to explore; what he calls 'an anticipative conversation with our practices' (1996: 149). This is a useful statement since it focuses attention onto the coach's modelling and evaluating of potential actions. Brehmer (1992) also uses the term 'feedforward' when he suggests the use of models to predict the state of complex systems.

What this shows is that coaches have mechanisms for trying to cope with the uncertainty of the future. Remember that this paper is largely concerned with hot action – decision making under time or complexity constraints. Coaches will try to anticipate by modelling what they think will happen, but then they have a continuing process of readiness to change by 'conversing' (monitoring) with the model. This may be thought of as hypothesizing about the future. Hypothesis generation is related to what is termed forward or backward reasoning. In rule-based problem solving, forward reasoning involves the use of given data to generate a hypothesis, and backward reasoning generates the data on the basis of a hypothesis. In non-deliberative or interactive situations, it is more likely that the coach is generating a hypothesis based on a recognition of the problem and is subsequently seeking confirmation of the hypothesis and its accompanying solutions as the situation unfolds. The hypotheses are generated from the coach's experience. When the coach has no link between observed data and hypothesis, it might be better termed guesswork. Much of this serial deliberation might be at a non-conscious level. In an interesting paper, Dougherty *et al.* (1997) examined the mechanisms by which individuals generated causal scenarios. They found that using a 'single path reasoning strategy' increased the individual's confidence in the scenario. The individuals created a few scenarios at the early stages of the problem, but quickly reduced these to one or two alternatives.

Models of decision making

The remainder of this chapter describes how coaches make decisions. It is based on what the literature has to say, and has been informed by research carried out by the author. This research, however, was focused on one sport, and would not permit significant generalization. The approach adopted, therefore, is to present the description and, in the context of a dearth of research in coaching, to invite students of coaching to use this as a resource for generating future research studies.

The most appropriate starting point is at a general level of understanding of cognitive activity. In a very valuable paper, Boreham (1988) elaborated on three models of cognitive organization: the rational model, the template model and the interactive model. The first of these, the use of theory and logic to work out solutions, is not appropriate in the coaching context. The template model is based on the use of schemata (context-specific knowledge structures). Recognition of the frame or schema automatically triggers off the appropriate response from the store built up through the trial and error of experience by the expert. His third model, termed interactive, allows for the individual to create a new 'diagnosis' from fragments of the earlier frames and the data from the contextual information, such as when injury happens during a game. This suggests a somewhat slower form of decision making than the automated response of the previous model. In a later paper,

Boreham (1994) proposes a 'dual cognitive architecture' to explain the intuitive, implicit practice of experts, which he contrasts with the rather more deliberative, analytical and explicit behaviour of the novice. Processing by the novice coach will be 'serial, slow, effortful, capacity limited, easily stopped and propositional' (1994: 174). The more automatic, unconscious implicit processing of the expert is fast, effortless and procedural. He suggests that this style is not available to introspection (cannot always be explained) and is under 'schematic' control. The individual coach may structure routines for everyday activity, but may not have the schemata to deal with irregularity, therefore employing the more explicit style for novel situations. This provides a useful distinction between routine responses and more analytical processes, but Boreham does not address how the individual responds to non-routine issues that are time-constrained.

There is another possibility, which is that the coach bases solutions less on a set of general propositions and more on specific cases: 'I recognize this as exactly like a previous case and this is what I did on that occasion.' Schmidt *et al.* (1990) describe how doctors move from memory-based knowledge structures to memories of specific illnesses and then to memories of specific patients as they become more expert. This reinforces the move to implicit behaviour, but stresses their recourse to 'illness scripts' based on particular instances from experience, diagnostic data, consequences and contexts. Unlike less experienced practitioners, experts recognize the similarity of cases and apply highly idiosyncratic 'recipe' solutions. Schmidt and co-workers' paper emphasizes, therefore, the idiosyncratic nature of theories of action, and the place of tacit knowledge structures in personal hypothesis testing, which closes down the range of options. There may be a difficulty here for the coach because of the many variables involved in each case. The coach may recognize a similar situation to a previous case, but the circumstances (including personnel) surrounding the case may be sufficiently different to render this a less viable way of making decisions. The coach recognizes similarities to previous cases, and then uses the previous solutions in the new problem. However, Caplan and Schooler (1990) identify difficulties in applying the analogy-based approach with complex problems that involve open-ended multiple decisions. The coach may retrieve examples that are similar, but which may differ in the characteristic that is essential for solving the problem. This points to the need for expert identification of the key features in the decision context.

At this point, four potentially useful models of decision making will be examined, summarizing with a fifth model that attempts to bring all of these together. A Rational Model can be dismissed. If such a model was relevant, the coach would react automatically to a logically computed analysis of all the factors involved, and the abstract schemata involved would calculate the optimum solution. However, rule-governed algorithmic responses of this sort cannot cope with the complexity of the decision task facing coaches. It will be valuable to note that schemata are mental models: knowledge structures made up of declarative and procedural knowledge, which are sensitive to coaches' current perceptions. It is through these that we store our representations of the world around us. They can be elaborate or simple, accessed through automatic pattern recognition or more deliberative memory-based analytical cognitions, and are based on our experiences. The interesting issues in decision making are how the coach can access these schemata and the problem solutions that are attached to them.

The Schema Model

The Schema Model uses domain-sensitive knowledge structures, which are activated by pattern recognition from the environment. It is dominated by production rules, which in turn trigger executive command solutions. It derives from a recognition model of decision making, and assumes (in a similar way to motor theories of behaviour) that the recognition of appropriate situations triggers a pre-selected response. The coach will feel that particular decisions 'have to' be made; that they are imperative. When thinking about the 'rules', the language used will be 'I should ... if ...'. In their working environments, coaches will recognize situations and, if the threshold on key factors is breached, an automatic response will be generated. An example of this might be the basketball coach who recognizes that the difference in the scores between the teams has reached a critical stage and calls a time-out. However, many coaches may feel uncomfortable in reacting automatically to stimuli, and may wish to exercise more deliberative control if possible. They may also be limited by the number of decisions possible.

The Script Schema Model

With the Script Schema Model, the coach recognizes an instance that is the first or early part of an unfolding event or process. Reading the 'enabling conditions' of the instance leads to a recognition not only of what is happening, but also of what is likely to happen. Expert coaches will read the conditions earlier and more accurately than the novice, although there will also be the problem of trying to decide too early with uncertain conditions. The recognition is not of a holistic snapshot (as in the Schema Model), but of the combination of enabling conditions. These will require technical knowledge and insight, and will be categorized by words such as faults, causes, trends, circumstances and conditions. An important part of the script is that the instance and enabling conditions have consequences attached to them. These then also have solutions or actions attached where necessary. Examples of this model in action will centre on technical analyses or relationship problems between performers. For example, a coach may recognize an aspect of a warm-up that indicates that a performer is not mentally focused. The coach has seen this script before, and knows that a number of technical, physical and attributional consequences will follow. The script also has built into it the solution, and the coach will therefore act at the early stage of the script before it unfolds too far.

The Script Schema Model recognizes a condition in which decisions or solutions are also implied. Rapid scanning, recognition and awareness of solutions will give the appearance of intuitive decision making. To this extent the script is merely another form of schemata-based knowledge framework, which can be accessed by the recognition of the appropriate cues. An important point is that, to change the problem, the coach must change the underlying 'enabling conditions'. Novice coaches will focus on the outcomes rather than the underlying causes and will, therefore, be less effective. The script has the potential to move from a fairly instantaneous recognition to a merely rapid one, since a threshold effect may again be involved. This might be explained as: the swimmer's second or third similar failure to complete a set correctly invokes a recognition that there may be a problem. The coach knows what the consequences of this might be, but has to consider the advantages and disadvantages of an alternative course of action, and the more medium-term state of training at the time. Although the coach has a non-deliberative option, which to the outsider may appear intuitive, it may be more prudent to apply a conservative approach and seek some confirmation of the problem. Once again, firming up the perception may come too late, but the coach may have learned that some caution is often effective (meaning that the problem is resolved without further intervention).

The Case Script Model

In the Case Script Model, the coach recognizes in the pattern a similarity to a previously experienced example. This triggers a repeat of the previous (providing it has not been a negative outcome) decision behaviour. Although there would be some benefit in using specific case recollections to provide shortcuts to solutions, the complexity of most interactive coaching contexts precludes this form of decision making. It does seem likely, however, that coaches dealing with, for example, the problematic behaviour of individual performers will be able to make use of previous instances of such behaviour.

The Slow Interactive Script Model

Decision behaviour in the Slow Interactive Script Model is governed by an interaction with the environment (what is termed a serial deliberation). This produces a slower, less reactive version of a script, which is capable of constant amendment. This approach assumes that there are limited decision choices available to the coach; previously determined strategy; the impact of the opposition; and the possibility of the coach attempting to minimize the non-deliberative element of the process. The Interactive component, therefore, assumes some of the characteristics of deliberative decision making. This model is less about the time-pressured decisions of competition and more about the management of training sessions. A direct parallel is teaching a class. Nevertheless, an interactive model is a valuable way of representing the coach's contest management. In most sports, the coach has a limited number of options during competition either because of the rules or because of the effect of constant change on the performers. A constant recognition process feeds at a non-conscious level the appropriate script, which the coach has modelled. The coach then monitors the situation to spot deviations from the outcomes anticipated by the model. Students of coaching will recognize that these models have to be capable of constant amendment as a competition progresses: perhaps another mark of the expert coach.

Coach's decision making

Before suggesting a model that embraces each of these types or stages in decision making, we will review some facets of the coach's decision making in summary form:

1. Coaches have to contend with the dilemma of making mistakes by deciding too soon, or being ineffective by delaying too long. In non-deliberative contexts this has to be accepted as inevitable, although the coach may try to reduce uncertainty.

2. A loss-minimization heuristic (a device for helping to choose between options) could be employed. This can be interpreted as conservatism – a reluctance to take chances (perhaps non-consciously acknowledging the uncertainties involved). In a very interesting paper, Lipshitz and Bar-Ilan (1996) identified three heuristics for problem solving: do not rush into action; diagnose as early as possible prior to taking action; and choose solutions with a wide range of 'coverage'. Although these are unrealistic in non-deliberative contexts, they might be useful guiding principles in naturalistic settings.

3. Schemata or scripts are accessed via 'trip' patterns or markers. Schemata, however, are acknowledged to be idiosyncratic. There are important implications for coach education in identifying and developing the key factors that will trigger responses.

4. A useful concept is that of 'decomposition'. This reinforces the notion that the dynamic chaotic stimuli in, for example, a game sport may not be easily decomposed (or broken down) by any but the expert coach and, even then, the room for error (perhaps, simply variation) must be considerable. Either the coach will use heuristic approaches with built-in biases and unreliability (for example, focusing on the last incident, or the most prominent one), or will attempt to regain the (illusion of) control by employing a degree of deliberation and analysis – and risking a delay in remedial action.

5. It might be expected that the different models would work together. In game sports, one explanation might be that coaches create individual match scripts that are informed by their existing knowledge and solution frames and are built up of enabling conditions as they develop. Mental models are created, which provide a synoptic overview of the game. Because of the limited options available (both human resource and game structure), it is necessary to wait until a threshold (individually constructed?) has been reached. This may be breached immediately in a crisis situation, in which case immediate action is taken. The coach has the capacity to react with a Schema (automated) approach if the pattern recognition is sufficiently strong, but it may be that even this is tempered by the knowledge of a limited range of actions.

6. There is a strong suggestion of 'anticipatory reflection' in coaches' cognitions. As the flow progresses and the options are narrowed, the coach has (subconsciously, using existing knowledge frames) modelled and scanned the potential variations in outcome which may arise. This allows the coach to have the solutions ready (again within a tacit data bank). This recognition of context has to be tempered or moderated by

the (perhaps conscious) acknowledgement of the limited resources available at any time, and by conscious strategic considerations.

7. Coaches will attempt to bring control to a very fluid and dynamic situation. This may be achieved by delaying their decisions if possible, in order to be sure of their reading of the problem (confirming their hypothesis). Of course, it may be that confirming a major problem is less valuable than acting proactively to prevent it from occurring. This may be another difference between novice and expert coaches.

8. One of the most significant factors in sports coaching decision making is that the decisions taken will often be contested by an opposition coach, who is attempting to achieve a similar objective. Part of the coach's dilemma is that the intentions of the opposition performers and coach are an unknown and have to be inferred from observations. Judgements of the relative technical capacities of the performers may be relatively easy to make for expert coaches, and these judgements will inform the solutions adopted. However, any action decision will be countered by the other coach (who is assumed also to be an expert). It must be assumed, therefore, that the decision problem may not be a static phenomenon and, indeed, may be made deliberately difficult to judge by the opposition. There are two important consequences of this. First, the situational analysis element of the decision problem is likely to assume very great importance. It is also easier to understand a common rule-of-thumb suggestion for coaches to focus on their own team's performance rather than the opposition to attempt a measure of control. Secondly, a coach might make a correct assessment, which brings with it the appropriate solution, but this has no effect because the opposition changes the problem space.

9. The coaches' key attractors will be sport-specific. For example in volleyball, playing rhythm, mental focus, clusters of points, key scores and momentum swings were identified as the key attractors in the game.

10. It is instructive to imagine the questions going through the mind of the coach as action is contemplated. 'I understand the problem at the moment, but how serious is it in relation to problems that might arise later? Is the problem likely to impact significantly on the target performance? The solution is obvious but will it work? If I make changes, will this restrict my freedom and flexibility to make more important changes later on? If I don't change now, will this problem continue to grow and become insurmountable? Do I have any other strategic/developmental plans in mind, which might supersede my interpretation of the current situation?' It is easy to appreciate why the coach has little time to deliberate on all of these issues and needs a decision making model, which has more shortcuts.

11. One way to shortcut the 'choice narrowing' is to anticipate what might happen. Because of the dynamic circumstances, the coach can anticipate rather than predict what the situation will become. The coach uses reflective anticipation (what would happen if?) to imagine the variations in the progress of the competition. The coach will use potential scripts (i.e. those they have modelled) to understand the anticipated future. Expert coaches will model better, and will choose a smaller number of likely scenarios because they can predict more accurately.

The impression of intuitive behaviour is maintained because the coach has already understood the implications of the future outcomes as they happen. Accompanying this recognition is the appropriate action decision (if triggered). Clearly there are a number of assumptions built into this explanation, but it certainly merits further research.

12. The forward modelling of options also helps to explain how action decisions may seem to be routine (and made deliberately this way to characterize expert behaviour). Some action decisions will already have been built into the coaches' modelled scenarios. Providing these scripts progress as expected, the action decisions (strategic substitutions, for example) can go ahead.

An Integrated Model

Klein's (1998) model, which will be described shortly, has an obvious appeal. The naturalistic setting characteristic of NDM fits very appropriately the coaching context. However, before describing the model there are a number of relevant propositions from this emerging field of study that will help us to gain a further insight into coaches' decision making.

Dealing with uncertainty is one of the coach's principal problems. In the NDM tradition, this can be dealt with by assumption-based reasoning and sound situational assessment. Lipshitz and Strauss (1997) suggest that individuals extrapolate from the available information, filling in gaps by assumption-based reasoning. They explain this as the use of mental simulation (Klein and Crandell, 1995) and scenario building (Schoemaker, 1995): 'imagining possible future developments in a script-like fashion' (Lipshitz and Strauss, 1997: 153). The most significant elements of their proposals are the use of delaying tactics and assumption-based reasoning models to reduce uncertainty. The coach would make sense of the situation and select an option, which is monitored. If the coach failed to make sense of the situation, perhaps because it was too complex, a decision would be delayed or the number of key variables in the environment would be reduced.

One of the interpretations of the coaches' cognitive organization suggested at an earlier stage in the chapter was that there was a strategic schema, which could be imposed in some way on the recognition-primed action choice. Cohen and colleagues (1996) propose a Recognition/Metarecognition Model, which has some potential explanatory power for this issue. The authors suggest that individuals adopt a two-tier process; following the recognition activation and its associated responses, there is an optional process of critiquing and correcting. They describe an empirically based model of the critiquing and correcting, which emphasizes metarecognition. For many coaches the issue of time pressure is problematic, and the authors suggest that individuals engage in a 'quick test'. This is used to judge if there is time before commitment to a decision is necessary, the consequences of an error are high, or the situation is unfamiliar. In such situations, the quick test inhibits the automatic response and allows for a critique of the situation. It could be speculated at this point that coaches might use a threshold trigger mechanism as part of the quick test stage. If the threshold was not breached, coaches would decide that, because of the limited decision resources and their knowledge of the strategic issues, they may choose to enter a process of metarecognition using mental simulations or other more deliberative processes.

A useful distinction is that between story building and mental simulation. Kaempf *et al.* (1996) investigated command-and-control decision making by naval personnel. Their study emphasized the importance of situational awareness, and stressed that this was more important than choices between different options. Individuals used feature matching (referred to earlier as recognizing key attractors) and story building if the situation was novel or complex. Story building was different to mental simulation in that it referred to analysis and interpretation of previous rather than subsequent states. There is no doubt that coaches build up pictures of what has happened. This story telling is required to make the diagnosis and hypothesize about the situation. The coach then mentally simulates the outcomes of the preferred solution. However, and most importantly, coaches must take into account what they predict will happen as the competition unfolds. Coaches in an interactive context must therefore simulate a number of scenarios with a number of solutions (the most obvious of which is action or no action).

Klein's model is illustrated in Figure 11.1 (Klein, 1998: 27).

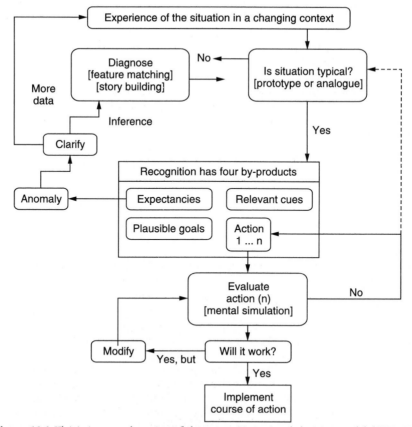

Figure 11.1 Klein's integrated version of the recognition-primed decision model (1998: 27). Reproduced with kind permission of MIT Press.

His model is termed the recognition-primed decision model, and pervades NDM literature. In its initial form, it is described as a pattern-recognition leading to a known schemata-based response. However, it has been extended in scope by Klein, and now encompasses the possibility of explaining how the individual might cope with a situation that is not immediately recognized and which, therefore, requires greater diagnosis. If the coach recognizes the situation as typical, four by-products are produced: expectancies, relevant cues, plausible goals and actions. In its simple form, a 'strong' recognition leads to one action, which is implemented. If the situation is not recognized, the coach builds a diagnosis by matching the key features until the situation is recognized. If, as a result of monitoring, the expectancies are violated, the coach will check the diagnosis. Where the coach has a choice of actions, mental simulations are evaluated until an appropriate outcome can be expected. This description perhaps underplays the need for hot action decisions, but is a useful starting point for coaching research. NDM identifies the making of decisions that are 'good enough' in the context of time pressure and limited data, rather than more optimal decisions, which imply some greater consideration. It also demonstrates that, in naturalistic contexts, non-compensatory decision making (i.e. without evaluating each option before acting) is the norm. The model has the potential to explain short-loop decisions (instant recognition and action) and the more interactive, serial decisions (monitoring a process as it emerges).

Klein's terminology is different to the traditional judgement decision making research literature, but it is an attractive agenda for understanding coaches' cognitions. Towards the end of his book, he summarizes what he terms the individual's sources of power in decision making, and cites the following:

- Intuition (pattern recognition, having the big picture, achieving situation awareness)
- Mental simulation (seeing the past and the future)
- Using leverage points to solve ill-defined problems
- Seeing the invisible (perceptual discrimination and expectancies)
- Story telling
- Analogical and metaphorical reasoning
- Reading people's minds (communicating intent)
- Rational analysis
- Team mind (drawing on the experience base of the team).

At this stage these say nothing about the cognitive organization underlying these assumptions about decision making in naturalistic settings, but they hold some promise for understanding the dynamic and contested situations in which coaches find themselves.

Educating the decision maker

What appears to be intuitive (and what feels intuitive to the decision maker) is an element of expertise that can (presumably) be trained. The question is, how can this best be done? Practical measures can be adopted. For example, experience of the task environment can be provided, but within a structured learning approach. Thus, the development of the procedural capacity (the actual 'doing') has to be complemented by a continuous process of support-ing declarative and (abstract or generic) propositional knowledge.

In conditions of risk, it has been necessary to simulate the task environ-ment. Examples include battlefield and aviation research (Klein, 1997: 6). However, with most sport contexts the coach will experience at first hand the training or competition environment. Nevertheless, the simulation of games in structured exercises is one possible training procedure. This might be video-based, and examine real-life examples commentated on by the expert concerned, or be in interactive-video format. Another suggestion is that coaches should experience difficult problems and be guided to appro-priate solutions. Although it may be likely that coaches would experience these in any event, through time, the embryonic expert would be given difficult cases to manage in a controlled and supportive environment.

Identifying critical cues is an important capacity. Once again, this requires simulation exercises with which to train perception for pattern recognition. A very important training mechanism is to help the coach to review prior experiences. Although this may happen in non-conscious ways, the learning process will be much enhanced by a structured approach that focuses on some of the stages identified above and requires the coach to reflect on the judgements made during the game. Clearly this might best be accompanied by a video recording and expert mentor notes, although this is a procedure that the coach can learn.

A further issue is the question of generic versus specific training. Should – or could – training in decision making be improved by studying the decision making process out of context and on more abstract problems? Lipshitz and Strauss are in no doubt about the specificity of the training material (1997: 160): 'training programmes should aim at teaching novices and mediocre performers the strategies and tactics that are used by experi-enced decision makers in the same domain'. This reinforces the need for research into the practice of our best coaches. An interesting issue, but one that can be resolved, is that the coach's expertise must deal with a different set of human resource factors on each occasion (numbers of players, cur-rent form, opposition strength etc.). To some extent, therefore, the coach's expertise in decision making should be thought of as a process in which default values (evaluations of current resources) are assessed at the begin-ning of the competition. These are then absorbed within the short-term memory structures.

More specific examples of the decision making components can be gleaned from the earlier parts of the chapter. It is obvious that situation assessment (including pattern recognition), key attractors and diagnostic hypothesizing, mental simulation involving assumption-based reasoning, knowledge frames or schemata with a range of appropriate solutions, development of threshold triggers, impact-forestalling tactics and meta-recognition capacities (judgement of threat and advantage) need to be developed within the coaches' repertoire. Abraham and Collins (1998) have already indicated that coach education is deficient in the development of propositional and procedural knowledge, but they failed to specify the training strategies to be adopted. It seems clear that experience alone will be insufficient, although it is likely to have an incremental effect on knowl-edge structures and performance.

Many of these suggestions are best implemented by expert mentors. This gives the coach an opportunity for some focused 'situated learning' (see Lave and Wenger, 1991) and diagnostic feedback. Interpretation of the mentoring role stresses the active contribution made by the expert coach mentor and goes beyond the guiding/monitoring role. Given the earlier arguments about the central role of decision making for the performance coach, it is obvious that one of the principal needs is for mentors to understand coaches' decision making processes and how they might be enhanced.

Summary

The intention was to convince the reader of the importance of effective decision making for the sports coach and to suggest an explanation of how coaches make decisions. It is worth stressing that the emphasis was on largely non-deliberative decision making, and this will be more relevant to games sport coaches and in competition.

A descriptive summary of a coach's decision making might be as follows. During action, coaches engage in decision framing and diagnosis based on the important stage of situation assessment. If the situation is sufficiently threatening to the competition objective, this will lead to a decision point. The solution to be adopted will have been generated by the pattern recognition process, and is one that has been used successfully in the past. If the situation is untenable but too uncertain, a default decision solution (one that usually works in such situations but is not specific to this problem) may be adopted. The diagnosis will have hypothesized the probable progress of the competition, and this is monitored in the next, on-going situation assessment. This in turn can lead to a decision point, a new diagnosis based on a threshold trigger, or the continuation of the original hypothesis. This process is continually repeated, and is fed by a constant awareness and monitoring of the situation.

The decision framing and diagnoses are based on cognitive schemata. In the context of time pressure, rapid diagnosis (particularly recalling that this will involve many potential hypotheses and solutions) is similar to the concept of script schemata. The diagnosis involves two sub-processes. One is a retrospective story telling, which provides an explanation for the development of the situation and associates, therefore, with the solutions adopted. The other is a reflective anticipation or mental simulation, which provides the expectancies against which progress can be evaluated.

The task environment is inherently uncertain because of the reliance on relatively fragile performer qualities and the contested nature of sport. For this reason, diagnoses, hypotheses, simulations and solutions are all inherently weak. Further research is required to assess the expertness of these judgements. The coaches' cognitive capacity to engage in such an effortful cognitive process has yet to be established. It seems likely that the coaches will seek further problem reduction strategies, for example, by employing favourite solutions. A further example is the routinization of some decisions within the game.

Coaches' monitoring processes involve some form of metarecognition, which is not yet fully understood. In critiquing progress, coaches will engage in judgements of the sort that balance impact of action against estimation of threat and desire to confirm the hypothesis. The putative heuristics mentioned earlier, such as 'don't be hasty' and 'don't judge early', might prove to be apt. The notion of intuition in coaching judgements seems very likely to be borne out of our general ignorance of the processes involved rather than to be an inexplicable phenomenon. The coach's cognitive organization is not fully theorized, but it seems likely that the mix of non-deliberative and more-deliberative processes has a basis in understandable and accessible neural states.

References

Abraham, A. and Collins, D. (1998). Examining and extending research in coach development. *Quest*, **50**, 55–79.

Adelson, B. (1984). When novices surpass experts: the difficulty of a task may increase with expertise. *J. Exp. Psychol.: Learning Memory Cognition*, **10(3)**, 483–95.

Beach, L. R. (1997). *The Psychology of Decision Making*. Sage.

Beckett, D. (1996). Critical judgement and professional practice. *Ed. Theory*, **46(2)**, 135–49.

Bloom, G. A., Durand-Bush, N. and Salmela, J. H. (1997). Pre- and post-competition routines of expert coaches of team sports. *Sport Psychol.*, **11**, 127–41.

Boreham, N. C. (1988). Models of diagnosis and their implications for adult professional education. *Studies Ed. Adults*, **20**, 95–108.

Boreham, N. C. (1994). The dangerous practice of thinking. *Med. Ed.*, **28**, 172–9.

Brehmer, B. (1992). Dynamic decision making: human control of complex systems. *Acta Psychologica*, **81**, 211–41.

Brehmer, B. and Allard, R. (1990). Dynamic decision making: the effects of task complexity and feedback delay. In *Distributed Decision Making: Cognitive Models for Co-operative Work* (B. Rasmussen, B. Brehmer and J. Leplat, eds), pp. 313–29. Wiley.

Byra, M. and Sherman, M. A. (1993). Pre-active and interactive decision-making tendencies of less and more experienced pre-service teachers. *Res. Q. Exer. Sport*, **64(1)**, 46–55.

Cannon-Bowers, J. A., Salas, E. and Pruitt, J. S. (1996). Establishing the boundaries of a paradigm for decision making. *Human Factors*, **38(2)**, 193–205.

Caplan, L. J. and Schooler, C. (1990). Problem solving by reference to rules or previous episodes: the effects of organized training, analogical models and subsequent complexity of experience. *Memory Cogn.*, **18(2)**, 215–27.

Chi, M., Glaser, R. and Farr, M. (eds) (1988). *The Nature of Expertise*. Lawrence Erlbaum Associates.

Claxton, G. (1998). Knowing without knowing why. *Psychologist*, **11(5)**, 217–20.

Cohen, M. S., Freeman, J. T. and Wolf, S. (1996). Metarecognition in time stressed decision making: recognising, critiquing and correcting. *Hum. Fact.*, **38(2)**, 206–19.

Cote, J., Salmela, J., Trudel, P. *et al.* (1995). The coaching model: a grounded assessment of expert gymnastic coaches' knowledge. *J. Sport Exer. Psychol.*, **17(1)**, 1–17.

Cratty, B. J. (1970). Coaching decisions and research in sport psychology. *Quest*, **13**, 46–53.

Cross, N. (1995a). Coaching effectiveness in hockey: a Scottish perspective. *Scot. J. Physical Ed.*, **23(1)**, 27–39.

Cross, N. (1995b). Coaching effectiveness and the coaching process. *Swimming Times*, **LXXII(3)**, 23–5.

Devine, D. J. and Kozlowski, S. W. J. (1995). Domain-specific knowledge and task characteristics in decision making. *Org. Behav. Hum. Decision Proc.*, **64(3)**, 294–306.

Dougherty, M. R. P., Gettys, C. F. and Thomas, R. P. (1997). The role of mental simulation in judgements of likelihood. *Org. Behav. Hum. Decision Proc.*, **70(2)**, 135–48.

Dreyfus, H. L. and Dreyfus, S. E. (1986). *Mind over Machine: The Power of Human Intuition and Expertise in the Era of the Computer.* Basil Blackwell.

Duke, A. and Corlett, J. (1992). Factors affecting University women's basketball coaches' timeout decisions. *Can. J. Sport Sci.*, **17(4),** 333–7.

Easen, P. and Wilcockson, J. (1996). Intuition and rational decision making in professional thinking: a false dichotomy? *J. Adv. Nursing*, **24,** 667–73.

Eraut, M. (1994). *Developing Professional Knowledge and Competence.* Falmer Press.

Fischhoff, B. (1996). The real world: what good is it? *Org. Behav. Hum. Decision Proc.*, **65(3),** 232–48.

Flin, R., Salas, E., Strub, M. and Martin, L. (eds) (1997). *Decision Making under Stress: Emerging Themes and Applications.* Ashgate.

Franks, I. M., Sinclair, G. D., Thomson, W. and Goodman, D. (1986). Analysis of the coaching process. *Sci. Period. Res. Technol. Sport*, January.

Goldstein, W. M. and Weber, E. U. (1995). Content and discontent: indications and implications of domain specificity in preferential decision making. In *The Psychology of Learning and Motivation. Volume 32. Decision Making from a Cognitive Perspective* (J. R. Busemeyer, R. Hastie and D. L. Medin, eds), pp. 83–136. Academic Press.

Gould, D., Giannini, J., Kane, V. and Hodge, K. (1990). Educational needs of elite U.S. National Team, Pan American and Olympic coaches. *J. Teach. Physical Ed.*, **9(4),** 332–44.

Griffey, D. C. and Housner, L. D. (1991). Differences between experienced and inexperienced teachers' planning decisions, interactions, student engagement, and instructional climate. *Res. Q. Exer. Sport*, **62,** 196–204.

Hammond, K. R., Hamm, R. M., Grassia, J. and Pearson, T. (1993). Direct comparison of the efficacy of intuitive and analytical cognition in expert judgement. In *Research on Judgement and Decision Making: Currents, Connections and Controversies* (W. M. Goldstein and R. M. Hogarth, eds), pp. 144–80. Cambridge University Press.

Housner, L. and Griffey, D. (1985). Teacher cognition: differences in planning and interactive decision making between experienced and inexperienced teachers. *Res. Q. Exer. Sport*, **56,** 45–53.

Jones, D. F., Housner, L. D. and Kornspan, A. (1995). A comparative analysis of expert and novice basketball coaches' practice planning. *Annual Appl. Res. Coach. Athletics*, **10,** 201–26.

Jones, D. F., Housner, L. D. and Kornspan, A. S. (1997). Interactive decision making and behaviour of experienced and inexperienced basketball coaches during practice. *J. Teach. Physical Ed.*, **16,** 454–68.

Kaempf, G. L., Klein, G. A., Thordsen, M. L. and Wolf, S. (1996). Decision making in complex command-and-control environments. *Hum. Fact.*, **38(2),** 220–31.

Karlsson, G. (1988). A phenomenological psychological study of decision and choice. *Acta Psychologica*, **68,** 7–25.

Kersholt, J. H. (1994). The effect of time pressure on decision-making behaviour in a dynamic task environment. *Acta Psychologica*, **86,** 89–104.

Klein, G. A. (1990). Knowledge engineering: beyond expert systems. *Inform. Decision Tech.*, **16,** 27–41.

Klein, G. A. and Crandall, B. W. (1995). The role of mental simulation in naturalistic decision making. In *Local Applications of the Ecological Approach to Human–Machine Systems* (P. Hancock, J. Flach, J. Caird and K. Vincente, eds), pp. 324–58. Lawrence Erlbaum Associates.

Klein, G. A. (1997). The current status of the naturalistic decision-making framework. In *Decision Making Under Stress: Emerging Themes and Applications* (R. Flin, G. Slaven, M. Strub and L. Martin, eds), pp. 11–28. Ashgate.

Klein, G. A. (1998). *Sources of Power: How People Make Decisions.* MIT.

Lave, J. and Wenger, E. (1991). *Situated Learning: Legitimate Peripheral Participation.* Cambridge University Press.

Leet, D., James, T. and Rushall, B. (1984). Intercollegiate teams in competition. A field study to examine variables influencing contests results. *Int. J. Appl. Sport Psychol.*, **15,** 193–204.

Lipshitz, R. and Bar-Ilan, O. (1996) How problems are solved: reconsidering the phase theorem. *Org. Behav. Hum. Decision. Proc.*, **65(1),** 48–60.

Lipshitz, R. and Strauss, O. (1997). Coping with uncertainty: a naturalistic decision-making analysis. *Org. Behav. Hum. Decision Proc.*, **69(2),** 149–163.

Lyle, J. (1992). Systematic coaching behaviour: an investigation into the coaching process and the implications of the findings for coach education. In *Sport and Physical Activity: Moving Towards Excellence* (T. Williams, L. Almond and A. Sparkes, eds), pp. 463–9. EFN Spon.

Lyle, J. (1996). A conceptual appreciation of the sports coaching process. *Scot. Cent. Res. Papers Sport Leisure Soc.*, **1(1),** 15–37.

Orasanu, J. and Connolly, T. (1993). The reinvention of decision making. In *Decision Making in Action: Models and Methods* (G. A. Klein, J. Orasanu, R. Calderwood and C. Zsambok, eds), pp. 3–20. Ablex Pub.

Pennington, N. and Hastie, R. (1993). Reasoning in explanation-based decision making. *Cognition*, **49,** 123–63.

Randel, J. M., Pugh, H. L. *et al.* (1996). Differences in expert and novice situation awareness in naturalistic decision making. *Int. J. Hum. Comp. Stud.*, **45,** 579–97.

Rasmussen, J. (1997). Merging paradigms: decision making, management and cognitive control. In *Decision Making under Stress: Emerging Themes and Applications* (R. Flin, E. Salas, M. Strub and L. Martin, eds), pp. 57–81. Ashgate.

Salmela, J. H. (1995). Learning from the development of expert coaches. *Coach. Sports Sci. J.*, **2(2),** 3–13.

Schmidt, H. G., Norman, G. R. and Boshuizen, P. A. (1990). A cognitive perspective on medical expertise: theory and implications. *Acad. Med.*, **65(10),** 611–21.

Schoemaker, P. J. H. (1995). Scenario planning: a tool for strategic thinking. *Sloan Management Rev.*, **36(2),** 25–50.

Schon, D. A. (1983). *The Reflective Practitioner: How Professionals Think in Action.* Basic Books.

Schon, D. A. (1987). *Educating the Reflective Practitioner.* Jossey Bass.

Strack, F. and Neumann, R. (1996). 'The spirit is willing, but the flesh is weak': beyond mind–body interactions in human decision making. *Org. Behav. Hum. Decision Proc.*, **65(3),** 300–304.

Svenson, O. (1996). Decision making and the search for fundamental psychological regularities: what can be learned from a process perspective? *Org. Behav. Hum. Decision Proc.*, **65,** 252–67.

Teigen, K. H. (1996). Decision making in two worlds. *Org. Behav. Hum. Decision Proc.*, **65(3),** 249–51.

Zsambok, C. and Klein, G. A. (eds) (1997). *Naturalistic Decision Making.* LEA.

12

Coaching and the management of performance systems[1]

John Lyle

- The contemporary development of performance sport
- The nature of performance sport
- Four levels of the performance sport system
- The characteristics and cohesion of a system
- Modelling the performance sport system
- Key features of the system
- Inputs, treatments and outputs
- Soft systems analysis
- Performance sport systems and the coaching process
- The role of the coach in management

Introduction

The inception of a British Academy of Sport in 1995, re-designated the UK Sports Institute (UKSI) in 1997, was the catalyst for an introspection of British sports policy and provision, which did little to enhance its credibility. This came at a time when the reorganization of the Sports Councils had exposed their self-interest (see Pickup, 1996). The nascent UK Sports Council (UKSC) has had to battle against the influence of the English Sports Council and the positioning of the Celtic Councils. At the same time, in the vacuum created by the neglect of performance sport by successive Sports Councils and the National Coaching Foundation, the British Olympic Association has been growing in stature as it moves from ticket agency to technical agency. Meanwhile, National Governing Bodies (NGBs) of sport have tried to exploit their influence to the extent that professionalization, sponsorship or public subsidy has allowed them to focus on the pursuit of international success. As developments have taken place within and between these umbrella agencies, those bodies responsible for sports medicine, sports science, coaching and higher education have monitored the situation and anticipated the resulting market opportunities. For example, a number of higher education establishments (most notably the University of Bath) have taken advantage of the

[1] The initial development of these ideas appeared as 'Managing excellence in sports performance' in *Career Development International*, **2(7),** 314–23 (Lyle, 1997).

coincidence of lifestyle focus, age range of performers, staffing expertise, facilities and the desire for a higher profile to develop centres of excellence.

There is no doubt that the acceleration in development has been fuelled by the proceeds of the National Lottery. Despite a faltering start, when money was channelled solely to capital projects, the National Lottery has transformed the financial structure and with it the aspirations of those sports selected to benefit most from the cash injections. The most significant development is the United Kingdom Sports Institute. This was originally conceived of as a replica of the Australian Sports Institute in Canberra, and perceived as the panacea for the ills of British performance sport (Hawkey, 1997). A combination of costs, a change of Government in 1997 and the outcome of a consultation exercise within sport has led to the reconceptualization of the UKSI as a network hub site. This is to operate through an integrated provision of local support services and facilities, a series of regional institutes, and sport-specific centres of excellence. It could be argued that the UKSI and its regional network have so far been cloaked in a miasma of financing, politics and self-interest.

This may seem a rather negative introduction to the chapter. However, the purpose is not to decry in any way the developments taking place, but to focus attention on the absence of a national strategy and the multiplicity of agencies involved in delivering performance sport in the UK. No great leap of imagination or detailed argument is required to appreciate that the 'system', such as it is, is neither efficient nor effective. The Government's intermittent interest and attempts to distance itself from the minutiae of sports policy formulation and the strong autonomy exercised by the British voluntary and professional sectors have resulted in a largely uncoordinated and undirected strategy and infrastructure. National Lottery finance has rekindled sports agencies' interest in performance sport. However, a significant problem is that the existing agencies have had very limited experience of operating within these new parameters. In this context, it is reasonable to ask questions about the management of the system: indeed, whether a 'system', in the true sense of the word, exists at all. The development of the UKSC, the UKSI and the World Class Performance Plans of the major NGBs are products of the system as it is, and have become constituent parts of its operations. How was the UK performance sport system analysed and evaluated at the time when change was being considered? How would it be evaluated at this moment in order to assess its effectiveness?

This chapter suggests that the sport performance system in the UK needs to be treated as a system and analysed as a system. It will be argued that this is the most appropriate way to understand its operation. However, it will be obvious to the reader that the space available will not permit a detailed analysis of each of the parts of the system. The focus will be on the method of systems analysis and the component parts of the performance sport system. Although the chapter embraces the performance sport system as a whole, the purpose of the book is to shed light on the principles and practice of coaching. The chapter is linked to coaching in two ways. First, the place of coaching in the performance sport input–output system is examined and evaluated. Secondly, the potential for understanding the coaching process from a system perspective is considered. Before moving on to consider the system approach, it will be valuable to examine the concept of performance sport in more detail.

Performance sport

There may be an absence of a national strategy for sport in the UK, but the externalities accruing from performance and excellence in sport have been recognized by successive Governments (Department of National Heritage, 1995; English Sports Council, 1997). The achievements of international representatives in sport provide sufficient justification for developing and nurturing talent in sport. The nation's image of itself and its profile abroad are influenced by the successes and failures of performers at this level. Sport is part of the cultural life of the nation and a significant focus of media attention. In addition, it provides a pinnacle to the ladder of opportunity to which younger performers can aspire and a catalyst for the beginner or more general recreationalist. These externalities have found their way into the rhetoric of the policy statements of Government and non-government organizations, but have not been matched by political will. In some ways this is surprising, given the scrutiny afforded to the success or otherwise of our international representatives. In Canada (see Kikulis *et al.*, 1995) and Australia (see Westerbeek, 1995), a perception of national failure in world level sport led to a significant change to their sport systems. The UK's response to limited achievement in Wimbledon, the World Cups or the Olympic Games has been to question our image of ourselves, but to be less effective in bringing about significant change. Part of the argument in this chapter is a suggestion that the undoubted importance of achievement in performance and excellence sport is not reflected in the level of analysis or research devoted to it. This may be the result of an absence of conceptual tools with which to analyse and understand the system. It is difficult to believe that the scale, scope and dynamics of the performance sport system can be adequately appreciated without a mechanism for developing a clear conceptual understanding of the structure and processes involved.

It can be argued that the lack of a critical and synoptic overview of the sports delivery system has prevented it being dealt with as a problematic issue. With or without attention to systems, sport will always produce good performers. The pyramidal competition structures currently in place will inevitably produce some good athletes. However, competition structures alone will not maximize levels of achievement or match those from other systems. Perhaps the failure to deal with performance development in a systematic way has helped to fuel the 'natural ability' ethos in sport. However, a reasonable assumption to make is that an unorganized and disaggregated system is unlikely to result in comparative excellence. If excellence is required, the systems in place need direction and control, and this must be effectively and efficiently managed.

The nature of the performance sport system has to be understood in the context of the nature of performance sport itself. The special demands made by performance sport differ significantly from participation and recreation sport. Performance sport is characterized by its intensity of commitment, its instrumental approach to achievement in competition, the scale and intensity of the activity required, and the level of technical and other areas of knowledge involved. It can also be related for the most part to its level of achievement in competition sport, although this is not necessarily a defining feature. When the level of achievement is of the highest order, the term 'sporting excellence' is used. Performance and excellence sport, therefore, is composed of the system that embraces those at the highest performance levels in sport and those who are in the development stage of this ambition. It also comprises the greater majority of those who may never reach the highest levels themselves, but who are intensely committed to their sport and form part of the competition structure which supports the elite.

Intrinsic to competition sport is a process of meritocratic deselection; that is, competition structures are designed to gradually winnow out those with the greatest ability. Of course this has to be handled carefully, and competition should be available for all levels. Nevertheless, the use of labels (such as good, excellent, international, representative) and the identification of ability (and latent ability) are problematic issues. Inevitably, any comparison of performance is fraught with difficulty, and it may be that the system or context within which the performance is produced has to be taken into account in the evaluation. Evaluation in sport is bedevilled by the distinction between relative and absolute measures of performance, by age-group excellence and by the issue of the resources available. In the context of this chapter, this might be termed the 'richness of the system'. Since we are interested in the management of the system, the extent to which developing nations and others with limited means have exploited their sporting resources is a valuable source of information. Once again, such awareness will only be optimized if the analysis is conducted, interpreted and comprehended at the level of the performance sport system as a whole.

This introductory section on defining performance sport has important ramifications for a systems analysis of the performance sport system. A number of key elements have already emerged:

1. The output from the system will be measured by competition performance achievement. To some extent this also defines the purpose of the system, and will have a strong influence on the values and culture exhibited within the system.
2. There will be a relationship between the performance sport system and other sport systems – for example, school, developmental and recreational. This is largely unexplored territory. What is clear is that the simplistic notions often expressed, such as 'higher standards will be achieved by expanding the base of the introductory pyramid', need much more detailed attention. Specific sports have to examine very carefully how the input from schools or developmental systems finds its way into the performance system. It will need to be a managed process – and cannot be based on an assumption of natural transfer.
3. The performance system is not large in comparison to the number of recreational participants in most sports. However, the range of performance levels and performer aspirations is considerable. It is useful, therefore, to conceptualize it as three sport sub-systems: (a) the development of excellence; (b) the pursuit of excellence; and (c) the practice of performance. The terms may seem tortuous, but it is important to

identify the characteristics (and therefore the needs of the participants) at each level. The development of excellence embraces those individuals, usually younger, whose current performance standards and potential suggest that they might become part of the very small proportion of the sports population that might be said to display excellence. They are likely to be part of age-group squads and to be dealt with in special development squads and/or centres of excellence. There is also a small proportion of performers who are pursuing excellence. This implies that they are at the top of their sport, and includes the elite group. Although defining boundaries is difficult, these might be thought of as internationalists or national squad members. These performers are likely to receive particular attention, since they constitute 'medal potential'. In addition to these categories, it must always be remembered that there is a large group of performers who have not and will not reach the excellence category, but who display the intensity of commitment, desire for competition achievement, and the preparation for improved performance that is characteristic of the performance sport system. The most important implication from identifying distinctive sub-sets within the system is that they require different structures, process and resources.

4. Sporting achievement is inherently normative; that is, it involves comparison between performers. Although a level of excellence will, therefore, always be achieved by the best at any given time, it is important to note that further comparison may be invited with standards from other countries. Resource allocation, and perhaps therefore the scale and scope of the performance system, may be based on an evaluation of standards in the context of overseas performances. This has been the basis of the Sports Councils' identification of target sports, to which a greater share of resources will be allocated (for example, Scottish Sports Council, 1998).

Simply drawing the boundaries of the performance sport system is beginning to sketch in some of the essential elements, which will have implications for management of the system. The most important to date has been the need to be precise about sub-sets of performers within the system in order to ensure that needs are matched to appropriate sub-processes and resources. However, it is also important to examine the nature of the coaching process which is characteristic of the sport performance system. In an earlier chapter, a clear distinction was drawn between participation and performance coaching. In the first, short-term horizons, the immediacy of objectives, lack of control over the variables influencing performance and a much-reduced emphasis on competition involvement or success leads to an episodic emphasis, which reflects the participants' lesser intensity of involvement or commitment. On the other hand, the performance coach will be required to direct a coaching process that displays characteristics of more intensive commitment to competition involvement, longer-term horizons, more non-intervention contact and a preparation programme which is planned, progressive and carefully monitored. In addition, the performers' lifestyles are more likely to be dominated by their commitment to sport and have to be managed accordingly. Readers will recall that it was indicated in the introduction that an argument would be further developed proposing that the performance coach's role mirrors that of a manager.

This then is performance sport. In the introduction, it was suggested that the contemporary development of performance sport was being accelerated by the funding made available by the National Lottery, but that the piece-meal, largely serendipitous, structures and processes of the past had not yet been superseded by an effective, co-ordinated system. Although the term 'system' has been assumed to this point, it is necessary now to explore what this term actually implies.

Performance sport as a system

Sport structures and processes can be managed most appropriately if they are conceived of as systems. The basis of this argument is that a system has a conceptual structure, which can then be applied to an analysis of any system. However, for our purposes, an important question is whether the collection of agencies, interaction of resources and performers, the delivery and provision structures, and the administrative, organizational and technical personnel constituting performance sport in the UK can collectively be considered to be a 'system'.

In order to answer this question, a model of a system will be presented against which a performance sport system can be compared. It will be demonstrated that this might be used to analyse the collective national system and sub-units within it. It will then be argued that the simplistic input–treatment–output model currently in vogue requires a further level of analysis. The performance sport system is a particular form of system, both an 'open system' and what Checkland (1989) calls a 'soft system'. This has special properties and requires a particular form of analysis. As these models are examined, there is a danger of falling into the trap of presenting a 'should be' description of a system – this is not a model 'for' a performance sport system (e.g. the current UK sport performance system). The target is to analyse and evaluate an existing system (i.e. a model 'of'). Only once this has been accomplished will it be possible to construct an ideal system (i.e. a model 'for').

Let us begin by recognizing the four levels of system likely to be present (see Figure 12.1). These will reflect the stages at which specific objectives are set.

Strategic level

Strategic management is exercised at the national level. This level within the system will be responsible for the setting of overall policy, strategy, targets and resource allocation. Although this is not a delivery stage, the strategic overview of the component parts necessary for the integrating and complete delivery of the system will be demonstrated at this level. Issues at this level will centre on Government direction and intervention, and the presence or absence of a national strategy or consensus on performance sport. It seems likely that major professional sports will be most strongly influenced by market forces, but periodic government interest in the national (media led!) perceptions of success and failure may prompt policy intervention. It is more likely that 'intervention by incentive' will be offered

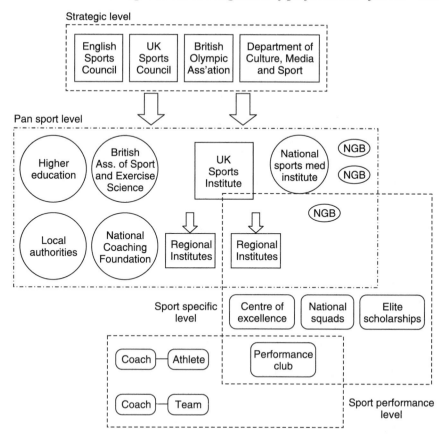

Figure 12.1 Parent and sub-system levels

to provide initiatives at the school/developmental system levels. Examples of this are the school initiatives (e.g. SportsMark) outlined in *Sport: Raising the Game* (DNH, 1995) and the programmes operationalized by the Youth Sport Trust (e.g. Top Sport, Coaching for Teachers). Occasionally, however, there may be a national initiative, and the UKSI is the best example of this. From an analysis of the system perspective, the interesting point has been the difficulty in integrating the UKSI into the existing elements of the performance sports system. In the context of the UK's liberal democracy and mixed economy, the strong autonomy of non-governmental bodies, the absence of one all-sport organizing body, the traditional primacy of sport-for-all policies, 'home nation' rivalry and a rather weak national ethos for supporting excellence in sport, it is hardly surprising that there has been no all-embracing national strategy for performance sport. Nevertheless, the dependence of many sports on National Lottery funding seems likely to lead to a centralization of policy direction. Future research may conclude that National Lottery distribution of sports resources has acted as a *de facto* national strategy.

Pan-sport level

Pan-sport structure and delivery is the first level at which active sportspersons are found. This is the level at which national and regional multisport agencies and provision is intended to cater for all or, in some cases, a number of targeted sports. The most obvious example is the UKSI and its network of regional institutes. However, there are a number of other agencies involved; those responsible for sports medicine, sports science, sports coaching and higher education. At a more localized level, Local Authorities may make specific provision for performance sport. As a collective entity, the National Governing Bodies of sport are also to be found at this level.

This is the level at which proactive management is most necessary and yet most difficult. The degree of integration and co-ordination required from so many disparate bodies – each with its own agenda but with the capacity to make a contribution to the whole – is extremely challenging. The lengthy process currently under way to develop both the UKSI and a network of regional institutes has demonstrated not only the enormity of the task of integrating so many organizations, but also has exposed the political ambitions which exclusion or inclusion can confer.

Sport-specific level

Sport-specific performance systems form the groups at the next level of analysis. Individual sports will have particular patterns of provision through which their performance sport is organized and developed. The elements of these systems may include performance sports clubs (remembering that not all clubs will have this ambition or capacity), centres of excellence, national squads (including age-group/school squads), specific higher-education institution elite programmes, and the relevant competition programme. Although there is a national pattern of provision in support services (or at least an emerging one), each NGB is likely to develop provision to satisfy its own scale of needs.

Given the more manageable scale and the complementarity of purpose within the different sports, one would imagine that managing this system would be easier than those systems above it. However, there have traditionally been a number of challenges to effective and efficient provision at this level: the availability of finance, the voluntaristic nature of provision, variable reward systems, and the expertise available within the system both to manage and to deliver. Once again, the demands dictated by the National Lottery funding and the increased understanding of models of performance planning may assist this level of management of the system.

Sport performance level

Performance system is the term given to the basic building block element in the system. This is the configuration of structures, personnel and processes within which the coaching process is enacted. At its most basic, this could be an athlete and coach operating in isolation. However, this is unlikely at performance levels. A more likely scenario would be the athlete within a top squad in a club in which the coach has assistance from a number of specialist services (physiotherapists, administrators etc.). Similar pictures could be conjured up for team sports players, the full-time athlete in a centre of excellence, or the tennis player operating with a full-time coach and making use of NGB-provided services.

There are many different variations of this sub-system. The most essential element is the direction given to the performer's development programme by the coach. The coaching process for the top-level performer may involve complete lifestyle management and integration into the systems levels above – that is, NGB provision structures and services and/or national pro-gramme provision (e.g. UKSI or BOA training camps). The management of this system should be individually tailored and strictly controlled. Traditionally again, the availability of finance and, as a result, competition access, training volume, sports science assistance and the availability of the most expert coaches, have been a problem. As finance becomes more readily available and there is greater commonality in treatment, it may be that other elements of the system, the input (e.g. recruitment) rather than treatment parts, become more limiting.

An obvious point to make, but very important nevertheless, is the integra-tion of all of these systems. Each is dependent on the other, and an evaluative measure of the collective performance sport system is the degree of integra-tion and co-ordination at all levels. There is a presumption that the integra-tion and co-ordination could be better in the UK system; in complex, multi-agency systems this is likely always to be the case. What is required is research to expose the implications of any lack of co-ordination in provision (other than simply assuming that results could be better!). Before moving on to suggest a possible mechanism for analysis, it is necessary to say a little more about what a system is, and the dangers of focusing on structures rather than processes.

A system is defined by the (usually purposeful) integration of interrelated elements into an entity that is intended to achieve an identifiable and con-sensual purpose. The system operates more effectively in achieving its objec-tives by operating as a whole rather than as a collection of parts. The characteristics of a system might be listed as:

- Common purpose
- Control strategy
- Structure
- Process (in our case this is sport performance, and assumes many sub-processes)
- Shared values and mores
- Integration
- Environmental influence (perhaps most often referred to as open or closed).

Systems may be tightly knit processes within organizations or, as has become obvious in our example, a rather looser coalition of agencies and processes. The defining features of the degree of 'tightness' of the system are:

- The locus of control (centralization/decentralization)
- The intensity of commitment to the common purpose
- The specificity of the objectives

- The diffusion of shared values
- The number of layers/levels within the system
- The adaptability/flexibility of response to the environment
- The effectiveness of communication between agencies.

As a result, some systems will be more closed or open than others. The question of whether UK performance sport actually constitutes a system may not yet have been fully answered, but there is no doubt that, if it does, it will be open in nature. It may also be worth noting that the systems being discussed involve human beings. The term 'system' may be used to describe manufacturing processes or physical features (e.g. drainage systems) in which human agency is much less of an issue. As noted later, a human system is more difficult to analyse.

There is no doubt that the term 'system', when applied to sport, has a common currency. This is evident in analyses of various national systems. For example, Riorden (1993: 43) uses the term 'elite sports system'. In a recent article, Gene Schembri of the Australian Coaching Council (1998: 7) assumes the 'sum of the parts' when he says, 'the strength of the Australian system is in its diversity'. He also states that 'social, cultural, historical and political factors are all important considerations in shaping the architecture of a country's sport system' (1998: 7). Despite this evidence of usage, the issue remains whether, after analysis and evaluation, the use of the term is justified by adherence to defining characteristics, rather than being used merely as a convenient descriptive term.

There is a danger that systems come to be represented by structures rather than functions. Perhaps this is part of a tendency to represent systems by drawing diagrams of interconnected stages and elements. Cole (1994) identifies a number of key elements that are required to implement strategy; a structural framework, leadership, financial and physical resources, an organizational culture, and an infrastructure of personnel and expertise. The implication is that, while a structural diagram may be a convenient form of shorthand, the strength of a system is measured by the extent to which the interdependence of structure, function and processes allows it to achieve its objectives. Identifying these constituent elements – leadership, a strategy, resourcing, supportive culture etc., in addition to the system characteristics outlined previously – begins to map out an analytical framework.

An illustrative example is to be found in an article by Frank Dick (1998). In what is effectively a blueprint for a performance sport system, Dick uses at least four diagrams in which various elements are connected by arrows to explain his thinking. However, it is not as clear as it might be. It is a little unfair to criticize the presentation when the ideas are very sound and the article was obviously not intended to have the depth to explain fully how the diagrams, or rather the systems and processes they represent, would operate. Nevertheless, it is a common situation to find the structure emphasized at the expense of the function. A second example is the debate that has surrounded the UKSI and a network of regional sports institutes. Considerable attention is paid to structural diagrams, but the functions and processes are merely listed (Sports Council, 1995; Scottish Sports Council, 1998). However, at the implementation stage, the integration of functions is often the most problematic issue. This is also the case with analysis. In order to provide a mechanism for analysing systems, it is important to look beyond structure.

Modelling the performance sport system

The input–treatment–output system

It has been suggested that the performance sport system can most appropriately be conceptualized as an input–treatment–output (ITO) system (see Figure 12.2) and managed and analysed accordingly. It remains, of course, an open question as to whether the national system is characterized sufficiently strongly by the criteria already identified to be thought of as a system at all. A further means of analysis will be necessary to understand fully the 'looser' system at national level. For the moment, it would be more helpful to use a National Governing Body or a performance sport club as an exemplar when describing the input–treatment–output model.

The model (see Figure 12.2) suggests that a number of input resources are sufficiently interdependent in their effect that they impact on the treatment phase and, in turn, on the output. This implies that the inputs, even when aggregated, will not of themselves produce the desired effect. This means that the treatment process is therefore both important and inherently problematical.

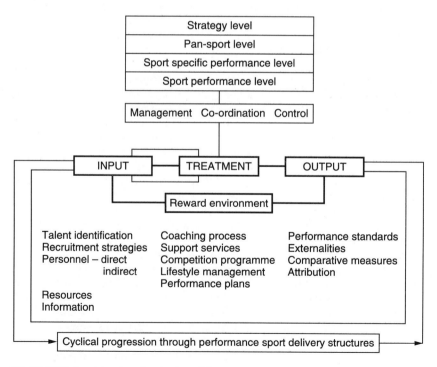

Figure 12.2 Input–treatment–output model

It may be a useful step to isolate a number of features of the model before elaborating to some extent on a number of the key elements:

1. A central feature is the reward environment. This can be thought of as a constant which influences the equation represented by each input–treat-ment–output example. The reward environment is created by the social/cultural status afforded to the system's outputs. For example, the outputs from a professional soccer club are highly valued within UK culture (similarly to basketball in the USA), and therefore the reward environ-ment is very positive. In such circumstances it should not be difficult to attract input resources to the system, and to expect the treatment process to be extensive and sophisticated. On the other hand, even international competitors in, for example, fencing are less well valued, and the reward environment will be less positive. In these sports, recruiting performers may be much more difficult, and the scale of the 'treatment' necessary for achievement-orientated outputs may not be justified by the reward envir-onment. Nevertheless, we should not underestimate the intrinsic reward environment that intense commitment to a sport brings. It is also very important to note that the advent of World Class Performance National Lottery grants have encouraged commitment to a larger-scale treatment process (i.e. more full-time training and coaching) in a large variety of sports, and are keeping athletes in sport for longer.
2. The input–treatment–output model is generic and can be applied to all levels of the sport system, whether club, NGB, regional or national orga-nization/system. This is an appropriate point to reinforce the fact that the delivery system levels (pan-sport, NGB, club, performance) should be inter-related and interdependent. The pan-sport system will not be effec-tive unless the NGB systems are effective, and so on.
3. The performance sport system, whether it is a club or national squad, is in competition with other similar systems. However, the performance sport system is also inherently competitive because the inputs are oper-ating in a reward environment in which resources are allocated inequi-tably. In theory, opportunities to take advantage of resources and support are available to all performers who wish to access them. However, those who manage the system must attempt to control the effects of intrinsic competition between individuals in order to ensure that it does not harm the integrated nature of the system and the outputs which should therefore be enhanced by it.
4. The input–treatment–output process is progressive over time. The input–treatment relationship is constantly renewed, and there is a strong feed-back mechanism which will certainly be activated if the outputs are less than anticipated. More important for achieving the system's outputs, however, is a structural progression as the performer moves through the 'ladder of opportunity'. The throughput (the athletes) in the system is constantly recycled. This may involve moving to another system, being renewed for a period of time within the system, being withdrawn from the system, or seeking new inputs to the system. In its simplest form, performers will move from club to club as their output improves and reaches target threshold levels. These levels are extremely difficult to set and measure, and may be based on even less reliable estimates of

potential. In most cases, the structure will be complex and may involve age-group squads, clubs, centres of excellence, performance clubs, national squads, etc. In this model, the very gifted performer progresses along a 'fast-track'. Others may progress so far, and then find that their individual performance output is insufficient to classify them as appropriate inputs for the next system. From our perspective, an important factor is that each system should itself be managed effectively, and the combination of systems should also be managed effectively. The simplistic and naïve models of sport development stages most often employed in development planning (e.g. foundation, participation, performance, and excellence: see English Sports Council, 1998) cannot disguise a lack of knowledge of the individual and collective systems in operation. The major criticism of these models is their lack of attention to the progression between stages. Attention to these mechanisms should characterize the integrated system.

These features of the model illustrate how it operates, and go some way to addressing the criticism of attending to structures rather than processes. Remembering that the purpose of the model is to provide a vehicle for analysis, the major components of the model will now be elaborated on.

System inputs
The performance sport system is centred on the improvement of competition sport performances. The inputs to the system, therefore, would be expected to be characterized by their contribution to this process. The basic unit is the individual performer, and this reinforces the need for *talent identification* and *recruitment strategies*. It is tempting to offer an evaluation of each of these elements, but the purpose of the chapter is to identify the components and to acknowledge their value for analysis. Talent identification is a current buzzword in performance planning, but there is little or no evidence of any systematic procedures which truly predict achievement (rather than sift and select very efficiently). The current competition sifting process, along with coaches' judgements, is much more common, although also inexact and often inaccurate. Recruitment strategies may be dependent on talent identification, but are more likely to result from the hierarchical recycling within system levels. Individuals are recruited into a performance system from another (feeder) system. This apparently simplistic process masks a range of issues of selection, poaching, partiality, buying, timing and equity. The specific reward environment may well be a significant attractor.

Personnel to implement the input and treatment stages also have to be recruited. The range of personnel will be dependent on the scale and scope of the system. The most important of these is the coach, but there may also be a need for assistant coaches, trainers, physiotherapist, performance managers, sport psychologists, administrators, etc. These can usefully be subdivided into those who have direct contact with the performer and who implement the treatment stage, and those who act in a more facilitating capacity. However, it is possible for the coach to fall into both camps.

A third group of input elements consists of *resource* or material factors. It will be clear that the scale of the resources available, particularly the finance to be deployed, will influence the treatment stage. Material resources encompass much more than finance. Facilities, and major specialist items of equipment, will also affect the quality of the treatment stage. Another input is the level of *information* available. This can range from awareness of opportunities, contacts with appropriate agencies and statistical data, to the technical sophistication available within the sport and reflected in coaching knowledge and technical resources.

System treatments

In aggregate form, this is the stage at which the above inputs are managed and manipulated in such a way that they result in improved sport performance. The essential feature is the *coaching process* – indeed, this might be argued to be the whole of the treatment stage. The coaching process is dealt with in greater detail at a later point in the chapter. From what we know already about coaching effectiveness, the coaching process will not be evaluated as effective solely on the competition output of the performers. However, it must also be recognized that the success of the coaching process is associated with the performers' success. In terms of an input–treatment–output model, the success of the treatment stage will be very dependent on the quality of the inputs – the performer, the coach and the technical and material resources available.

However, there is much that can be done at the treatment stage to assist the coaching process, and a number of these elements can be identified in isolation. A major influence will be the *competition structure*, which the system can access. There would be little disagreement that the quality of the competitions, both domestic and international, is a major factor in enhancing performance, since it allows the coach/performer to devise the most appropriate schedule. Increasingly, *sports science support* is becoming commonplace in performance sport. The range and quality of such support is an important element. Another current buzzword is *lifestyle management*. For many performers, sport is their central life interest. They may be full-time performers. This brings with it the need to ensure that performers are not only able to focus exclusively on the coaching process, but that their welfare is protected at the same time. Lifestyle management, therefore, addresses some of the potential pressures and stresses by advising and educating, and by making services available on matters such as time management, financial management, dealing with the media, career guidance, vocational training, higher education opportunities and strategies for disengaging from sport.

It is perhaps significant that the treatment stage is important enough to warrant special attention by grant-awarding agencies. NGBs are required to submit *performance plans* to demonstrate that the process is not haphazard and that basic principles are being adhered to. The performance plan is the system's way of focusing or targeting its energies. It is time- and context-bound, and is directed to achieving specific and identified outputs. This is a good example of planning to manage and regulate the system in a meaningful way.

System outputs

For performance sport systems, the outputs are measured in increased *performance standards*. These are likely to be translated into comparative achievements, such as medals, league positions, championship placings etc. It is worth pointing out that the output system is linked in a feedback loop to the other stages. A failure to achieve output goals may be reflected in a revised treatment stage, or in a change of inputs. (This second possibility may be a polite way of saying sack the coach and get some new performers!) Another alternative, however, is that the expectations generated within the system were over-ambitious and these have to be tempered – particularly if the flexibility to manipulate input and treatment stages is limited. Therefore, it is important that outputs are evaluated in the context of both realistic *comparative measures* and realistic goal setting. It is equally important that a systems perspective is adopted and output achievement is *attributed* correctly to specified elements within the input and treatment stages. It is necessary to identify the elements acting as constraints, and to have an awareness of their effect on related elements.

Remember that identifying a limiting factor and remedying that limitation are two quite distinct stages. It has already been noted that sport systems are inherently competitive and that resources, including talented performers, are a scarce commodity. There is a temptation to imagine that a sports system – a club or NGB – will always be able to progress at an acceptable rate. The key word is 'acceptable', or 'appropriate'. However, the system may become efficient and internally effective without achieving comparative success. Despite this, there will be an *externalities* effect. Particularly at national level, performance sport produces role models for other sport sub-systems, provides an enhanced level of national prestige when successful, provides opportunities for spectators as a leisure product, and contributes significantly to the local and national economy.

Summary of the input–treatment–output system
A number of concluding points can be made about the input–treatment–output system:

1. The model is intended to be a tool for analysis. To some extent, however, it can also act as a model for development inasmuch as it establishes relationships between elements of the system.
2. The model can be applied to all levels – from club, though individual NGBs to the national sport system.
3. It is self-evident that the system, at any level, will be more efficient and effective if it is co-ordinated and integrated. Sport systems have to be managed, and the quality of the management is likely to have a not insignificant influence on its efficacy. The management and control of the system at strategic and pan-sport levels in the UK is currently problematic.
4. A potential value of the input–treatment–output model is its capacity for analysing and comparing systems. This can be carried out at club or national system levels. One of the shortcomings of analyses of sport systems abroad, e.g. previous Eastern-Bloc state bureaucracies or the US Collegiate system, is that they have failed to identify the main features in system terms, and therefore to understand their effect on the operation of the system itself. Only in this way can the lessons learned be transferred appropriately to the development of new systems.

5. A particular approach has been adopted in this chapter to emphasize performance sport as a system. This may have seemed to depersonalize the performers and the other individuals involved; also perhaps, to ignore the social, cultural and ethical context in which the system is situated. This is merely a matter of emphasis. There is no doubt that performance systems operate within – indeed, may contribute significantly to – a set of values. It has already been noted that social and cultural values contribute to the status of performance sport. The reward environment and the limited access to success can lead to problematic behaviour. This may be evidenced as a general means-ends culture in which ethical standards are sacrificed for competitive advantage, or individualized as over-stressed athletes and burn-out. The most obvious example is the use of performance enhancing substances, which may be at an individual or endemic level within the system.

The ITO model is best suited to circumstances in which there is a closely integrated system with a clearly defined structure, a readily identified common purpose and a mechanism for integration. It is for this reason that it has been suggested that the model could best be exemplified in a sports club or NGB context. At the level of the national or pan-sport system, the system is more complicated and diffuse and, although the ITO analysis would be useful, it may appear to assume a degree of integration that actually does not exist. An alternative method of analysis is to use the soft systems methodology (SSM), which is more applicable to looser systems (Checkland, 1989; Checkland and Scholes, 1990).

Soft systems methodology

In systems analysis, the soft systems methodology grew out of a realization that the rational, 'hard' systems approach was much less applicable in human organizational contexts in which consensual objectives were problematical, structures and relationships were 'messy' rather than well-defined, and there were significant issues of perspective, politics and power. However, any approach to systems analysis is open to criticism when dealing with social change (see Ellis, 1995 for a brief review of different approaches to systems analysis and their development).

There is something of a paradox in our analysis of performance sport systems. The coaching process itself has traditionally been approached in scientific or pseudo-scientific terms–at least as far as the performance itself is concerned. However, the performance sport system is clearly a much less well-defined entity. There is a need, nevertheless, to investigate this system, not least because of the need for financial accountability. The SSM has a number of principles that can be applied with some advantage to the analysis of performance sport systems. The following description has been developed from Checkland's work (Checkland, 1989; Checkland and Scholes, 1990).

The performance sport system is a combination of a human activity system and a designed system. It has the properties of a conventional system but is inherently multi-perspective, having power relationships both within the system and with other systems. SSM can be applied to this system with the

purpose of both understanding and improving it. The process goes something like this:

1. Enter the process. In this case, assume that performance sport systems
   are under-performing and could be improved (or have simply not been
   subjected to analysis).
2. Define the problem situation. In this case, performance sport systems are
   under-theorized and there is a lack of knowledge and research.
   Investigation is never entirely neutral, and we must be aware that findings can have repercussions for the main players in the system.
3. Construct 'root definitions'. This involves restating the purpose of the
   system and its basic premises. The mnemonic CATWOE is used for this:
   C: *Customers.* A difficult question to start with. Who are the beneficiaries
      of the purposeful activity within the system? Probably the performers,
      but there are other beneficiaries too because of the externalities
      involved. (A current term is 'stakeholders'.)
   A: *Actors.* Who carries out the activity? This would be an extensive listing
      and includes agencies and groups of individuals.
   T: *Transformation process.* This draws upon our ITO model. The trans-
      formation in this example is sports competition performance, which is
      improved because of the 'treatment' stage.
   W: *Weltanschauung.* Clearly a borrowed term – simply put as cultural or
      organizational values that bring some meaning to the system. Perhaps
      needs to encompass competition, excellence in sport, rational
      approaches, accountability, efficiency etc.
   O: *Owner.* This is normally explained as 'who could stop this activity?'
      Once again, a difficult question. Could anyone? Is this a government
      system at national level? The issue is more easily understood at per-
      formance club level.
   E: *Environmental constraints.* Which aspects of the environment are
      relevant, but not under the direct control of the system? Because of
      the expansive, loose nature of the performance sport system, the
      answer could be lengthy, from legislation to competitors.

(Obviously this is not intended to be an example of the analysis itself but
merely an indication of the categories to be identified.)

4. The next stage is to construct a model of the system as it should be, and
   which satisfies the purpose described above. This can be a fairly simple
   process diagram, which will address the operational system and a monitoring and control system. It should also address the measures of effectiveness, efficacy and efficiency (sometimes ethics and elegance are
   added) to be used. The elements of the ITO model would be a useful
   start. The modelling is a conceptual stage, and there is a deliberate level
   of abstraction (or reduction) in the process.
5. This model is now compared to the reality of the existing system.
   Obviously this reality has to be modelled/described for this comparison
   stage. The differences between the conceptual and the actual are recognized to be noteworthy and are recorded for analysis and evaluation.

As a result of the analysis at stage 5, a number of changes are indicated. At a
further stage of analysis (if the analysis is by a group of stakeholders with its

own agenda and not simply for understanding), discussions have to take place about the desirability, feasibility, practicality and potential impact of any changes.

At the NGB, pan-sport and strategic national levels, performance sport systems are very complex human, organizational and inter-agency phenomena. It is not even clear if the system as a whole is recognized as such in the minds of the stakeholders. To date, there has been no comprehensive strategy with which to realize the benefits of such a system. The system may operate efficiently and effectively, or it may be disorganized and fragmentary. Either way, there is certainly a good case for further analysis. There is no doubt that any analysis is a challenging task, but the purpose of this section has been to demonstrate that some tools are available (ITO and SSM) to assist in this process.

Performance sport systems and the coaching process

The central theme of this chapter is that the management of performance sport systems will be more effective if understood and treated as a formal system. In terms of the coaching process, the broader context (what we might call the parent systems) is important because it will influence, directly or indirectly, coaching practice. Both politically and practically, a culture, structure and material context will be created within which the coach/performer or coach/team relationship has to operate. One of the purposes of this chapter is to demonstrate that an analysis of the various parent systems, systems and sub-systems is necessary to appreciate fully the coaching environment.

Arguments have been presented elsewhere to suggest that the quality of coaching is central to the quality of performance sport. It has also been suggested that the coaching process is a much more all-embracing process than the narrower technical delivery model would imply. The important contribution of the coach to standards of performance sport and a recognition of the wider definition and scope of the coaching process is not seriously in doubt. Nevertheless, the systems themselves may have voluntary coaches operating, even with top-level performers, within difficult constraints. This is a good example of the need to change the supporting culture within the system. A further example is the way that the national performance sport system has increased inputs as the funding to performers has increased, but lagged behind in implementing the necessary system adjustments in the provision of sufficient coaches with appropriate working conditions and professional contracts.

The coaching process is another name for the transformation or treatment phase of the input–treatment–output model. In fact, it may be the appropriate parent term for the whole of the sub-system structure supporting the treatment stage. The effectiveness, efficiency and efficacy (to borrow SSM terminology) of the coaching process is influenced by system decisions at all levels. At the strategic level, has the system provided a career structure for performance coaches? At the pan-sport level, has there been sufficient integration between sports science and coaching? Were elite athletes' coaching needs the central focus of the debate about the establishment of the UKSI? At the NGB level, have centres of excellence and higher education elite squads paid sufficient attention to the provision of suitable coaches? Have NGBs paid sufficient attention to the recruitment and education of those coaches likely to become performance coaches (implying, of course, that the entry pathways for performance coaches do not reflect the existing coach education stages)? Whatever the answers, the point being made is that system provision at all levels influences the ultimate quality of the coaching process.

At the sport performance level in the system, the interaction between the inputs and the treatment is at its most obvious. Elements such as talent identification and recruitment, access to facilities, finance for competitions, and, in particular, the reward environment significantly affect the implementation of the coaching process. If it is the control of variables influencing performance that is the principal distinction between participation and performance coaching; do the inputs and the reward environment provide the context within which control is both feasible and apparent? The coach will be very close to the performer, both physically and metaphorically, at the output performance (the competition). Indeed, in some sports the coach is part of the performance itself. The picture emerging is that of the coach as a manager of performance, one who has to manage all of the variables that influence the final output. This management role was already proposed in the first chapter, when a distinction was made between the coach's direct intervention, indirect responsibilities and management of the external environment roles. This is simply an extension of that argument, with a rather more extensive set of responsibilities identified. An issue that is raised by this is whether the coach can cope, or should have to cope, with the extensive control/management function.

One way of conceptualizing this issue is to distinguish between creating the conditions for the coaching process and managing those conditions. In the former, the individual coach may have little control of the wider system. In the latter, there may be a useful description of the coach's role – technical performance development within the management of the conditions applying to that particular coaching process. This can be encapsulated in the phrase 'the coach as a manager of performance'. This has at least three sets of implications – for role analysis, for role conflict, and for education and training.

Consider the following action verbs: planning, monitoring, regulating, controlling, crisis managing, directing, facilitating, leading, and motivating. This set of role descriptors would not be out of place when describing either managing or coaching. However, the balance between technical delivery and the management of the overall process is one that will differ with the scale and complexity of the coaching context. In performance sport, particularly when the coaching process reflects a full-time, sophisticated coaching context, the coach may be part of a larger team. A US football head coach may be the most pertinent example. Dick (1998) also describes a pan-sport system in which there is a need for 'cross-functional teamwork'. In a useful article by MacLean and Chelladurai (1995), six dimensions of coaching performance are identified: team products, personal products, direct task behaviours, indirect task behaviours, administrative maintenance behaviours and public relations behaviours. Although these were devised for the career coach in US education establishments, the recognition of the wider system is a helpful contribution.

Lack of clarity in role definition can lead to role conflict. Such situations develop when responsibilities, for example, between managers and coaches of representative teams appear to overlap or conflict. If the coach is accepted as the manager of sport performance, then all matters that influence performance need to be controlled by the coach. This does not imply, of course, that the coach should necessarily carry out all functions. Managers, administrators, assistants, trainers and support staff all have their roles to fulfil. This may be at odds with the traditional circumstances within some NGBs. It must also be recognized that many coaches have encouraged situations in which they have been relieved of what they perceive to be administrative tasks (e.g. organizing transport), but this may also have resulted in them being distanced from decision making which influences the coaching environment. In many sports, the coach's role has less status than that of the manager, who may or may not have the technical competence to distinguish between those decisions which impinge on performance and those which are other-directed. We may have to recognize that the all-embracing description of the coach's status is an ideal and partisan approach. In many instances, the coach will have a quite sharply defined set of responsibilities within the performance sport system, and these may be quite limiting. In such cases, the coach's influence will be restricted and the issue of effectiveness and accountability becomes relevant. In analysing sport performance systems it is important to establish who is responsible for what!

There is no doubt that the qualified and experienced coach is a craftsperson – very skilled and knowledgeable about performance sport and the strategies and environment required to bring about improvements in sports performance. These skills extend not only to technical matters, but also to the range of interpersonal skills required to 'manage' the relationships with the performers. In addition, this chapter has identified that the coach will have some responsibilities for managing and influencing the elements of the input–treatment–output model. This has significant implications for coach education, which has traditionally been focused on technical matters. The interpersonal skills required for successful management have largely been ignored by formal coach education training. Even less attention has been paid to the knowledge and understanding of the management of the performance system.

Summary

A case has been argued that performance sport can be understood, and consequently managed, most appropriately if it is recognized to be a system. Systems have distinctive characteristics, and a set of criteria was suggested by which the integrity of a system could be assessed. The purpose of the chapter was to make the case for a systems approach and to identify a useful model for analysis. An input–treatment–output model was described in which inputs to the coaching process, such as performer recruitment and material resources, had to be understood in the light of the reward environment operating within the system. Some attention was given to the soft systems approach first proposed by Checkland (1989). In this regard, if the performance sport system is insufficiently structured or defined, it may be necessary to adopt an analytical approach that first identifies the objectives of the intended system and compares this to existing practice.

An analytical approach to systems will be useful at all levels, from the strategic national level and pan-sport level to the individual NGB and sport performance levels. Although it was not the purpose of this chapter to carry out an analysis of the UK system, it is apparent that a rather loose form of soft system applies. The re-organization and re-shaping (and political re-positioning) which has attended the establishment of the UKSC and the UKSI, and the sudden focus on World Class Performance Plans, has once more demonstrated that the strategic national system is neither effectively nor efficiently managed. However, this chapter has suggested that the advent of the National Lottery rules and regulations for supporting sport provision may have imposed a *de facto* management system.

Given the orientation of the book, it is not surprising that the chapter has concluded with an examination of the coach's role in performance sport systems. It was acknowledged that the transformation process is focused on improving sport performance, and that this is synonymous with the coaching process. We speculated, therefore, that the coach should be perceived as a 'manager of sport performance'. However, the coach's influence on the various levels of the performance sport system may be somewhat limited, and is often restricted to the technical sport performance level. This limits the coach's accountability for system outputs, although this is not always acknowledged by employers. The coach is a significant player in the performance sport system, but too little attention has been paid to the system and to the coach's role within it.

References

Checkland, P. (1989). Soft systems methodology. In *Rational Analysis for a Problematic World* (J. Rosenhead, ed), pp. 71–99. John Wiley and Sons.

Checkland, P. and Scholes, J. (1990). *Soft Systems Methodology in Action*. John Wiley and Sons.

Cole, G. A. (1994). *Strategic Management*. DP Publications.

Department of National Heritage. (1995). *Sport: Raising the Game*. Department of National Heritage.

Dick, F. W. (1998). Winning coaches in the game of change. *Coaching Focus*, **37**, 21–3.

Ellis, R. K. (1995). Critical considerations in the development of system thinking and practice. *Systems Practice*, **8(2)**, 199–214.

English Sports Council. (1997). *England, the Sporting Nation: A Strategy*. English Sports Council.

Hawkey, I. (1997). A £100M school for scandal. *The Sunday Times*, 23 February, p. 10.

Kikulis, L. M., Slack, T. and Hinnings, B. (1995). Does decision making make a difference? Patterns of change within Canadian National Sport Organisations. *J. Sport Man.*, **9**, 273–99.

Lyle, J. W. B. (1997). Managing excellence in sports performance. *Career Dev. Int.*, **2(7)**, 314–23.

MacLean, J. C. and Chelladurai, P. (1995). Dimensions of coaching performance: development of a scale. *J. Sport Man.*, **9**, 194–207.

Pickup, D. (1996). *Not Another Messiah: An Account of the Sports Council 1988–93*. Pentland Press.

Riorden, J. (1993). Soviet-style sport in Eastern Europe: the end of an era. In *The Changing Politics of Sport* (E. Allison, ed.), pp. 37–57. Manchester University Press.

Schembri, G. (1998). Australian Institute of Sport: copy at your PERIL! *Supercoach*, **2,** 6–7.
Scottish Sports Council. (1998). *The Scottish Institute of Sport*. Scottish Sports Council.
Sports Council. (1995). *The British Academy of Sport: a Discussion Paper*. The Sports Council.
Westerbeek, H. (1995). The Australian sports system: its history and an organisational overview.
    Eur. J. Sport Man., **2(1),** 42–58.

Index